Atlas of Multiparametric Prostate MRI

Joan C. Vilanova • Violeta Catalá • Ferran Algaba
Oscar Laucirica
Editors

Atlas of Multiparametric Prostate MRI

With PI-RADS Approach and Anatomic-MRI-Pathological Correlation

Springer

Editors
Joan C. Vilanova
Department of Radiology
Clínica Girona
Institute Catalan of Health-IDI
University of Girona
Girona, Spain

Ferran Algaba
Department of Pathology
Fundació Puigvert
Universitat Autònoma de Barcelona
Barcelona, Spain

Violeta Catalá
Department of Radiology
Fundació Puigvert
Universitat Autònoma de Barcelona
Barcelona, Spain

Oscar Laucirica
Department of Urology
Hospital Sant Joan Despi Moises Broggi
Sant Joan Despí
Barcelona, Spain

ISBN 978-3-319-61785-5 ISBN 978-3-319-61786-2 (eBook)
DOI 10.1007/978-3-319-61786-2

Library of Congress Control Number: 2017953531

Printed on acid-free paper

This Springer imprint is published by Springer Nature
The registered company is Springer International Publishing AG
The registered company address is: Gewerbestrasse 11, 6330 Cham, Switzerland

To my wife, Cris, and our children, Cristina and Eduard, for their love and support

Kai

To Sim, Cande, and Lluís (they know why ...)

Violeta

To the prostate cancer patients

Ferran

To my wife, Pili, and our seven wonderful children.
This book would not be possible without their never-ending encouragement and unwavering support.

Oscar

Foreword

Prostate magnetic resonance imaging (MRI) has tremendously evolved in recent years. Initially consisting of purely anatomy-based T2- and T1-weighted sequences, it has gradually incorporated functional tools such as dynamic contrast-enhanced MRI in the evaluation of angiogenesis, spectroscopic imaging in the evaluation of metabolic processes, and diffusion-weighted imaging in the evaluation of cell density. The combined use of anatomical and functional imaging has been named multi-parametric MRI (mpMRI) and with the recent advent of robust sequences and powerful hardware, diffusion-weighted imaging has become its dominant sequence.

Several promising validation studies in expert centres have sparked the interest of many urologists all over the world, ubiquitously increasing the demand for high-quality mpMRI. To facilitate this, the European Society of Urogenital Radiology (ESUR) issued technical and reporting guidelines for standardization of mpMRI in 2012. This first version of the Prostate Imaging Reporting and Data System (PI-RADS) was updated in 2015 in collaboration with the American College of Radiology and now serves as a touchstone for high-quality mpMRI all over the world.

The availability of such a touchstone, however, needs to be complemented with appropriate teaching and reference material for anyone performing prostate MRI. In this respect, the authors have added to their book an impressive amount of useful reference material. They highlight the correlation between mpMRI observations and histopathological findings, and provide comprehensive and nicely illustrated chapters on prostatic and periprostatic anatomy, technical requirements, and PI-RADS reading. Furthermore, the reader is updated about the use of MRI in staging and recurrence detection.

The authors must be commended for the tremendous amount of work they have dedicated to this project. I am confident that the *Atlas of Multiparametric Prostate MRI* will become an invaluable tool in the daily practice of many radiologists and other specialists involved in the diagnosis and management of prostate cancer.

Geert M. Villeirs
Division of Genitourinary Radiology
Ghent University Hospital, Ghent, Belgium

Preface

Magnetic resonance imaging (MRI) has played a minor role to manage prostate cancer until nearly a decade ago. With the development of advanced MRI techniques, MRI is increasingly playing a main role in the clinical pathways of detection, local staging, active surveillance and posttreatment follow-up for prostate cancer.

The possibility of including multiparametric MRI, especially using T2-weighted imaging (T2WI), diffusion-weighted imaging and dynamic contrast-enhanced imaging, in the diagnostic management to improve the detection of aggressive cancer while reducing the overdiagnosis of indolent cancer represents a change in the diagnostic management. This new paradigm can be achieved performing the acquisition, interpretation and reporting of a standardized multiparametric MRI with a Prostate Imaging Reporting and Data System (PI-RADS) guide.

The purpose of this book is to provide a useful multiparametric MRI manual to be used by a wide range and variety of disciplines involved in the management of prostate cancer, including radiologists, urologists, pathologists, oncologists and radiotherapists. We have provided and covered all the information related to prostate cancer using multiparametric MRI. The first chapter is dedicated to MRI technique, providing all the technical information from the bases through the most advanced sequences of functional MRI. The second chapter deals with the anatomy and its correlation with MRI in order to understand the MRI findings of the prostate and pelvic structures. The third chapter addresses the pathology of prostate cancer, providing the histological information of the Gleason grading system. The fourth chapter provides a systematic reading model using the PI-RADS v2 guide to perform an appropriate structured report for diagnosis of clinically significant cancer. The fifth chapter provides useful tips and tricks to avoid the common pitfalls while reading the multiparametric MRI of the prostate. The sixth chapter is focused on the prostate cancer local staging on MRI with anatomical drawings correlated with MRI and pathology. The seventh chapter is focused on the MRI findings from normal MRI after different treatments and the MRI signs of recurrence, as well as the recommended management of MRI on active surveillance, using the useful information to be reported on the follow-up MRI studies.

This book has been possible due to the generous effort of all contributing authors. All of them are well-known experts in their respective fields such as radiology, pathology and urology. They have made possible to compile and integrate all the information to correlate the anatomy, the pathology and the MRI imaging in order to facilitate the interpretation of multiparametric MRI.

It has been challenging to coordinate such a great team from different disciplines, making editing this book a learning and enjoyable process.

Finally, we would like to express our thanks and appreciation to all the patients and our gratitude to Seila Ballerini, for her efficient support to adapt the formal aspects of the manuscript; Ricard Pellejero, for his support in the bibliographic searches; and Carles Fernández and Sònia Sala, for their collaboration with the graphic material.

We hope this book can be helpful for all those who are interested in prostate cancer multi-parametric MRI interpretation and can make it a little bit easier for the readers and as exciting as it was for us.

Girona, Spain	Joan C. Vilanova
Barcelona, Spain	Violeta Catalá
Barcelona, Spain	Ferran Algaba
Barcelona, Spain	Oscar Laucirica

Contents

Prostate MRI Technique

1

Lidia Alcalá Mata, M. Álvaro Berbís, and Antonio Luna Alcalá

Contents

1.1 Introduction

Prostate cancer (PCa) is the most common solid tumor in the male patient, with 220,800 new cases and 27,540 deaths in the USA in 2015 [1]. In Europe, the incidence of PCa was close to 23% in 2012, with a yearly direct mortality of over 92,000 [2]. However, the 5-year survival rate of PCa has steadily increased to reach 83.4% in 2005–2007 in this continent [3].

Today, PCa is considered a generally multifocal disease, with a dominant focus (index lesion) and one or more separate low-volume foci. From the clinical viewpoint, it has to be discriminated between two subtypes of PCa: indolent or clinically insignificant (Gleason ≤6) and clinically significant (Gleason ≥7), which can compromise the patient's quantity and/or quality of life if not properly treated [4]. Now, it is under discussion if Gleason pattern 3+4 can be also considered as low-risk disease [5]. In order to improve patient stratification, a new grading system has been proposed to address the confusion inherent in the Gleason system [6].

Currently, the clinical suspicion of PCa is established by prostate-specific antigen (PSA) blood test and digital rectal examination (DRE).

DRE has a very low sensitiveness and can only detect tumors with a volume over 0.2 mL. Moreover, PSA is elevated in benign conditions other than PCa, such as benign prostatic hyperplasia (BPH) and prostatitis. A recent study has pointed out that, although PSA-based screening increases diagnosis of PCa in early stages of the disease (when it is confined to the gland), it does not show a significant benefit neither in PCa-specific survival rate, nor in averaged survival rate of the screened patients. Moreover, this screening is associated with overdiagnosis and overtreatment [7, 8].

However, and despite its low specificity, PSA can be used as an independent variable for PCa diagnosis [9]. Higher levels of this blood marker, and especially a progressing elevation thereof, are correlated with an increased probability of

L. Alcalá Mata, M.D.
SERCOSA, Health Time, Carmelo Torres, 2, 23007 Jaén, Spain
e-mail: l.alcala.o@htime.org

M. Álvaro Berbís, Ph.D.
Health Time, Av. del Brillante, 106, 14012 Córdoba, Spain
e-mail: a.berbis@htime.org

A. Luna Alcalá, M.D., Ph.D. (✉)
SERCOSA, Health Time, Carmelo Torres, 2, 23007 Jaén, Spain

Department of Radiology, University Hospitals of Cleveland, Case Western Reserve University, Cleveland, OH, USA
e-mail: aluna70@htime.org

J.C. Vilanova et al. (eds.), *Atlas of Multiparametric Prostate MRI*, DOI 10.1007/978-3-319-61786-2_1

clinically significant PCa. In this manner, blood levels of PSA between 3 and 4 ng/mL are associated with a PCa risk of 27% and a Gleason >7 tumor risk of 6.7%.

Multiparametric MRI (mpMRI) has demonstrated to be a useful tool to discriminate between PCa of high and low aggressiveness, and thus it is suitable for stratification of patients with clinically significant PCa, especially in cases of previous negative TRUS [10]. Due to this, the 2015 European Association of Urology (EAU) guidelines on PCa acknowledge the role of this approach in cases involving negative biopsies and persisting clinical suspicion of PCa [11]. The development of targeted biopsies to the suspicious areas on mpMRI by means of either MRI-ultrasound fusion systems or in-bore biopsy in the magnet with an MRI-compatible guidance approach has definitely changed the diagnosis of PCa [12]. In this sense, recent data has shown the performance of targeted biopsy increased in 18% the number of clinically significant cancer in comparison to the standard diagnostic pathway of TRUS biopsy [13].

1.2 Multiparametric MRI (mpMRI)

Over recent years, MRI has provided an increasing impact in the management of PCa. By using a combination of morphologic and functional sequences, which allow for the analysis of several, differentiated tumor features. Besides, and more importantly, mpMRI can discriminate between clinically significant PCa (Gleason >7), which have to be treated, and clinically insignificant carcinomas, which do not require immediate treatment, in order to avoid undesired side effects associated with overtreatment.

1.2.1 Clinical Considerations

In general, it is accepted that the performance of mpMRI of the prostate gland for tumor detection purposes can be performed anytime. Only, if a TRUS-guided biopsy has been performed recently, the presence of hemorrhage, as areas with either high signal intensity on T1-weighted sequence or susceptibility artifact on diffusion-weighted imaging (DWI) and dynamic contrast-enhanced (DCE)-MRI, can disturb the interpretation of mpMRI. However, it is very unlikely that the presence of postbiopsy hemorrhage limits significantly the detection of significant PCa, particularly after a previous negative TRUS-guided biopsy. Conversely, the presence of hemorrhage may result confounding for the local staging of PCa and if it is recommended to delay the performance of the mpMRI 6 weeks after a positive systematic biopsy.

Another area of debate is the necessity to submit the patient to a specific preparation before the mpMRI. It is recommended that the rectum is clean, as the presence of air and stool can cause distortion artifacts on DWI or interfere the correct placement on an endorectal coil, if it is used. Normally, it is suggested the evacuation of the rectum just before the test and in some centers an enema is also administered just before the mpMRI. Further actions, such as emptying the rectum of air with a catheter or performing the study in the prone position, are rarely needed.

Also, the use of antispasmodic agents to reduce bowel peristalsis is under discussion, and it may be more necessary according to the used protocol (i.e., 3D fast spin-echo T2-weighted sequences are more prone to peristalsis than 2D ones).

1.2.2 Technical Considerations

1.2.2.1 Magnetic Field Strength

mpMRI of the prostate gland is usually performed in high-field magnets (1.5T or above). Three tesla magnets offer an obvious advantage over those with lower field intensities (1.5T), due to increased signal-to-noise ratio (SNR), which allow for improved spatial and/or temporal resolutions. In spite of this, both 3T and 1.5T fields are suitable for PCa detection, diagnosis, and staging, although the use of modern 3T fields, if available, is recommended, as it is specified in the Prostate Imaging Reporting and Data System (PI-RADS) version 2.0 guidelines [14].

One of the main drawbacks associated with 3T fields is their higher proneness to magnetic susceptibility artifacts, signal heterogeneity, and geometric distortion.

1.2.2.2 Coils

The use of endorectal coils is still a matter of debate, even after the advent of surface coils with a higher number of channels (16 channels or above). The endorectal coil, when used in combination with the surface coil, allows for increased SNR, thereby improving spatial resolution of morphological sequences and signal intensity in diffusion-based sequences and DCE-MRI. The combined use of both types of coils can be a useful approach when imaging large patients, for which the surface coil does not provide sufficient signal intensity for optimal sequence acquisition or in certain clinical scenarios such as staging. However, the use of endorectal coils presents several drawbacks, such as extended preparation and examination times. It also may cause deformities in the prostate gland and is uncomfortable for the patient, who may be reluctant to undergo the study. In order to minimize susceptibility artifacts associated with the endorectal coil, a careful positioning of the coil and the distension of the balloon with liquid perfluorocarbon or barium suspension instead of air are necessary.

Modern MRI scanners with high-field intensities and multielement surface coils enable successful acquisition of prostate studies without endorectal coils. It is accepted that mpMRI performed at 3T may obviate the use of endorectal coil, providing a similar image quality to studies performed at 1.5T magnets with endorectal coil. The need of endorectal coil for 1.5T magnets is more controversial and probably related to the specific characteristics of each machine, number and size of elements of the used phased-array coil and sequence design. The current tendency is to minimize the use of endorectal coils in both 1.5 and 3T magnets. Furthermore, a recent meta-analysis showed that the use of endorectal coil for local staging of PCa did not offer an additional benefit for extracapsular extension detection and only slightly improved sensitivity for seminal vesicle invasion detection [15].

1.2.3 mpMRI Sequences and Protocol

A typical mpMRI protocol consists of two groups of sequences: morphological (T1- and T2-weighted sequences) and different types of functional ones (DWI, DCE-MRI, and proton spectroscopy). The combination of sequences is defined by the clinical indication and acquisition time constraints. Nowadays, the use of proton MR spectroscopy (MRS) has declined. Furthermore, due to the fast increase in the number of performed mpMRI in the clinical setting and the constraints in magnet slots, biparametric MRI, only including a T2-weighted sequence and DWI, is being actively tested for detection and screening purposes. In this direction, PI-RADS version 2.0 also reduced the role of DCE-MRI in the detection of PCa [16].

PI-RADS version 2.0 includes technical specifications on how to perform a mpMRI protocol and makes recommendations on the design of the different sequences to warranty the quality of mpMRI.

1.2.3.1 Morphologic Sequences

T1-Weighted Sequences

Axial or coronal spin-echo (SE) or gradient-echo (GE) sequences, with or without fat suppression, with wide fields of view (FOV), are useful for ruling out postbiopsy hemorrhage in the prostate gland and seminal vesicles and for the detection of locoregional adenopathy and bone metastasis in PCa staging studies (Fig. 1.1). They are most commonly acquired in the axial plane using the same orientation as for the rest of the study. As previously discussed, their use for detection purposes is declining. Also, it has to be taken into account that the basal pre-contrast acquisitions of DCE-MRI can accurately detect the presence of hemorrhage, making not necessary to include specific T1-weighted sequences in detection-only protocols.

There is growing interest in the determination of the tissue T1 relaxation time, also known as T1 mapping, to differentiate PCa from normal prostatic tissue and other benign conditions, such as prostatitis. Preliminary data has shown lower T1 values from cancer than normal peripheral zone [17].

T2-Weighted Sequences

T2-weighted images permit to evaluate the prostate zonal anatomy (Figs. 1.2 and 1.3). The outer peripheral zone, due to its intrinsic high signal intensity, can be easily differentiated from the transition and central zones and anterior fibromuscular stroma. T2-weighted images are the dominant sequence for PCa detection in transition and central zones in PI-RADS version 2.0 guidelines. Also, significant PCa can be detected in the peripheral zone with T2-weighted sequences, although with a nonspecific appearance. Therefore, these acquisitions are not considered in PI-RADS version 2.0 guidelines for PCa detection in the peripheral zone. Also, T2-weighted images are key for local staging of PCa, as they allow the depiction of extracapsular extension, seminal vesicle invasion, and nodal involvement.

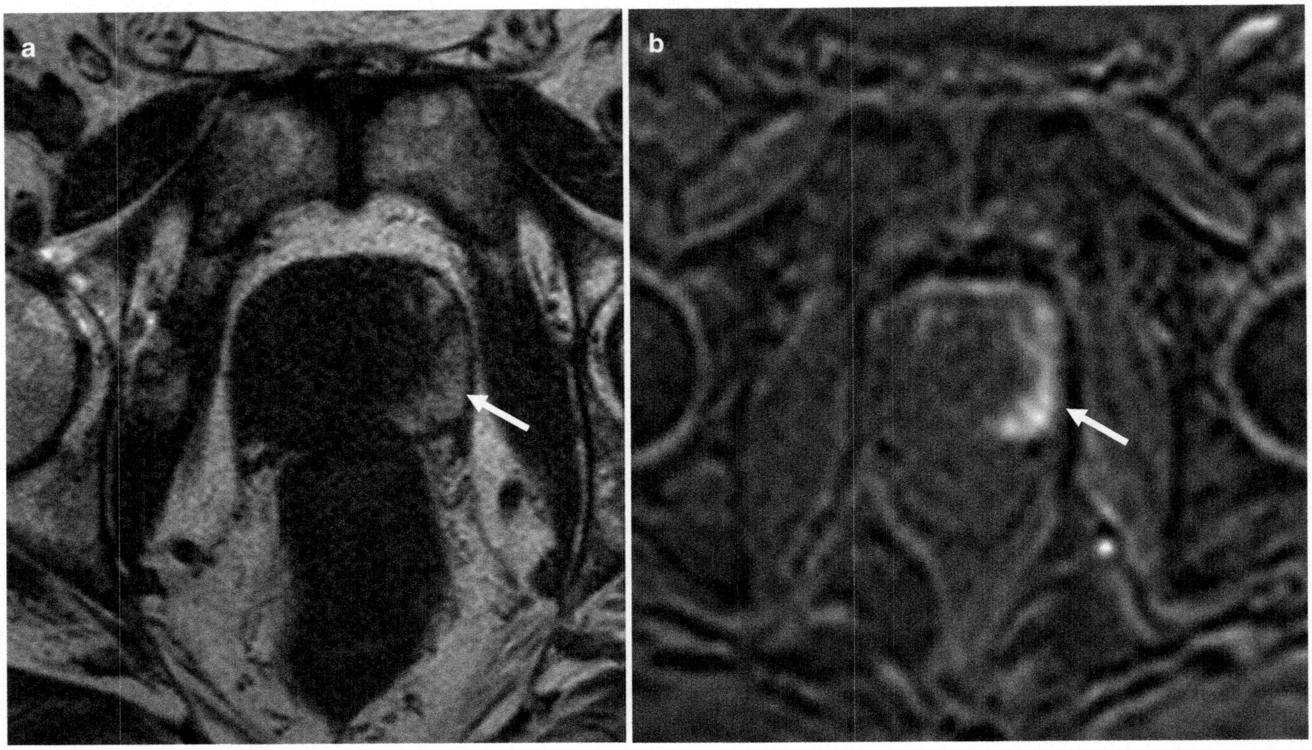

Fig. 1.1 Postbiopsy hemorrhage area showing hyperintensity in T1-weighted sequences: (**a**) axial TSE T1-weighted sequence (**b**) precontrast fat-suppressed fast-field-echo (FFE) T1-weighted image in the left central gland and peripheral zone

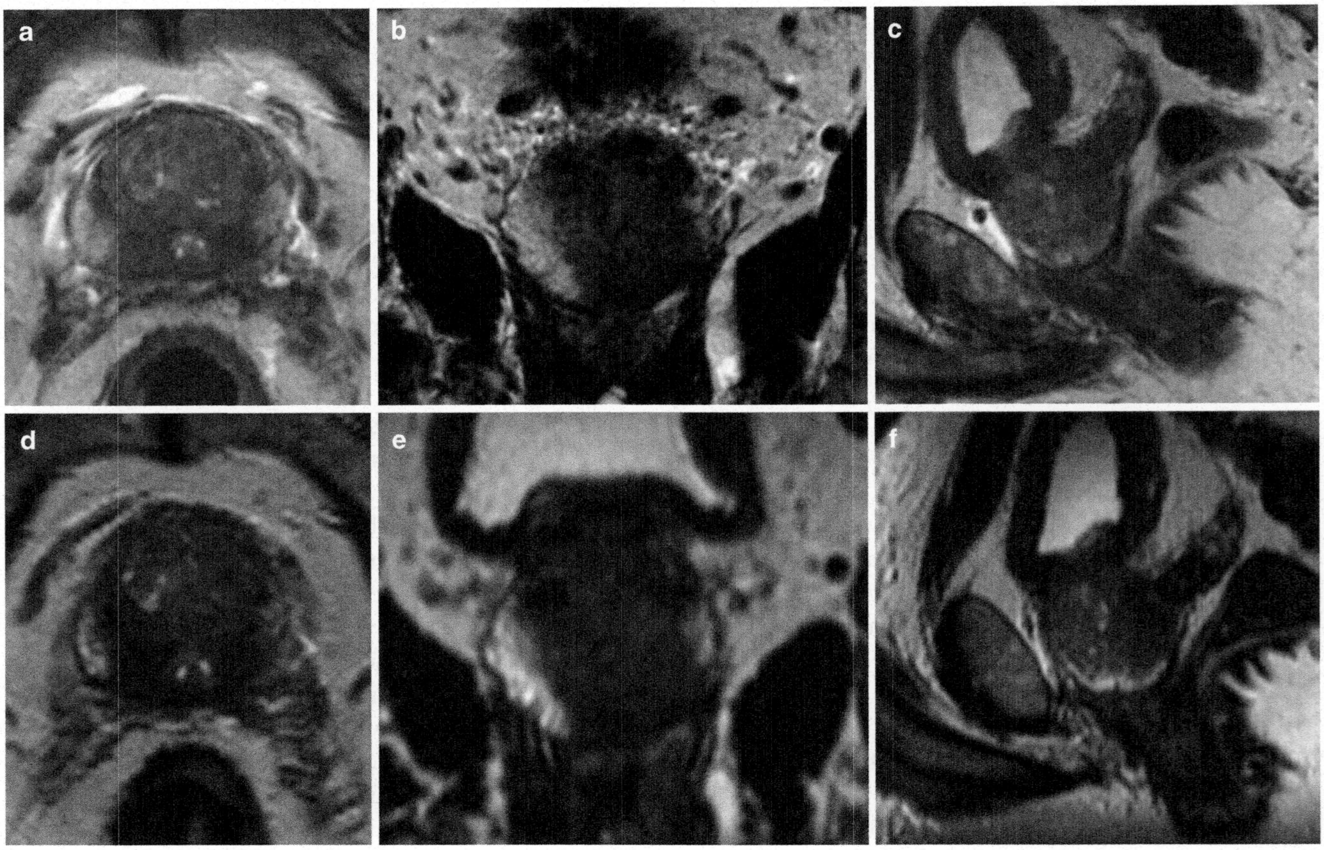

Fig. 1.2 2D TSE T2-weighted sequence acquired on the three planes: (**a**) axial, (**b**) coronal, and (**c**) sagittal. Similar image qualities are observed in the axial 3D TSE T2-weighted sequence (**d**) and MPR reconstructions in coronal (**e**) and sagittal (**f**) orientations of the same patient

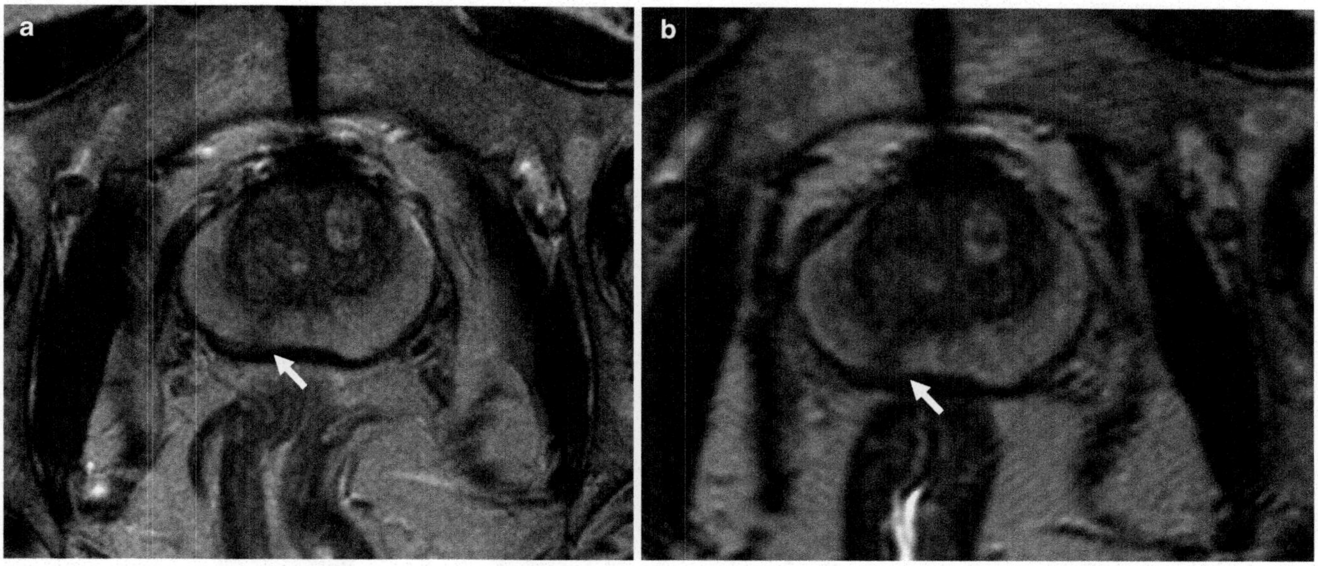

Fig. 1.3 3D TSE T2-weighted sequences display a better contrast for lesions in the peripheral zone and avoid partial volume artifacts, as shown in this case. In the 2D TSE T2-weighted sequence (**a**) it is difficult to detect the lesion located in the posteromedial right quadrant of the peripheral zone, which is better depicted in the 3D acquisition. (**b**)

Most commonly, T2-weighted images are acquired in the three orthogonal spatial planes, with high spatial resolutions and small FOVs.

Two approaches can be used:

- High-resolution 2D fast spin-echo (FSE), also known as turbo spin-echo (TSE) or rapid acquisition with relaxation enhancement (RARE), acquisitions with slice thickness ≤3 mm and no gap, with small FOV between 12 and 20 cm. FSE acquisitions were demonstrated in a meta-analysis [18] to significantly improve the local staging performance of mpMRI compared to protocols using spin-echo (SE) acquisitions. Optimal contrast for tumor detection is achieved with a TE between 90 and 120 ms [19]. More importantly, FSE sequences also reduce total acquisition time, which is around 4 min for each acquired plane. PI-RADS version 2 guidelines recommend at least an in-plane resolution of <0.7 mm (phase) × <0.4 mm (frequency). Long echo trains should be limited to avoid excessive image blurring.
- Single 3D FSE acquisition with isotropic voxel and contiguous thin-section slices ≤1 mm in the axial plane and reconstructions in the coronal and sagittal planes. This type of sequences is known as CUBE, VISTA (volume isotropic turbo spin-echo acquisition), SPACE (sampling perfection with application-optimized contrasts using different flip-angle evolution), 3D MVOX, or isoFSE, depending on the vendor. These sequences use a 3D acquisition with very long echo train and ultrashort echo spacing due to nonselective refocusing pulses and reduced flip angles. 3D images show a better contrast between tumor and the peripheral zone and an improved detection of anatomy and millimetric lesions, avoiding partial volume artifacts. In addition, this approach leads to shorter acquisition times, although at the expense of lower SNR and in-plane resolution vis-à-vis 2D acquisition sequences. They are also more susceptible to motion artifacts, potentially requiring the use of antiperistaltic agents to minimize bowel loop movement [20, 21]. However, a recent study showed that 2D or 3D FSE images are equivalent to delineate the zonal anatomy and detect PCa, although 2D images are significantly sharper than 3D images, and also significantly demonstrated non-motion artifacts [22]. Quantitative T2 mapping using multiecho, either GE or FSE, sequences has been tested for tumor detection and characterization. PCa shows shorter T2 values than normal peripheral zone [23]. According to the preliminary data available, T2* mapping in combination with T2-weighted sequences improves the diagnostic performance of PCa detection compared to T2-weighted images only [24] and demonstrates greater diagnostic accuracy than ADC mapping in the characterization of intermediate- and high-grade PCa but limited value in the characterization of low-grade PCa [25].

1.2.3.2 Functional Sequences

Diffusion-Weighted Imaging (DWI)

DWI is able to detect in vivo and noninvasively the Brownian movement of water molecules at microscopic level. As such, it is able to assess tissue microstructure reflecting cell membrane integrity and cellularity [26]. In tissues exhibiting an

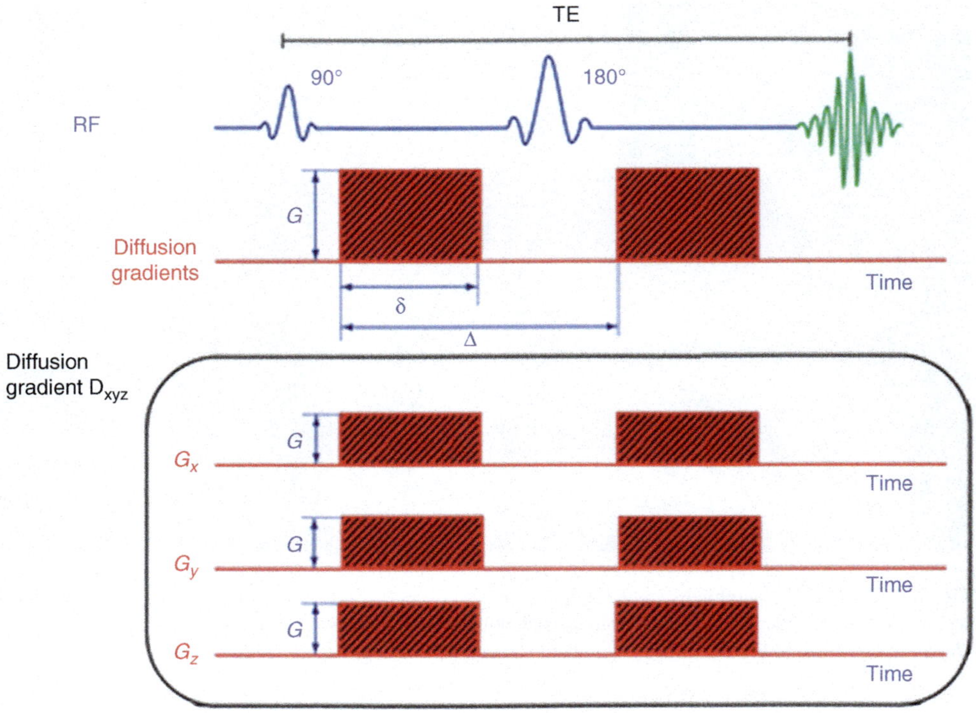

Fig. 1.4 DWI sequence diagram. This sequence is based on the use of two gradients with the same area between 180° radiofrequency pulses. The signal is obtained after dephasing of water protons sensitive to Brownian motion. The amount of diffusion weighting can be controlled by modifying the *b*-value, which is related with the gradient area as well as the separation between gradients, as discussed in the text. Reprinted with permission from [27]

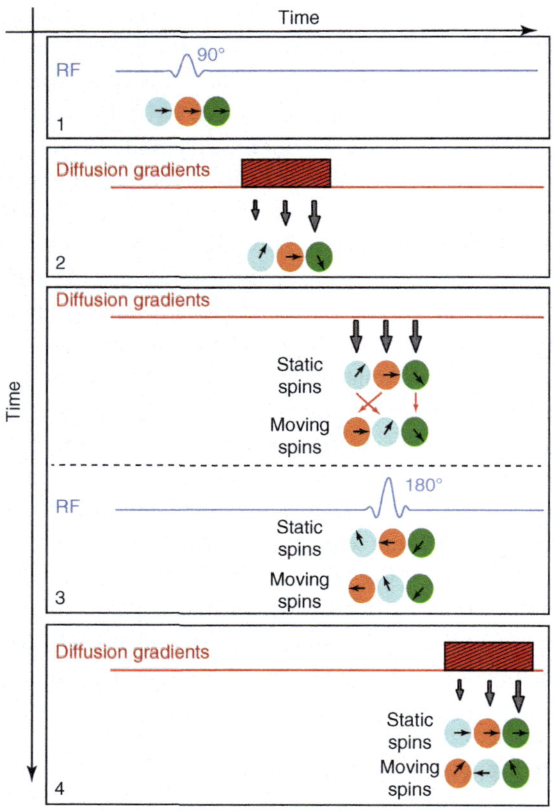

Fig. 1.5 Schematic representation of proton movement during the application of gradients and radiofrequency pulses in the DWI sequence. The first gradient induces dephasing of water proton spins, while the second gradient is applied to reverse spin dephasing. Spins belonging to water molecules that remain in the same location experience no net dephasing, while moving spins display a net phase shift, leading to signal loss in the MR image. Reprinted with permission from [27]

increased cellularity or occupancy and tortuosity of the interstitial space, such as tumor lesions, the free movement of water in the interstitial space is restricted in comparison with the normal tissue. Thus, DWI is an excellent oncologic biomarker, and it is used in detection and characterization of tumors, staging, and prognosis, as well as in treatment response and detection of recurrence studies, thanks to quantitation enabled by apparent diffusion coefficient (ADC) maps.

DWI sequences are based on the application of two magnetic field gradients with the same area and opposed polarity, around a 180° pulse (Fig. 1.4). The first gradient induces dephasing of water proton spins, while the second gradient is applied to reverse spin dephasing. Spins belonging to water molecules that remain in the same location experience no net dephasing, while moving spins display a net phase shift, leading to signal loss in the MR image (Fig. 1.5).

Current DWI protocols are normally based on single-shot spin-echo echo planar imaging (SS SE-EPI). As other EPI sequences, they are severely affected by motion and magnetic susceptibility artifacts and lead to poor spatial resolution and low SNR.

The amount of diffusion weighting depends on the *b*-value, a parameter which is related with the strength and duration of the applied gradients as well as the time spacing between them (Fig. 1.4). Usually, the highest *b*-value of the sequence is chosen as the maximum possible value yielding an image of sufficient quality, SNR, and absence of artifacts, since noise and signal decay increase exponentially as *b*-values increase. In prostate studies, maximum values of $b \geq 1400$ s/mm^2 are recommended for 1.5 and 3T fields to

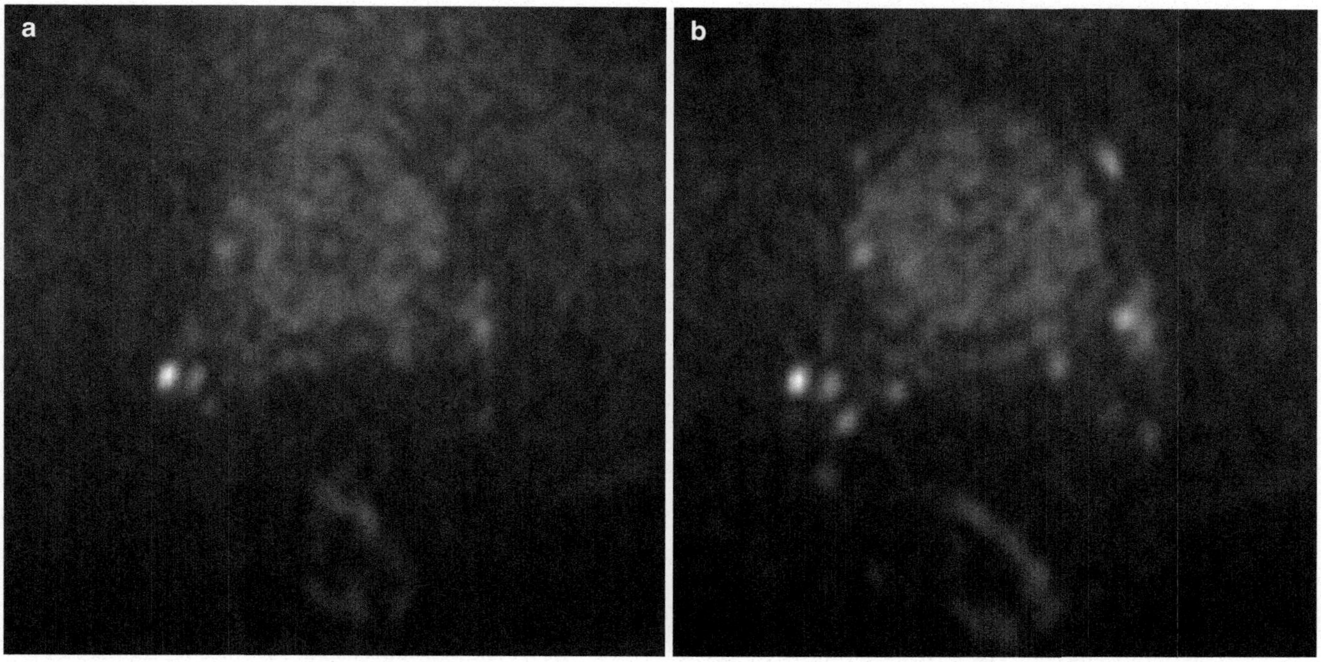

Fig. 1.6 By increasing the number of excitations (NEX), image quality is also increased, but so is the examination time. As shown in this case, DWI with b value of 1000 s/mm^2 (**a**), acquired with NEX = 3, shows more noise and less image quality than (**b**), same sequence but acquired with NEX = 4

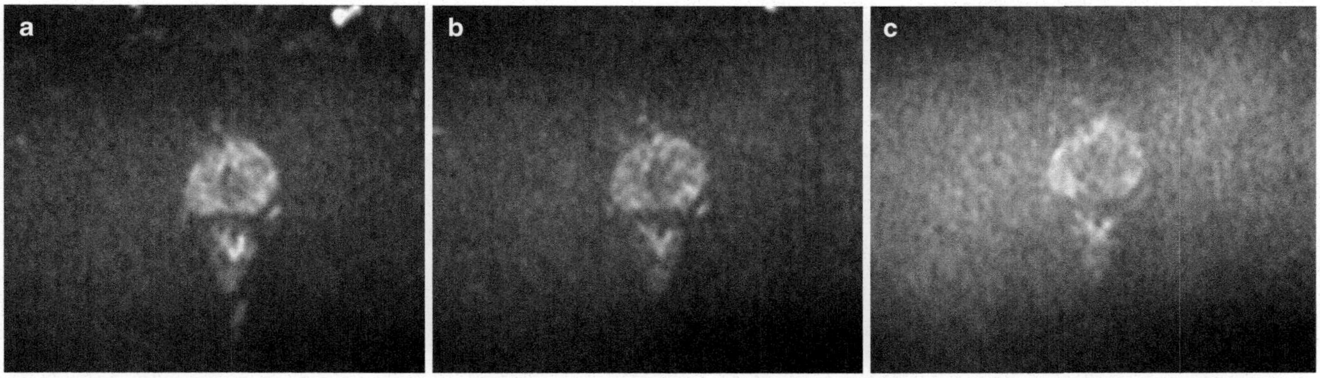

Fig. 1.7 A lower TE leads to an enhanced signal-to-noise ratio (SNR). DWI with b of 1000 s/mm^2 acquired with TE = 60 ms (**a**) shows a higher SNR than that using TE = 90 ms (**b**) and a much higher SNR than (**c**), with TE = 110 ms

enhance PCa detection, although *b*-values over 2000 up to 3000 s/mm^2 have been also used to increase the depiction of malignant areas [28].

The reduction of SNR as *b*-values increase also has implications for proper quantitation of water diffusion in tissues and hence on ADC maps. Thus, it is important to optimize SNR through different acquisition parameters:

- Number of excitations (NEX): NEX can be increased, thereby also increasing examination time (Fig. 1.6).
- Echo time (TE): TE increase causes signal reduction of tissues with short TEs, greatly hampering ADC calculations (Fig. 1.7). Thus, it is advisable to minimize TE, which can be achieved using the maximum gradient strength available and by combining the strength of all gradient axes simultaneously. Also, the use of parallel imaging and high bandwidth helps to shorten effective TE. PI-RADS version 2.0 recommends to keep TE under 90 ms.

To minimize the artifacts of DWI, two main strategies can be considered:

- Increasing acquisition bandwidth: tissue interfaces (air-soft tissue interfaces, i.e., as in the rectal wall-posterior

aspect of the prostate interface) lead to field inhomogeneities, which result in distortion artifacts. In this regard, applying a greater acquisition bandwidth has two consequences. First, frequency shifts between pairs of adjacent phase-encoding lines become larger, thereby minimizing the impact on final readout of error arising from the lack of field homogeneity. Secondly, spin dephasing caused by field inhomogeneity is reduced due to shorter acquisition times (Fig. 1.8).
- Using parallel acquisition techniques: parallel imaging reduces the number of phase-encoding steps, collecting spatial information from multichannel coils. This lowers the EPI factor of the sequence, reducing readout dephasing and image distortion [29] (Fig. 1.9).

Another problem arising from EPI sequences is related with fat chemical shift artifacts. The difference in the resonance frequencies of water and fat causes a water-fat shift in EPI readouts, resulting in fat signals overlapping with the region of interest. These effects, known as ghosting artifacts, are magnified at higher *b*-values and may seriously complicate proper quantitation of diffusion in ADC maps, due to superimposition of fat and tissue signals in the same voxels. For these reasons, inclusion of fat signal suppression modules is mandatory in DWI sequences. Several possibilities exist (Fig. 1.10):

- Short-tau inversion recovery (STIR): this approach uses a nonselective inversion pulse for fat saturation, achieving a good fat suppression in wide FOV acquisitions, since it becomes less affected by field inhomogeneities and causes less distortions. However, STIR sequences lead to lower SNR than those involving selective fat suppression, requiring higher NEX and thus longer examination times. Thus, they are rarely employed in diffusion applications other than whole-body studies.
- Frequency-selective fat suppression: these techniques are more suitable for the study of specific regions of interest, because they provide a higher SNR in soft tissues than STIR [27]:
  - Spectral presaturation with inversion recovery (SPIR) is an optimum technique at 1.5T fields, because the 120° inversion pulse reduces the inversion time (TI) required for fat signals to cross the zero line (no net magnetization), yielding good results in reasonable times.
  - Spectral attenuated inversion recovery (SPAIR) is the most common approach at 3T, since it produces a more homogeneous excitation of the adiabatic pulses, which reduce the effect of B1 inhomogeneities. Adiabatic pulses require long TIs and large flip angles, and they entail increased specific absorption rates (SAR) vis-à-vis normal excitation pulses, requiring longer repetition times (TR).

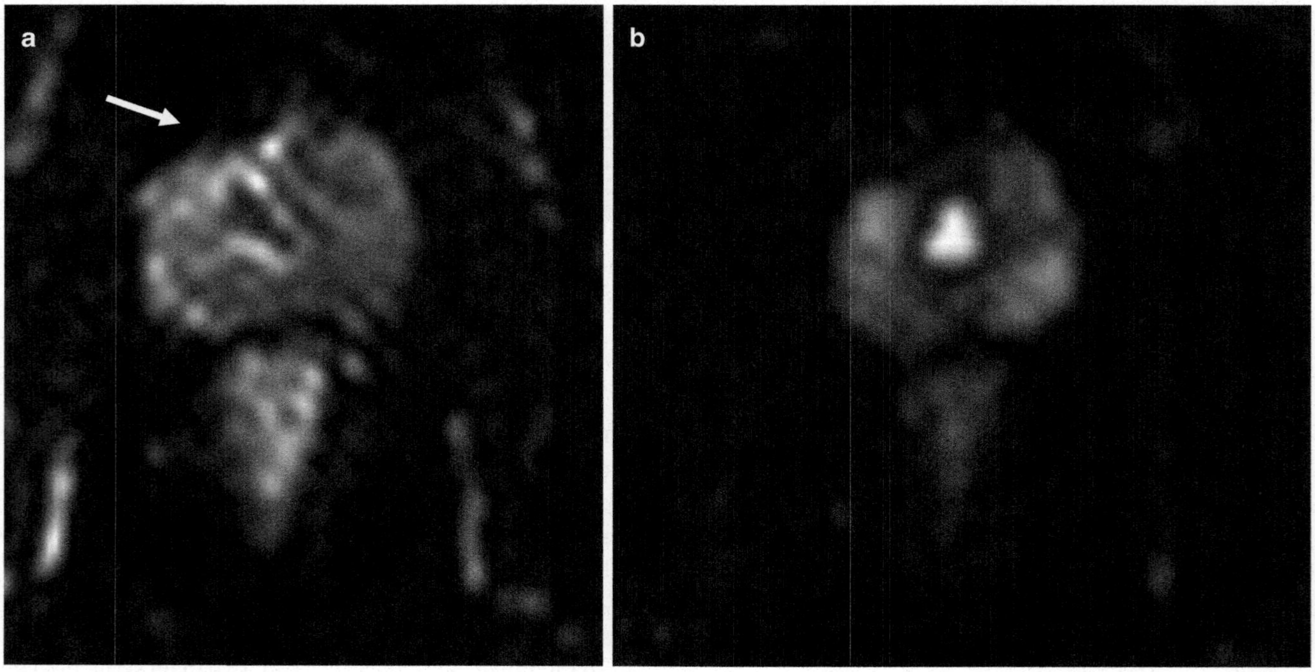

Fig. 1.8 By increasing acquisition bandwidth, geometric artifacts due to tissue interfaces are minimized. In this example, an important artifact arising between intraurethral liquid and the transition zone (*arrow*) in a patient treated with transurethral resection is apparent when acquiring DWI with high b value with a 13 Hz bandwidth (**a**). This effect disappears using an acquisition bandwidth of 20 Hz (**b**)

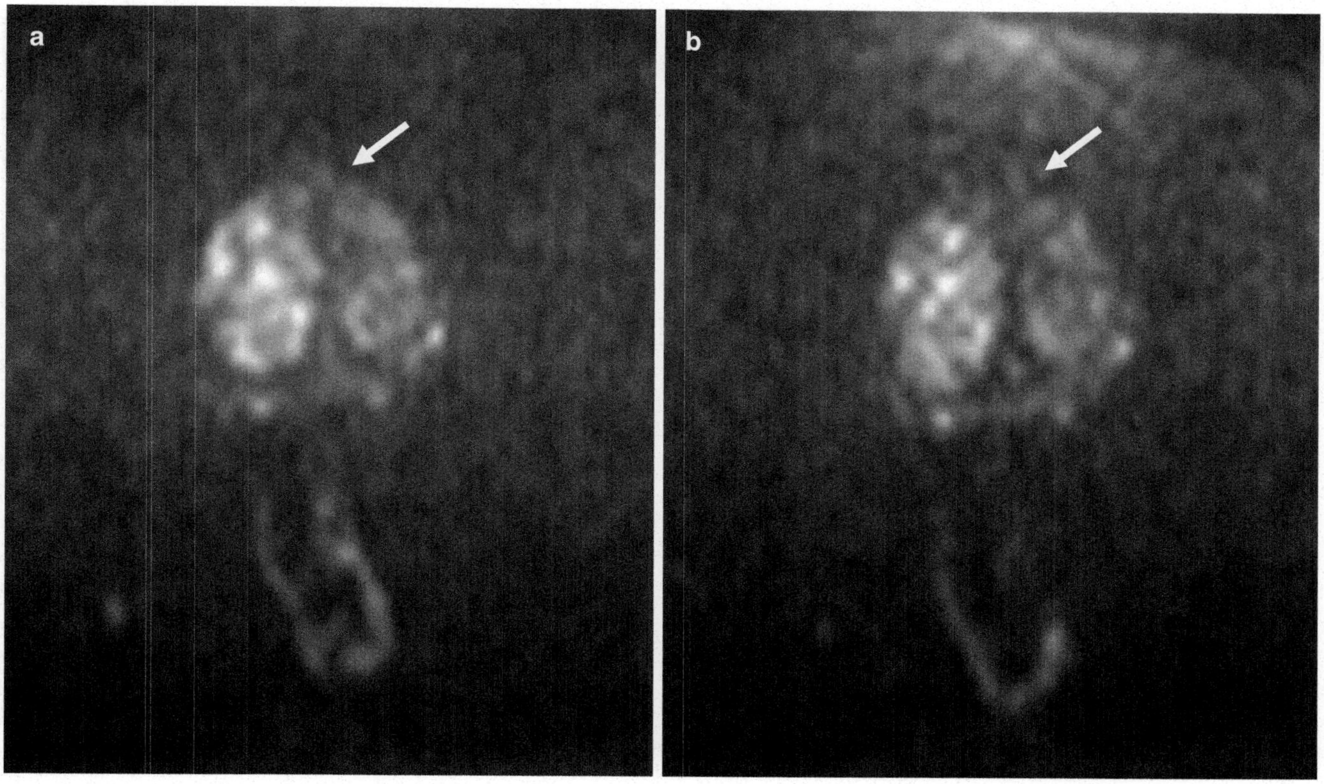

Fig. 1.9 The use of parallel acquisition techniques helps to avoid geometric artifacts in DWI (*arrows*). By increasing SENSE factor to 2 (**a**), geometric artifacts arisen in the anterior fibromuscular stroma using a SENSE factor of 1.4 (**b**) are drastically reduced

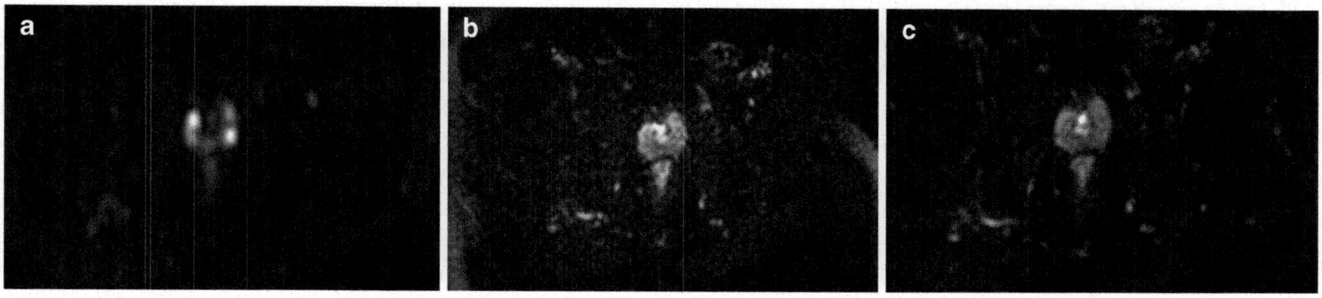

Fig. 1.10 Application of fat suppression techniques in DWI. (**a**) STIR: this method minimizes field inhomogeneity artifacts but leads to low SNRs, requiring increase the number of NEX and acquisition time. As a result, its use is not adequate for prostate examinations. (**b**) SPIR: this method is optimum for 1.5T fields. (**c**) SPAIR: this is the most adequate technique for 3T magnets, since it provides the best reduction of effects arisen from B1 inhomogeneities

Respiratory movement is also a common cause of artifacts and misregistration between *b*-values in body applications of DWI. Therefore, some kind of respiratory motion control is necessary. However, the prostate gland is located deep in the pelvis, and the effect of breathing movement on diffusion signal is not severe. Therefore, DWI of the prostate can usually be performed with free-breathing sequences.

One of the main problems with DWI of the prostate is its lack of standardization, which has limited the comparison between centers, due to lack of agreement on the election of the number and combinations of *b*-values to be used, and different sequence designs between manufacturers and quantification methods.

PI-RADS version 2.0 guidelines recommend the use of a free-breathing SS-SE-EPI with spectral fat suppression and high-resolution sequence (slice thickness ≤4 mm with no gap, reduced FOV between 16 and 20 cm, and in-plane resolution of 2.5 × 2.5 mm) in the axial plane. The number of *b*-values for ADC calculation is not clearly defined. At least, two *b*-values are needed for ADC calculation. The low *b*-value should be between 50 and 100 s/mm^2 to minimize perfusion contamination and the high *b*-value between 800 and 1000 s/mm^2.

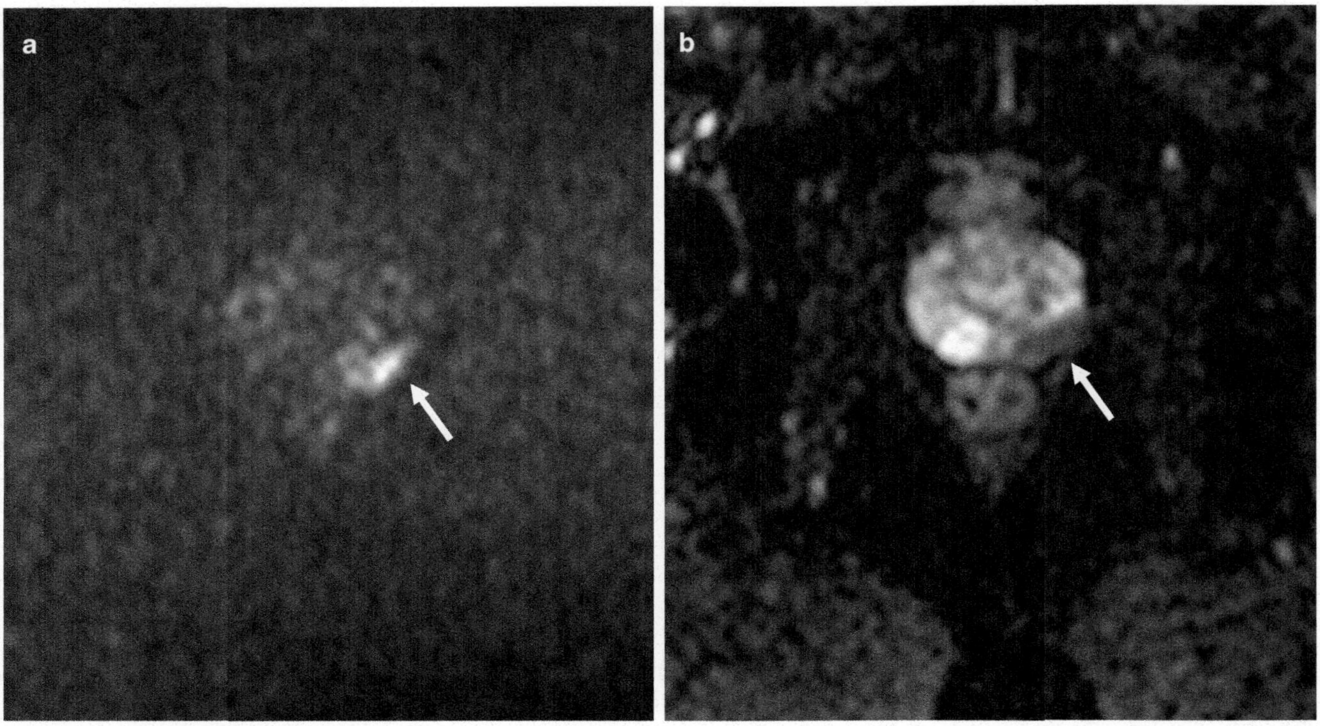

Fig. 1.11 Monocompartmental model of diffusion. The lesion located in the left posterior peripheral zone shows hyperintensity at ultrahigh *b*-values (*b*, 2000 mm^2/s) (**a**) and low ADC values (**b**), thus confirming diffusion restriction of this prostate cancer (*arrows*)

Analysis and Quantitation of Diffusion

DWI is an excellent method to detect pathology in the prostate. In addition, DWI can provide quantitative information about water motion by means of different biomarkers, depending on the diffusion model used for the analysis. The most usual one, involving ADC mapping, derives from the monocompartmental model. This model bypasses one of the most common problems arising from DWI: the T2 shine-through effect, which arises when tissues with long T2 values give rise to signal hyperintensity at high *b*-values, without corresponding to actual restriction of diffusion. In ADC maps, lesions exhibiting high signal intensities at high *b*-values due to actual diffusion present low signal and low ADC values (Fig. 1.11). In contrast, T2 shine-through artifacts remain hyperintense and show high ADC values. An opposite phenomenon, i.e., the T2 blackout effect, occurs in tissues with very short T2 or T2* values, like fibrosis or subacute hemorrhage. Such tissues display low signal intensities at high *b*-values and low ADC values, not as a result of actual restriction of diffusion, but owing to magnetic susceptibility artifacts.

Attention must be also paid to naturally restrictive structures for water diffusion, e.g., normal lymph ganglia, intestinal and rectal mucosae, or the sacral nerve roots in the pelvis, which can become confused with pathologic features in high *b*-value images.

Quantification of diffusion signal is mainly based on the monoexponential model, which assumes a Gaussian distribution of free water motion. However, other models of analysis of diffusion signal decay have shown that the monoexponential model is not completely adequate to evaluate in vivo tissues, as tissue complexity can hinder water diffusion. In this manner, non-Gaussian models such as intra-voxel incoherent motion (IVIM), diffusion kurtosis imaging (DKI), and stretched-exponential model (SEM) can show the in vivo deviation of water proton signal attenuation from the monoexponential model:

- Monocompartmental model: by acquiring only one low *b*-value (between 0 and 100 s/mm^2) and one high *b*-value, whose degree depends on the target anatomy, it is possible to quantify the movement of free water using ADC. In the prostate, a high *b*-value between 800 and 1000 s/mm^2 is recommended, as those *b*-values over 1400 s/mm^2 introduce noise in ADC maps. The use of ultrahigh *b*-values has shown to improve tumor conspicuity. Particularly interesting is their application in the differentiation of benign prostatic hyperplasia from transition zone malignancies or detection of lesions in atypical areas such as anterior fibromuscular stroma or apex [30]. A recent approach permits the calculation of synthesized ultrahigh *b*-value from the extrapolation of normal, acquired *b*-values. This method does not add acquisition time, although the obtained images can be analyzed only qualitatively to improve tumor detection, but should not be included in any quantification model [31].

- According to these guidelines, ADC can also be used to characterize malignant lesions, which appear as areas of decreased signal. However, DWI and ADC mapping are used as qualitative tools, without considering the quantitative information derived from ADC (Fig. 1.11). ADC represents the absolute line slope of the exponential decrease of signal intensities in diffusion images, and it has shown value in the differentiation of PCa from normal peripheral zone with high accuracy and reproducibility [32]. However, to define a threshold value is not possible due to differences in sequence design and set of *b*-values used for calculation [33]. Significant inverse correlation between ADC values and Gleason score has been observed but with important overlap in ADC values of tumors with different Gleason scores [34, 35] and benign prostatic hyperplasia. Also, inverse correlation of ADC with higher percentage of tumor load in biopsies and proliferation markers such as Ki-67 have been reported. However, ADC still presents limitations, such as overlap between ADC values of PCa and prostatitis and other benign conditions [36].
- DWI can help to identify the index lesion for staging purposes. Also, a low ADC value and high PI-RADS assessment category favor the presence of extraglandular extension [37–39].
- Tumor response is in general associated with increases in ADC. But the extent of this response is variable according to the type of therapy (e.g., hormonotherapy will induce a more limited increase in ADC than radiation therapy, RT) [40]. After RT, there is a decrease in ADC of normal peripheral and transition zones [41]. In responding tumors, there is an increase in ADC. Thus, ADC is not able to differentiate between responding tumor and normal prostate after RT [42]. The assessment of prostate after RT is challenging due to glandular atrophy and fibrosis, resulting in diffuse low signal on T2-weighted sequences. Recurrent tumor tends to appear at the site of the primary tumor, as areas of restricted diffusion signal [43]. The combination of DWI and T2-weighted images shows higher area under the curve than T2-weighted sequence alone, without incremental value with the addition of DCE-MRI [44]. Also, DWI, particularly with ultrahigh *b*-value, shows similar results to DCE-MRI in this task [45], and the combined use of DCE-MRI and DWI has a sensitivity near 100% to depict recurrent tumor after RT or prostatectomy [46].
- Finally, active surveillance is recommended in patients with low-grade tumors. DWI can help in the selection of patients and also in their follow-up, due to its ability to differentiate high- and low-grade PCa. In this group of patients, ADC can be used to identify changes in tumor phenotype and as a biomarker of tumor progression [47]. Furthermore, mpMRI improves risk stratification of patients since the development of MRI-TRUS fusion biopsy, which increases detection of clinically significant PCa while reducing detection of insignificant disease [48].
- Bicompartmental model or intra-voxel incoherent motion (IVIM): this model assumes that water movements not only occur in the interstitial spaces but also in vascular spaces. The signal decay kinetics is biphasic, with a fast decay at *b*-values between 0 and 100 s/mm^2, which corresponds to the vascular component, and a slower decay at higher *b*-values owed to conventional water diffusion inside the tissues. The bicompartmental model was initially described by Le Bihan to evaluate brain tumor microcirculation [49], but it has also proved useful for applications in other well-perfused organs, such as the liver, pancreas, kidney, and prostate [50–54].
- In the bicompartmental model, diffusion and perfusion measurements are heavily dependent on the choice of *b*-values. Typically, several *b*-values below and above 100 s/mm^2 are acquired, although faster methods, involving only three *b*-values, have also been proposed.
- The bicompartmental model can be mathematically described by the following equation:

$$\frac{S_b}{S_0} = (1-f)\exp(-bD) + f\exp\left[-b\left(D+D^*\right)\right]$$

where S_0 represents the signal intensity at each *b*-value, also including T1 and T2 relaxation, f represents the perfusion fraction, D is the diffusion coefficient of the tissue, and D^* is the pseudo-diffusion coefficient, which reflects microcapillary perfusion (Fig. 1.12).

Scarce reports have evaluated the role of IVIM in PCa assessment. D, D^*, and f are significantly different in PCa than in normal peripheral zone in the vast majority of series [55]. But they have not shown a clear advantage over ADC in this task [56–58].

Diffusion kurtosis analysis: the monocompartmental model presupposes a Gaussian behavior of free H_2O. Gaussian diffusion assumes a linear decay in the natural logarithm of the DWI signal intensity, but as *b*-values increase, the slope of the decay line (ADC) highlights a loss of linearity. Using ultrahigh *b*-values ($b > 1500$ s/mm^2), non-Gaussian effects of diffusion become apparent. These phenomena are related with a population of H_2O molecules of very slow motion, corresponding to intracellular and membrane-interacting water, and require a more sophisticated analysis, such as diffusion kurtosis imaging (DKI):

$$\frac{S_b}{S_0} = \exp\left(-bD + \frac{b^2D^2K}{6}\right)$$

DKI involves two additional variables in comparison with the monocompartmental model: D (or D^{app}) is the diffusion coefficient adjusted to consider the non-Gaussian

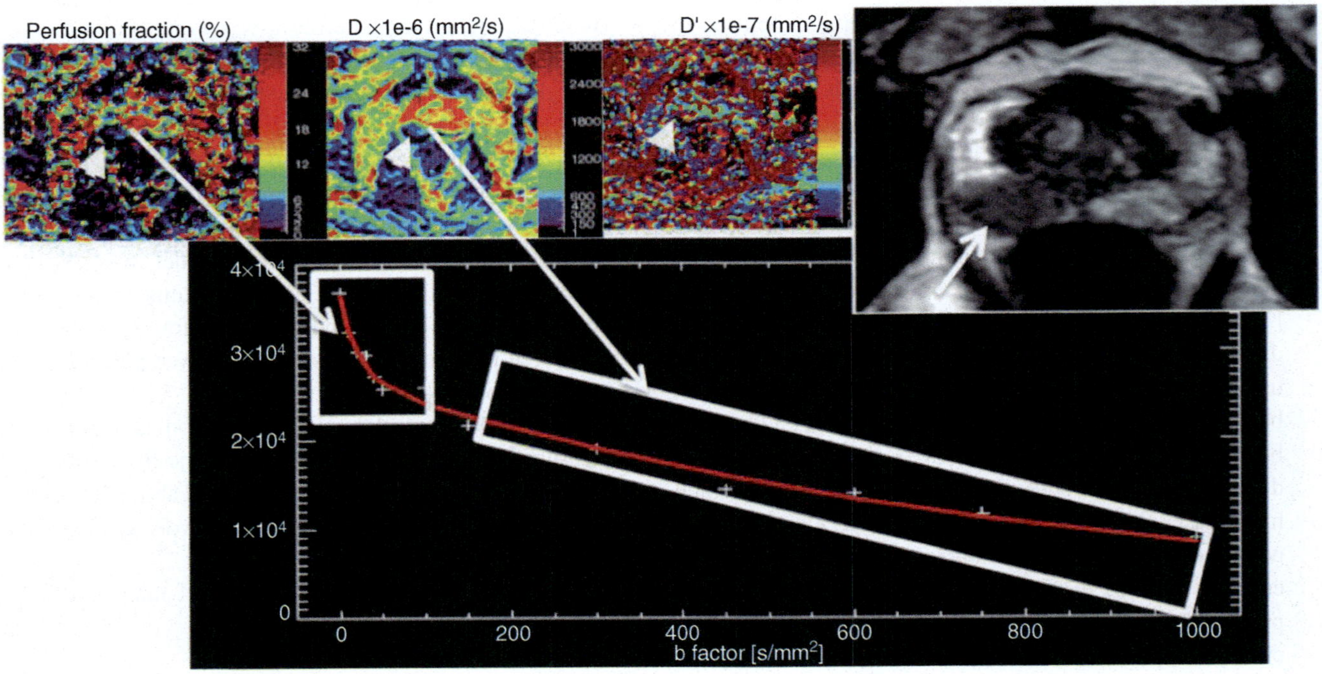

Fig. 1.12 Bicompartmental model of diffusion (IVIM) of prostate cancer of the right peripheral zone (*arrows*). Prostate cancer shows a rapid of diffusion signal for *b*-values between 0 and 100 s/mm^2, corresponding to water motion in the intravascular space representing increased tumor perfusion. It is possible to calculate values of perfusion fraction (*f*) and microcapillary perfusion (D^*). The lesion also shows a slower decay of diffusion signal with b values over 100 mm^2/s, due to restricted water movement in the extracellular space (D)

behavior of diffusion. Like ADC, it is measured in 10^{-3} mm^2/s units. K (or K^{app}) is a dimensionless parameter representing apparent diffusion kurtosis and does not have a direct biophysical basis (Fig. 1.13). Preliminary data evaluating the accuracy of kurtosis in detection of PCa have shown a better fitting of diffusion signal decay with kurtosis than monoexponential model, with improved results in the distinction of PCa from normal peripheral zone [59].

Stretched-exponential model: defines a single additional stretching term, which may represent an approximation either to the intra-voxel diffusion heterogeneity or non-Gaussian diffusion. This model allows the quantification of both Gaussian and non-Gaussian diffusion. Derived biomarkers are the distributed diffusion coefficient (DDC) and α, the heterogeneity index, which evaluates the deviation of the signal attenuation from the monoexponential behavior [60].

Another approach of DWI is diffusion tensor imaging (DTI). It is based on a multidirectional diffusion-encoded approach, through which water movement can be expressed as a matrix of 3 × 3, if a tensor of diffusion is performed. From a DTI point of view, the transitional zone is composed by organized ductal structures with smooth muscle fibers and stroma, which confers hindered diffusion and higher anisotropy, measured using fraction anisotropy (FA). However, the peripheral zone has a random structure and less cellularity, displaying facilitated diffusion of free water and lower anisotropy. Several in vivo studies have demonstrated to discriminate between CG and PZ in basis of both FA and ADC values. CG shows higher FA values and lower ADC values than PZ due to its major cellular component and tissue organization.

The value of DTI for PCa assessment is controversial. PCa with increased cellularity shows an increase of anisotropy, especially compared to normal PZ, with higher FA values than expected. Furthermore, FA values in the sextants found to harbor cancer have shown to positively correlate with the Gleason score, while the ADC values are negatively correlated [61, 62] (Fig. 1.14). In vivo increase in FA values of PCa may be due to low SNR of in vivo acquisitions rather than the presence of cancer, due to an overestimation of the FA values with decreasing ADC [63]. In addition, no significant differences have been found between prostatitis and PCa in basis only of FA values [64]. FA and ADC are useful for distinguishing PCa of CG from benign prostatic (stromal and glandular) hyperplasia nodules in a significant manner, with better diagnostic accuracy for ADC [65, 66].

Other clinical applications of DTI in the prostate are the evaluation of periprostatic nerve plexus through tractographic reconstructions and assessment of number and disposition of those fibers. This application allows to assess both morphological and functional infiltration of those nerve structures for treatment option decision [67] (Fig. 1.15). However, until now there is no evidence to support the systematic use of DTI for PCa evaluation.

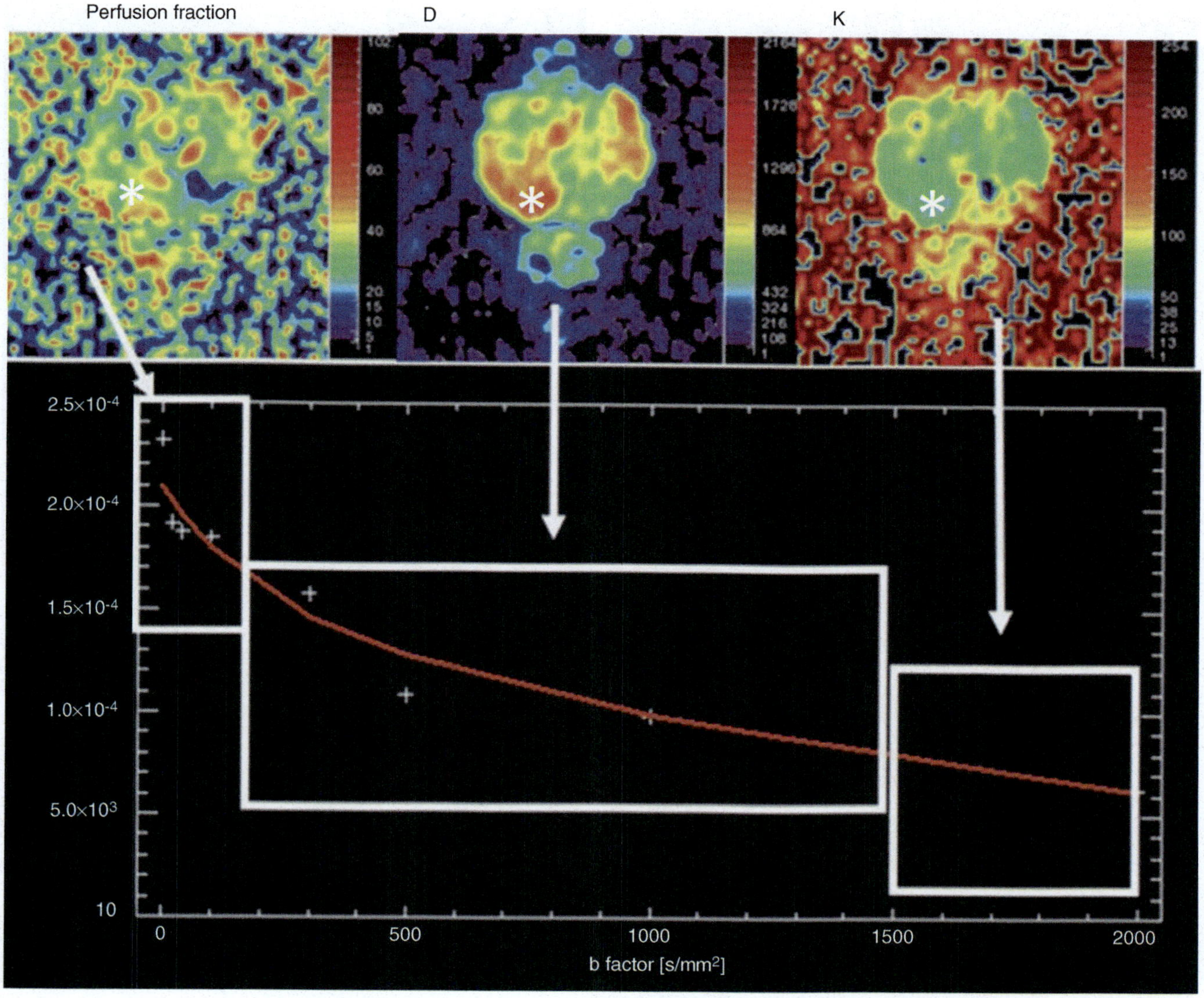

Fig. 1.13 Models of analysis of DWI of prostate cancer of the right peripheral zone. IVIM model provides information of tumor perfusion and tumor restriction. In this manner, the prostate cancer shows increased perfusion fraction calcuated from the fast initial signal decay of signal with *b* values under 100 s/mm^2 and decreased D value calculated with *b* values over 100 s/mm^2. However, the slope of the diffusion signal decay line highlights a loss of linearity at b-values higher than 1500 s/mm^2. Diffusion signal over these values is owed to the movement of water in the intracellular space and its interaction with membranes. As such, kurtosis is increased in irregular, heterogeneous environments as in the malignant lesion (*asterisks*)

DCE-MRI

DCE-MRI sequences, also known as perfusion MRI, were the first functional sequence to be included in clinical protocols of PCa. Neoangiogenesis is an essential process for tumor growth, which is triggered in response to the increasing demand of oxygen and nutrient supply by the tumor. In addition, neoangiogenesis allows the cancer to metastasize. In PCa, the production of antiangiogenic factors (VEGF, VPF) leads to an increase in the microvascular density and permeability of the tumor tissue. As a result, the contrast enhancement pattern of PCa in DCE-MRI studies is different from that of the normal tissue. Thus, dynamic sequences allow for an indirect evaluation of angiogenesis in vivo, in a noninvasive, quantitative manner.

DCE-MRI is based on lower spatial and higher temporal resolution acquisition of multiple scans before, during, and after intravenous contrast administration. The use of multiphasic imaging with high spatial resolution and low temporal acquisitions has been limited in prostatic imaging, as differences between benign and malignant regions in the prostate can be subtle. Therefore, DCE-MRI protocols are based on 3D GE T1-weighted sequences to improve resolution and coverage and minimize inhomogeneity artifacts, providing high temporal resolution. To achieve an appropri-

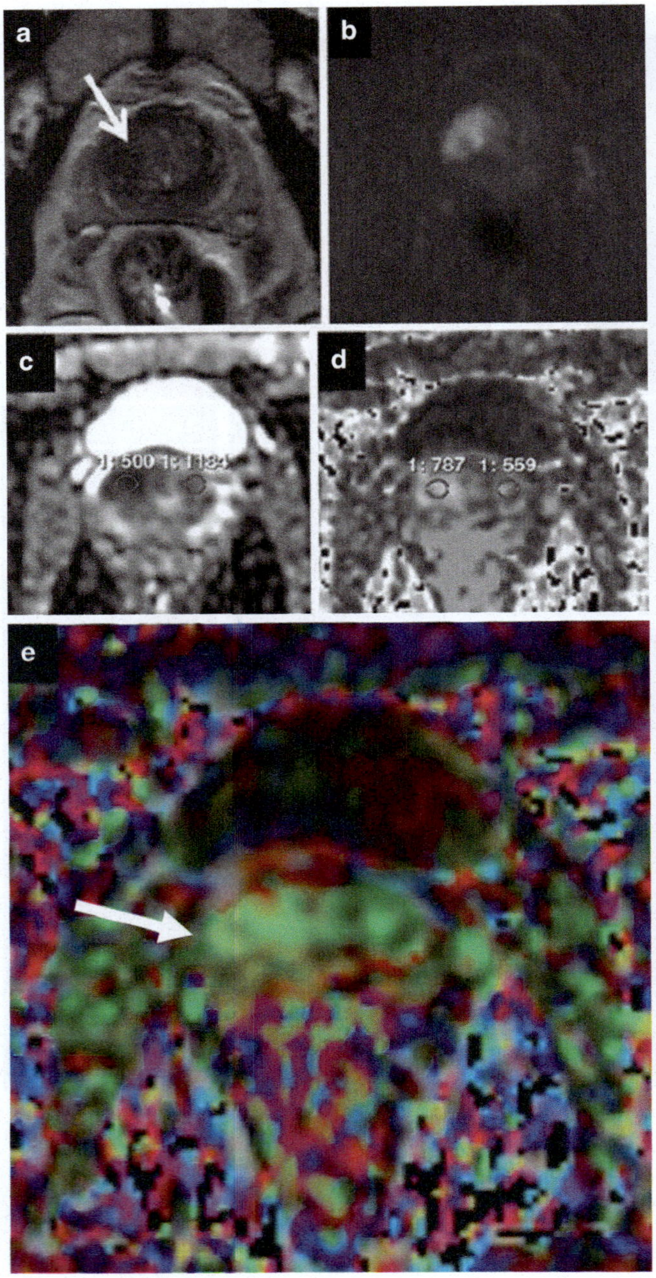

Fig. 1.14 DTI: a hypointense lesion is identified in axial TSE T2-weighted image (*arrow* in **a**) in the right anterior TZ, which shows highly restricted diffusion (**b**) on axial DWI (*b*, 2000 s/mm^2), consistent with clinically significant prostate cancer (Gleason 4+3). (**c**) MD map confirms low diffusivity within the malignant nodule, and (**d**) FA map shows higher FA values than contralateral healthy transition zone. (**e**) FA color-coded map also demonstrates an increased FA (more intense *green tone* at PCa, *arrow*)

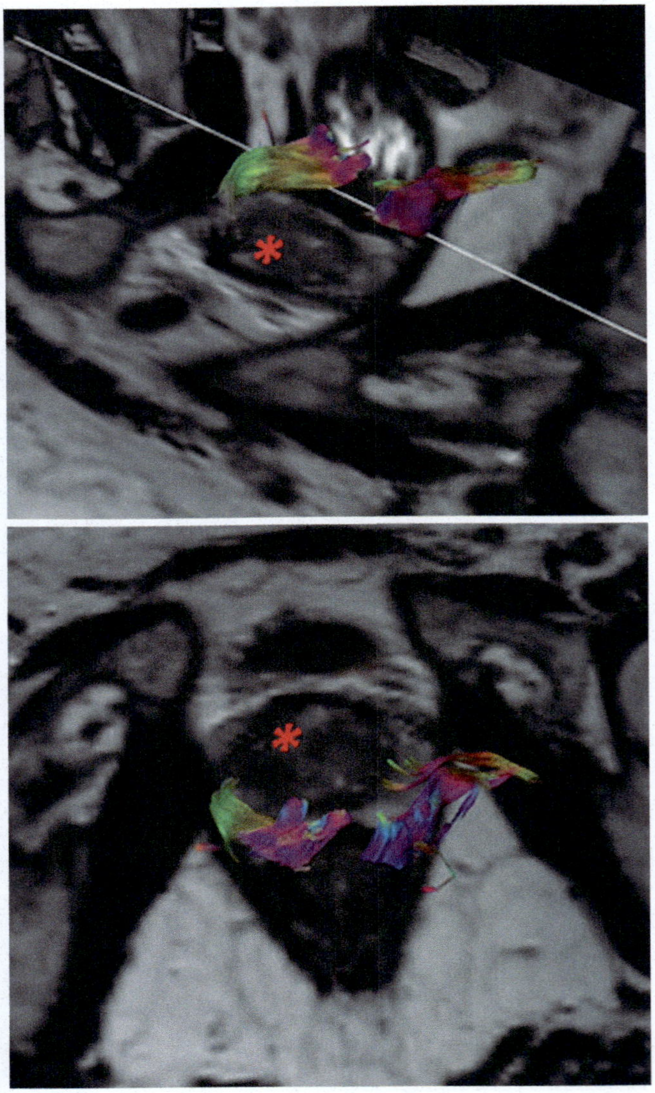

Fig. 1.15 Neurovascular bundle evaluation with DTI in the same patient as the previous figure. Neurography representation of periprostatic nerve plexus shows a marked change with decrease of anisotropy and color-coded tone at the right bundle, which is suspicious of nerve infiltration in close vicinity of the malignant nodule (*asterisk*)

ate spatial resolution needs slice thickness <3 mm with no gap, in-plane resolution ≤2 mm × 2 mm, and FOV adjusted to cover the prostate gland and seminal vesicles. Sequences involve short repetition times (TR) (<1000 ms) and parallel acquisition techniques, with the aim of minimizing the acquisition time of each dynamic dataset, since a high temporal resolution (ideally <3 s per dynamic) is needed. The TE used must also be short (<5 ms), as a means to reduce T2* effects induced by the contrast agent. Similarly, the flip angle must be small (15°). Dynamic images must be acquired over a range of 2 min at least, ideally over 5 min, in order to properly study lesion washout. New technical developments, such as phased-array coils with more elements, higher factors of parallel imaging, compressed sensing, and advanced acquisitions of K-space (i.e., golden radial sampling), are providing high spatiotemporal DCE-MRI, and improvements in image quality and lesion depiction are expected [68].

A dose of 0.1 mmol/kg of low-molecular-weight gadolinium chelates is normally used. The contrast bolus is

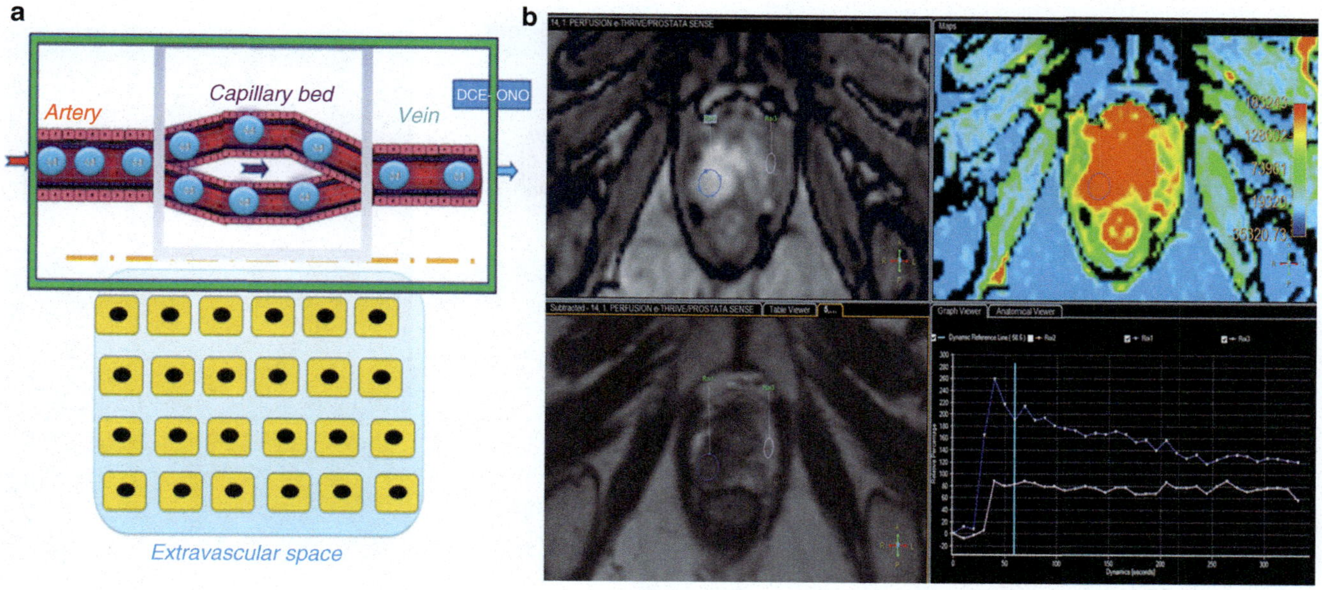

Fig. 1.16 Monocompartmental DCE model studies the passage of contrast only through the intravascular space (**a**). This permits the calculation of time-intensity curves, as well as obtaining parametric maps of tumor, such as relative enhancement (**b**). In this case, a hypervascular prostate cancer is shown in the right peripheral zone marked by a region of interest (blue ROI) demostrating fast initial enhancement and posterior washout (type III time-intensity curve) in comparison with normal left peripheral zone which demosntrates reduced initial enhancement and a delayed plateau (type II time-intensity curve)

intravenously delivered at a rate of 3–5 cc/s, followed by a saline flush of 20–30 mL, injected at the same rate as the contrast medium.

Analysis of DCE-MRI is also controversial. In clinical practice, the use of direct visual assessment of differences in contrast enhancement between prostate gland and suspicious lesions is the most extended. For this purpose, it is preferred to use subtraction techniques or fat-suppressed acquisitions. In order to standardize the analysis of DCE-MRI and improve the results of visual assessment, different software analysis approaches of DCE-MRI have been introduced in the clinical setting:

- Curve typing: this approach provides the analysis of the enhancing kinetics of lesions, by calculating signal intensity-time curves (TIC) and obtaining color parametric maps, generated voxel by voxel, in relation with the tumor blood volume (relative enhancement and maximum relative enhancement) and contrast wash-in (slope, peak enhancement) and washout times. Malignant tumors typically show a rapid contrast uptake and washout (i.e., a so-called type 3 curve), as a characteristic pattern of enhanced perfusion, paralleling the terminology used in breast MRI [69] (Fig. 1.16).
- Pharmacokinetic modeling, also known as compartmental modeling: this model takes into consideration capillary permeability, i.e., the passage of contrast agent from the vessels to the extravascular space. This type of analysis establishes quantitative measurements of constants related to the volume and blood flux through the vessels, using biomarkers, such as k^{trans} (passage of contrast from the vessel to the extravascular compartment), k_{ep} (passage of contrast out of the extravascular space to the intravascular compartments), and V_e (volume of extravascular extracellular space per unit volume of tissue) (Fig. 1.17). For an optimal analysis of the sequence, it is necessary to acquire two T1 maps with different flip angles (10° and 15°), using the same geometry and acquisition parameters as in the dynamic study, in order to calculate the baseline T1 value. Also, it is needed to calculate the arterial input function (Fig. 1.18). These sequences allow to objectify tumor vascular heterogeneity by means of quantitative biomarkers, which can be useful for active and therapeutic monitoring of PCa and for drug development trials. However, as is also the case for DWI sequences, lack of standardization of sequences and postprocessing methods has limited inter-center reproducibility of these analyses, and their use is uncommon in clinical practice [70].

For detection purposes, DCE-MRI has shown limited specificity, with important overlap in curve-type presentation of benign prostate conditions such as prostatitis and benign prostatic hyperplasia and PCa [71]. Therefore, owing to the marked vascular heterogeneity and variable behavior of PCa, the role of perfusion MRI is today secondary for the detection and characterization of the disease, according to the PI-RADS version 2.0 guidelines, where DCE-MRI is relegated to the assessment of indeterminate lesions in the peripheral zone. Thus, DCE-MRI is regarded as a secondary

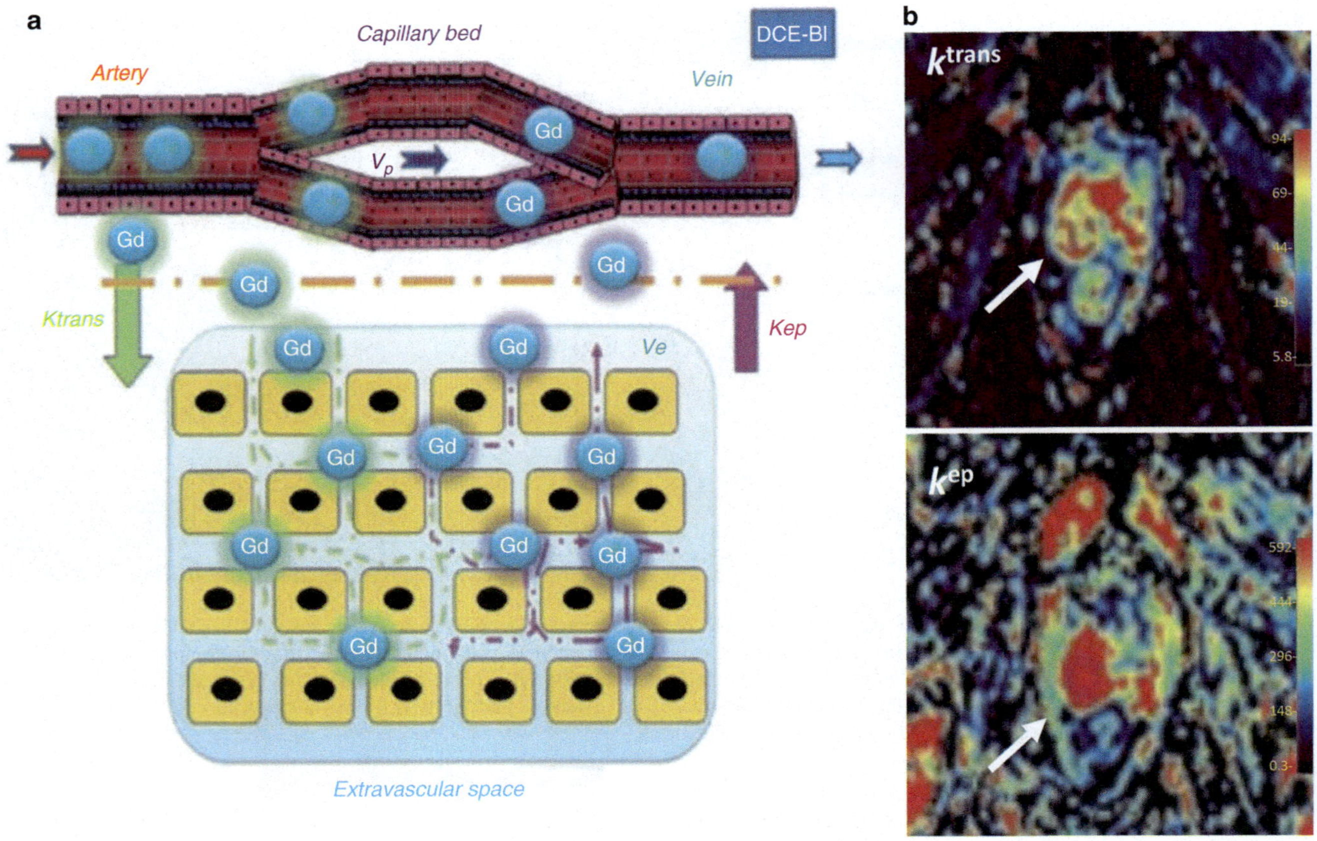

Fig. 1.17 Bicompartmental DCE model studies the passage of contrast through the intravascular space as well as the extravascular intercellular space (**a**). This permits the quantitation of capillary permeability and tumor blood volume. In this case, the PCa (*arrows*) shows increased k^{trans} and k^{ep} values (**b**)

modifier of DWI, the dominant sequence in the peripheral zone, only in cases where DWI depicts a lesion with uncertain features of malignancy (PI-RADS 3). However, DCE-MRI is helpful in cases where the quality of DWI is compromised or there are multiple suspicious lesions on T2-weighted sequence and DWI [16, 72].

DCE-MRI has also demonstrated a role in staging of PCa [73], guiding biopsy [74], planning treatment [75], and monitoring posttherapy recurrences [76]. In this last scenario, there are also data supporting the exclusion of DCE-MRI in the detection of recurrence after radiation therapy [46]. However, this approach is still needed in the assessment of patients treated with ablative focal therapy [71].

MR Spectroscopy (MRS)

MRS can provide metabolic information on the normal and pathologic prostate gland and has the ability to detect specific patterns suggestive of malignancy. The normal prostate gland shows elevated levels of citrate (Cit), which is synthesized and secreted by normal prostatic epithelial cells [77], and low levels of choline (Cho), the latter being a marker of cell proliferation. In malignant processes, this pattern is reverted, i.e., Cho is elevated and Cit levels are depleted, reflecting an increase in cell turnover and the loss of normal cellular function and luminal organization, respectively [19] (Fig. 1.19). Cit is centered at 2.6 ppm and Cho resonates at 3.2 ppm. Other relevant metabolites that can be found in the prostate proton MR spectrum are creatine, which is located at 3.0 ppm, and polyamines, particularly spermine, which are located between the Cho and creatine peaks. The polyamine peaks are usually broad and overlap Cho and creatine, being better depicted using 3T magnets. Also, polyamine levels typically decrease in CaP [78]. Relative indices have been proposed among these metabolites to be used as markers of malignancy, as the quantification of metabolites in the prostate is very challenging due to poor SNR and strong *J*-coupling of the citrate.

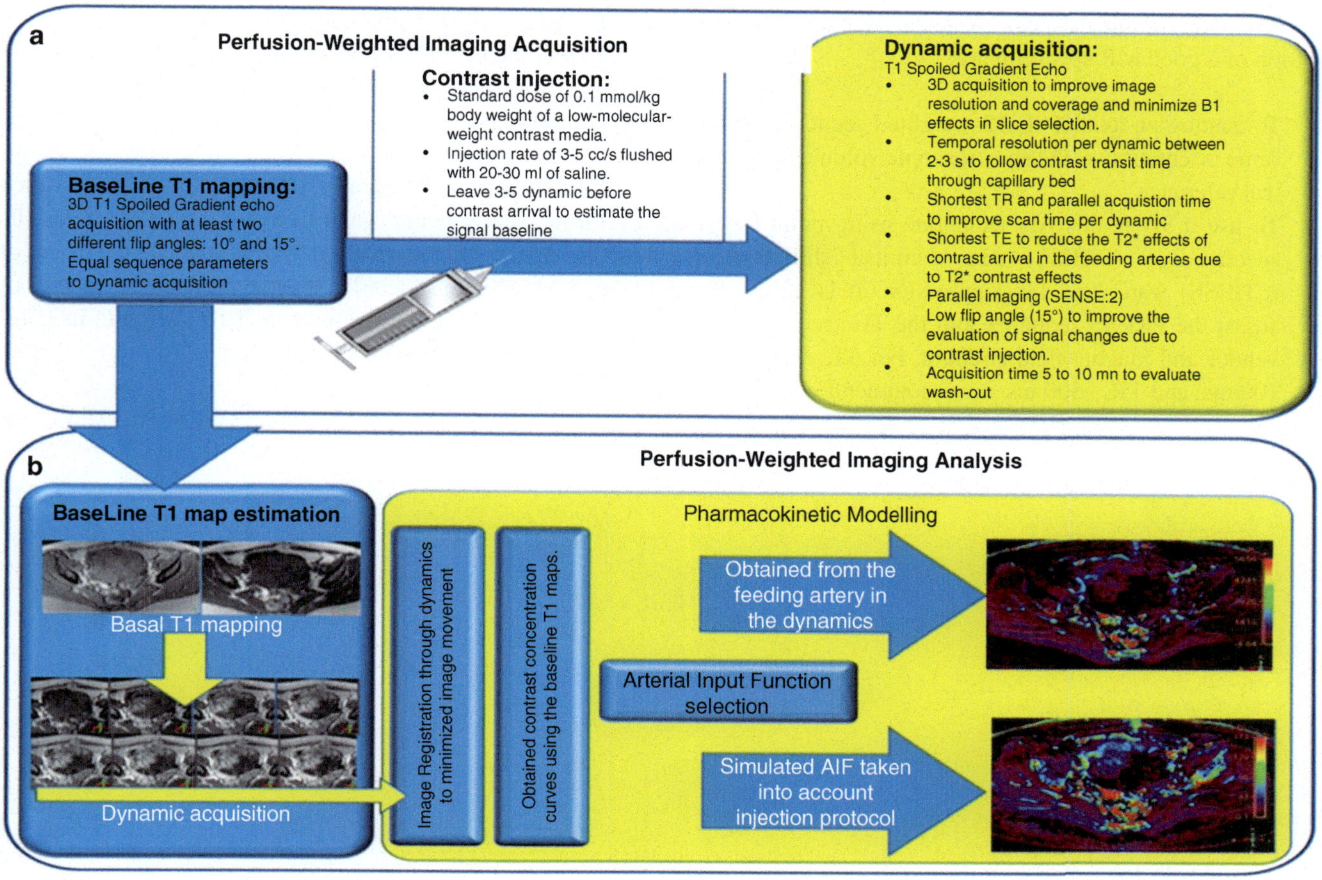

Fig. 1.18 Schematic representation of a perfusion sequence acquisition (**a**) and analysis thereof (**b**)

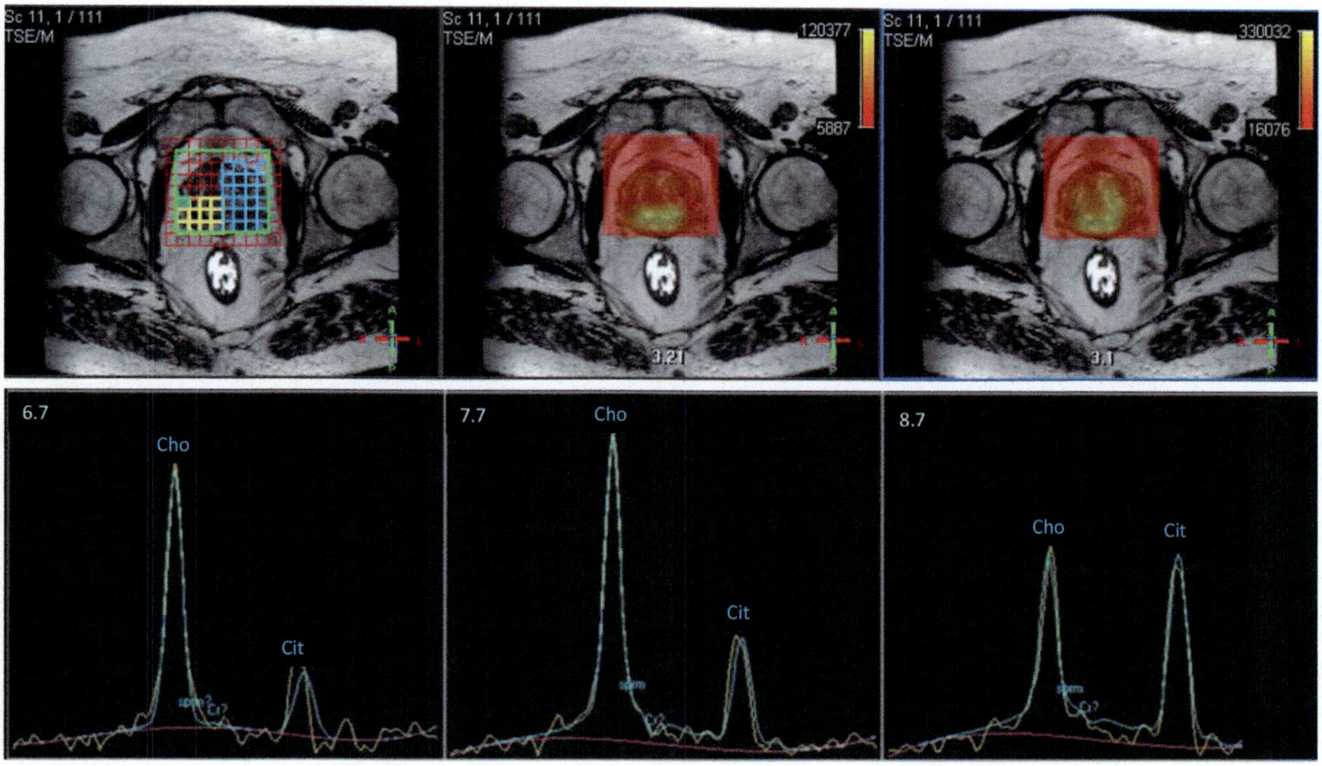

Fig. 1.19 Multivoxel MR spectroscopy study, showing increased levels of choline (Cho) and depleted levels of citrate (Ct)

The main technical aspects to be considered for the acquisition of a good MR spectrum are:

- To acquire an axial TSE T2-weighted sequence with the same orientation as the spectroscopic volume, as anatomical reference.
- To use a 3D multivoxel technique using point-resolved spectroscopy (PRESS) and chemical shift selective (CHESS) water and fat suppression. It is necessary to adjust the PRESS sequence and the TE according to the vendor and magnet field strength. For 3T, generally TE, 100 ms, and TR, 1500 ms, are recommended.
- To use automatic shimming for linewidth reduction.
- To include the entire prostate gland avoiding contamination from periglandular fat and seminal vesicles using saturation bands.

MRS is a very technically demanding technique, which performs clearly better when using 3T magnetic fields. Its use has dropped significantly in recent years, to the extent of being no longer considered in the recommended protocols of PI-RADS version 2.0 guidelines in 2015, owing to its complex acquisition and low reproducibility.

1.3 Advanced Analysis of mpMRI

Different types of *computer-aided diagnosis systems* (*CAD*) are clinically available. This type of software permits to automatically extract and evaluate imaging features, calculate prostate and lesion volumes, and integrate multiple quantitative parameters from functional sequences, improving lesion detection, diagnostic workflow, and reader accuracy, particularly for the less experienced ones [79, 80]. Also, CAD is usually needed to plan targeted biopsy or focal therapy of PCa. Furthermore, they have been evaluated for radiotherapy planning [81].

Prostate cancer is often multifocal and heterogeneous, and there are various analytic methods to measure intratumor spatial heterogeneity such as histogram analysis, texture-based analysis, or fractal analysis.

Histogram analyses study the distribution of signal intensity in a tumor for describing its composition and heterogeneity. In clinical practice, it is usually performed based on a region of interest (ROI), although volume of interest-based analysis is probably more accurate. ADC histogram analysis has been used in clinical studies to measure its impact in PCa management [82].

Texture-based analysis can identify imaging texture features, more commonly tactile, which describe and quantify the spatial distribution and heterogeneity of voxel intensities. It has been applied to the different sequences of mpMRI, demonstrating a potential role in the differentiation of PCa from normal prostatic tissue [83–85] and in the noninvasive stratification of patients with PCa according to their Gleason score [86, 87]. In a similar manner, *fractal analyses*, which assign a fractal dimension and other fractal characteristics to mpMRI, can also quantify the spatial heterogeneity in texture and intensity distribution associated with PCa on T2-weighted images [88, 89] (Fig. 1.20).

Radiomics and *radiogenomics* use complex computational algorithms of analysis to extract quantitative descriptors of PCa heterogeneity and phenotype from mpMRI and correlate them with clinical, analytical, or genetic data, respectively. Radiomic features using a specific peripheral zone classifier significantly improved the accuracy of PCa in the peripheral zone in a very recent multicenter study [90]. Also, a series correlating radiogenomic parameters of six PCa cases confirmed by MRI-guided biopsy showed significant correlations between three gene signatures associated with adverse outcome in aggressive PCa and quantitative imaging data, indicating the prognostic value of the radiomic features [91]. Finally,

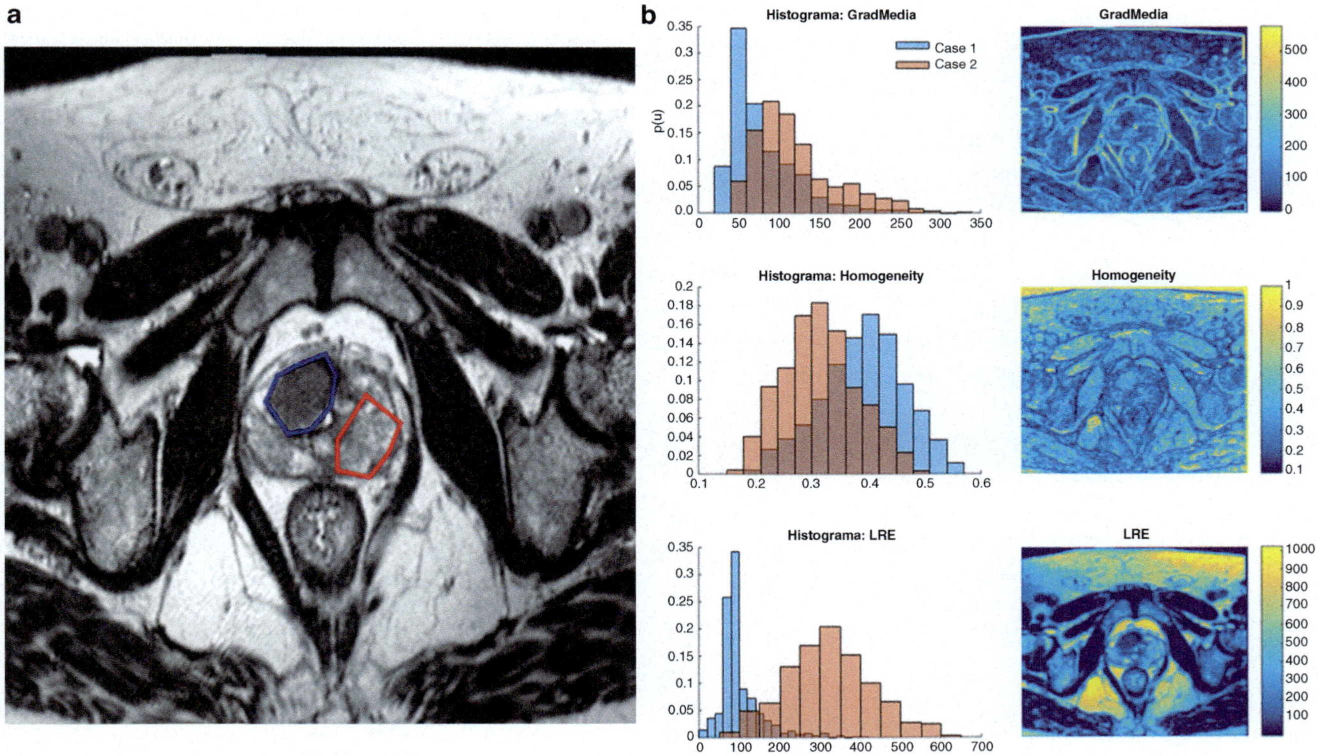

Fig. 1.20 Texture analysis. (**a**) Axial section corresponding to a TSE T2-weighted image, highlighting a tumor lesion (*blue ROI*) and a healthy tissue area (*red ROI*). (**b**) Histograms (*left*) and parametric maps (*right*) according to different texture analysis parameters corresponding to statistical (SGLD) and structural (run-length) methods. Histograms of the tumor ROI are shown in *blue*; histograms of the healthy ROI are shown in *brown*

other series showed weak but significant associations between K_{ep} derived from pharmacokinetic modeling of DCE-MRI and Gleason score with PTEN phosphatase and tensin homolog expression, an independent prognostic marker of biochemical recurrence and clinical outcome parameters [92].

Conclusion

mpMRI is a very useful tool in studies of PCa and has a real potential to change the management of the uro-oncologic patient for the better. It is gaining acceptance as the first test in patients with clinical suspicion of PCa. Through a palette of morphologic and functional techniques, including T1-weighted, T2-weighted images, DWI, and DCE-MRI, and thanks to hardware improvements such as high-field scanners and multichannel surface coils, mpMRI offers the possibility to detect and characterize clinically significant PCa with a high degree of sensitivity and specificity. Different adjustments in sequence design are required to optimize the results of mpMRI. Also, new sequences, such as T1 and T2 mapping, offer opportunities to improve the performance of mpMRI. Furthermore, non-Gaussian models of quantification of DWI and new mathematical methods of analysis of mpMRI representing PCa tumor heterogeneity, such as texture-based analysis, fractal analysis, and histogram analysis, will probably expand the applications of mpMRI in the future.

Key Points

- Multiparametric MRI (mpMRI) uses morphologic and functional techniques, including T1-weighted, T2-weighted images, DWI, and DCE-MRI to detect and characterize clinically significant PCa.
- Different adjustments in sequence design are required to optimize the results of mpMRI.
- New sequences, such as T1 and T2 mapping, offer opportunities to improve the performance of mpMRI.
- Non-Gaussian models of quantification of DWI and new mathematical methods of analysis of mpMRI representing PCa tumor heterogeneity, such as texture-based analysis, fractal analysis, and histogram analysis, will probably expand the applications of mpMRI in the future.

References

1. Siegel RL, Miller KD, Jemal A. Cancer statistics, 2015. CA Cancer J Clin. 2015;65(1):5–29.
2. Ferlay J, Steliarova-Foucher E, Lortet-Tieulent J, et al. Cancer incidence and mortality patterns in Europe: estimates for 40 countries in 2012. Eur J Cancer. 2013;49(6):1374–403.
3. De Angelis R, Sant M, Coleman MP, et al. Cancer survival in Europe 1999–2007 by country and age: results of EUROCARE--5-a population-based study. Lancet Oncol. 2014;15(1):23–34.
4. Ahmed HU, Arya M, Freeman A, et al. Do low-grade and low-volume prostate cancers bear the hallmarks of malignancy? Lancet Oncol. 2012;13(11):e509–17.
5. Musunuru HB, Yamamoto T, Klotz L, et al. Active surveillance for intermediate risk prostate cancer: survival outcomes in the Sunnybrook experience. J Urol. 2016;196(6):1651–8.
6. Epstein JI, Zelefsky MJ, Sjoberg DD, et al. A contemporary prostate cancer grading system: a validated alternative to the Gleason score. Eur Urol. 2016;69(3):428–35.
7. Dahm P, Neuberger M, Ilic D. Screening for prostate cancer: shaping the debate on benefits and harms. Cochrane Database Syst Rev. 2013;(9):ED000067.
8. Ilic D, Neuberger MM, Djulbegovic M, et al. Screening for prostate cancer. Cochrane Database Syst Rev. 2013;(1):CD004720.
9. Catalona WJ, Richie JP, Ahmann FR, et al. Comparison of digital rectal examination and serum prostate specific antigen in the early detection of prostate cancer: results of a multicenter clinical trial of 6,630 men. J Urol. 1994;151(5):1283–90.
10. van Hove A, Savoie PH, Maurin C, et al. Comparison of image-guided targeted biopsies versus systematic randomized biopsies in the detection of prostate cancer: a systematic literature review of well-designed studies. World J Urol. 2014;32(4):847–58.
11. Heidenreich A, Bellmunt J, Bolla M, et al. EAU guidelines on prostate cancer. Part 1: screening, diagnosis, and treatment of clinically localised disease. Eur Urol. 2011;59(1):61–71.
12. Kuru TH, Herden J, Zugor V, et al. How to perform image-guided prostate biopsy: in-bore and fusion approaches. Eur Urol Focus. 2016;2(2):151–3.
13. Ahmed HU, El-Shater Bosaily A, Brown LC, et al. Diagnostic accuracy of multi-parametric MRI and TRUS biopsy in prostate cancer (PROMIS): a paired validating confirmatory study. Lancet. 2017;389(10071):815–22.
14. Weinreb JC, Barentsz JO, Choyke PL, et al. PI-RADS prostate imaging - reporting and data system: 2015, version 2. Eur Urol. 2016;69(1):16–40.
15. de Rooij M, Hamoen EH, Witjes JA, et al. Accuracy of magnetic resonance imaging for local staging of prostate cancer: a diagnostic meta-analysis. Eur Urol. 2016;70(2):233–45.
16. Stanzione A, Imbriaco M, Cocozza S, et al. Biparametric 3T magnetic resonance imaging for prostatic cancer detection in a biopsy-naive patient population: a further improvement of PI-RADS v2? Eur J Radiol. 2016;85(12):2269–74.
17. Yu AC, Badve C, Ponsky LE, et al. Development of a combined MR fingerprinting and diffusion examination for prostate cancer. Radiology. 2017;283(3):729–38.
18. Engelbrecht MR, Jager GJ, Laheij RJ, et al. Local staging of prostate cancer using magnetic resonance imaging: a meta-analysis. Eur Radiol. 2002;12(9):2294–302.
19. de Leon AD, Costa D, Pedrosa I. Role of multiparametric MR imaging in malignancies of the urogenital tract. Magn Reson Imaging Clin N Am. 2016;24(1):187–204.
20. Rosenkrantz AB, Neil J, Kong X, et al. Prostate cancer: comparison of 3D T2-weighted with conventional 2D T2-weighted imaging for image quality and tumor detection. AJR Am J Roentgenol. 2010;194(2):446–52.
21. Cornud F, Rouanne M, Beuvon F, et al. Endorectal 3D T2-weighted 1mm-slice thickness MRI for prostate cancer staging at 1.5Tesla: should we reconsider the indirects signs of extracapsular extension according to the D'Amico tumor risk criteria? Eur J Radiol. 2012;81(4):e591–7.
22. Westphalen AC, Noworolski SM, Harisinghani M, et al. High-resolution 3-T endorectal prostate MRI: a multireader study of radiologist preference and perceived interpretive quality of 2D and

3D T2-weighted fast spin-echo MR images. AJR Am J Roentgenol. 2016;206(1):86–91.
23. Yamauchi FI, Penzkofer T, Fedorov A, et al. Prostate cancer discrimination in the peripheral zone with a reduced field-of-view T(2)-mapping MRI sequence. Magn Reson Imaging. 2015;33(5):525–30.
24. Wu LM, Yao QY, Zhu J, et al. T2* mapping combined with conventional T2-weighted image for prostate cancer detection at 3.0T MRI: a multi-observer study. Acta Radiol. 2017;58(1):114–20.
25. Wu LM, Zhao ZZ, Chen XX, et al. Comparison of T2(*) mapping with diffusion-weighted imaging in the characterization of low-grade vs intermediate-grade and high-grade prostate cancer. Br J Radiol. 2016;89(1063):20151076.
26. Le Bihan D. Apparent diffusion coefficient and beyond: what diffusion MR imaging can tell us about tissue structure. Radiology. 2013;268(2):318–22.
27. Vilanova JC, García-Figueiras R, Barceló J, et al. Diffusion-weighted imaging of prostate, bladder, and retroperitoneum. In: Luna A, Ribes R, Soto JA, editors. Diffusion MRI outside the brain: a case-based review and clinical applications. Berlin: Springer; 2012. p. 145–75.
28. Panebianco V, Barchetti F, Sciarra A, et al. Multiparametric magnetic resonance imaging vs. standard care in men being evaluated for prostate cancer: a randomized study. Urol Oncol. 2015;33(1):17 e1–7.
29. Pruessmann KP, Weiger M, Scheidegger MB, et al. SENSE: sensitivity encoding for fast MRI. Magn Reson Med. 1999;42(5):952–62.
30. Katahira K, Takahara T, Kwee TC, et al. Ultra-high-b-value diffusion-weighted MR imaging for the detection of prostate cancer: evaluation in 201 cases with histopathological correlation. Eur Radiol. 2011;21(1):188–96.
31. Taouli B, Beer AJ, Chenevert T, et al. Diffusion-weighted imaging outside the brain: consensus statement from an ISMRM-sponsored workshop. J Magn Reson Imaging. 2016;44(3):521–40.
32. Vargas HA, Akin O, Franiel T, et al. Diffusion-weighted endorectal MR imaging at 3 T for prostate cancer: tumor detection and assessment of aggressiveness. Radiology. 2011;259(3):775–84.
33. Turkbey B, Shah VP, Pang Y, et al. Is apparent diffusion coefficient associated with clinical risk scores for prostate cancers that are visible on 3-T MR images? Radiology. 2011;258(2):488–95.
34. Gibbs P, Liney GP, Pickles MD, et al. Correlation of ADC and T2 measurements with cell density in prostate cancer at 3.0 Tesla. Investig Radiol. 2009;44(9):572–6.
35. Hambrock T, Somford DM, Huisman HJ, et al. Relationship between apparent diffusion coefficients at 3.0-T MR imaging and Gleason grade in peripheral zone prostate cancer. Radiology. 2011;259(2):453–61.
36. Zhang J, Jing H, Han X, et al. Diffusion-weighted imaging of prostate cancer on 3T MR: relationship between apparent diffusion coefficient values and Ki-67 expression. Acad Radiol. 2013;20(12):1535–41.
37. Rud E, Klotz D, Rennesund K, et al. Detection of the index tumour and tumour volume in prostate cancer using T2-weighted and diffusion-weighted magnetic resonance imaging (MRI) alone. BJU Int. 2014;114(6b):E32–42.
38. Karavitakis M, Ahmed HU, Abel PD, et al. Margin status after laparoscopic radical prostatectomy and the index lesion: implications for preoperative evaluation of tumor focality in prostate cancer. J Endourol. 2012;26(5):503–8.
39. Baco E, Rud E, Vlatkovic L, et al. Predictive value of magnetic resonance imaging determined tumor contact length for extracapsular extension of prostate cancer. J Urol. 2015;193(2):466–72.
40. Vargas HA, Wassberg C, Akin O, et al. MR imaging of treated prostate cancer. Radiology. 2012;262(1):26–42.
41. Padhani AR, Gogbashian A. Bony metastases: assessing response to therapy with whole-body diffusion MRI. Cancer Imaging. 2011;11(1A):S129–45.
42. Song I, Kim CK, Park BK, et al. Assessment of response to radiotherapy for prostate cancer: value of diffusion-weighted MRI at 3 T. AJR Am J Roentgenol. 2010;194(6):W477–82.
43. Park JJ, Kim CK, Park SY, et al. Prostate cancer: role of pretreatment multiparametric 3-T MRI in predicting biochemical recurrence after radical prostatectomy. AJR Am J Roentgenol. 2014;202(5):W459–65.
44. Panebianco V, Barchetti F, Sciarra A, et al. Prostate cancer recurrence after radical prostatectomy: the role of 3-T diffusion imaging in multi-parametric magnetic resonance imaging. Eur Radiol. 2013;23(6):1745–52.
45. Roy C, Foudi F, Charton J, et al. Comparative sensitivities of functional MRI sequences in detection of local recurrence of prostate carcinoma after radical prostatectomy or external-beam radiotherapy. AJR Am J Roentgenol. 2013;200(4):W361–8.
46. Donati OF, Jung SI, Vargas HA, et al. Multiparametric prostate MR imaging with T2-weighted, diffusion-weighted, and dynamic contrast-enhanced sequences: are all pulse sequences necessary to detect locally recurrent prostate cancer after radiation therapy? Radiology. 2013;268(2):440–50.
47. van As NJ, de Souza NM, Riches SF, et al. A study of diffusion-weighted magnetic resonance imaging in men with untreated localised prostate cancer on active surveillance. Eur Urol. 2009;56(6):981–7.
48. Giles SL, Morgan VA, Riches SF, et al. Apparent diffusion coefficient as a predictive biomarker of prostate cancer progression: value of fast and slow diffusion components. AJR Am J Roentgenol. 2011;196(3):586–91.
49. Le Bihan D, Breton E, Lallemand D, et al. Separation of diffusion and perfusion in intravoxel incoherent motion MR imaging. Radiology. 1988;168(2):497–505.
50. Guiu B, Cercueil JP. Liver diffusion-weighted MR imaging: the tower of Babel? Eur Radiol. 2011;21(3):463–7.
51. Granata V, Fusco R, Catalano O, et al. Early assessment of colorectal cancer patients with liver metastases treated with antiangiogenic drugs: the role of intravoxel incoherent motion in diffusion-weighted imaging. PLoS One. 2015;10(11):e0142876.
52. Hectors SJ, Wagner M, Besa C, et al. Intravoxel incoherent motion diffusion-weighted imaging of hepatocellular carcinoma: is there a correlation with flow and perfusion metrics obtained with dynamic contrast-enhanced MRI? J Magn Reson Imaging. 2016;44(4):856–64.
53. Chandarana H, Lee VS, Hecht E, et al. Comparison of biexponential and monoexponential model of diffusion weighted imaging in evaluation of renal lesions: preliminary experience. Investig Radiol. 2011;46(5):285–91.
54. Dopfert J, Lemke A, Weidner A, et al. Investigation of prostate cancer using diffusion-weighted intravoxel incoherent motion imaging. Magn Reson Imaging. 2011;29(8):1053–8.
55. Shinmoto H, Tamura C, Soga S, et al. An intravoxel incoherent motion diffusion-weighted imaging study of prostate cancer. AJR Am J Roentgenol. 2012;199(4):W496–500.
56. Suo S, Chen X, Wu L, et al. Non-Gaussian water diffusion kurtosis imaging of prostate cancer. Magn Reson Imaging. 2014;32(5):421–7.
57. Roethke MC, Kuder TA, Kuru TH, et al. Evaluation of diffusion kurtosis imaging versus standard diffusion imaging for detection and grading of peripheral zone prostate cancer. Investig Radiol. 2015;50(8):483–9.
58. Rosenkrantz AB, Padhani AR, Chenevert TL, et al. Body diffusion kurtosis imaging: basic principles, applications, and considerations for clinical practice. J Magn Reson Imaging. 2015;42(5):1190–202.
59. Rosenkrantz AB, Sigmund EE, Johnson G, et al. Prostate cancer: feasibility and preliminary experience of a diffusional kurtosis model for detection and assessment of aggressiveness of peripheral zone cancer. Radiology. 2012;264(1):126–35.

60. Mazaheri Y, Afaq A, Rowe DB, et al. Diffusion-weighted magnetic resonance imaging of the prostate: improved robustness with stretched exponential modeling. J Comput Assist Tomogr. 2012;36(6):695–703.
61. Li C, Chen M, Li S, et al. Diffusion tensor imaging of prostate at 3.0 Tesla. Acta Radiol. 2011;52(7):813–7.
62. Li L, Margolis DJ, Deng M, et al. Correlation of Gleason scores with magnetic resonance diffusion tensor imaging in peripheral zone prostate cancer. J Magn Reson Imaging. 2015;42(2):460–7.
63. Uribe CF, Jones EC, Chang SD, et al. In vivo 3T and ex vivo 7T diffusion tensor imaging of prostate cancer: correlation with histology. Magn Reson Imaging. 2015;33(5):577–83.
64. Xu J, Humphrey PA, Kibel AS, et al. Magnetic resonance diffusion characteristics of histologically defined prostate cancer in humans. Magn Reson Med. 2009;61(4):842–50.
65. Park SY, Kim CK, Park BK, et al. Diffusion-tensor MRI at 3 T: differentiation of central gland prostate cancer from benign prostatic hyperplasia. AJR Am J Roentgenol. 2014;202(3):W254–62.
66. Gurses B, Tasdelen N, Yencilek F, et al. Diagnostic utility of DTI in prostate cancer. Eur J Radiol. 2011;79(2):172–6.
67. Panebianco V, Barchetti F, Sciarra A, et al. In vivo 3D neuroanatomical evaluation of periprostatic nerve plexus with 3T-MR diffusion tensor imaging. Eur J Radiol. 2013;82(10):1677–82.
68. Rosenkrantz AB, Geppert C, Grimm R, et al. Dynamic contrast-enhanced MRI of the prostate with high spatiotemporal resolution using compressed sensing, parallel imaging, and continuous golden-angle radial sampling: preliminary experience. J Magn Reson Imaging. 2015;41(5):1365–73.
69. Alonzi R, Padhani AR, Allen C. Dynamic contrast enhanced MRI in prostate cancer. Eur J Radiol. 2007;63(3):335–50.
70. Vilanova JC, Luna-Alcala A, Boada M, et al. Multiparametric MRI. The role of MRI techniques in the diagnosis, staging and follow up of prostate cancer. Arch Esp Urol. 2015;68(3):316–33.
71. Barrett T. Contrasting opinions: biparametric versus multiparametric prostate MRI. Diagn Interv Radiol. 2016;22(3):299.
72. Thestrup KC, Logager V, Baslev I, et al. Biparametric versus multiparametric MRI in the diagnosis of prostate cancer. Acta Radiol Open. 2016;5(8):2058460116663046.
73. Dickinson L, Ahmed HU, Allen C, et al. Magnetic resonance imaging for the detection, localisation, and characterisation of prostate cancer: recommendations from a European consensus meeting. Eur Urol. 2011;59(4):477–94.
74. Franiel T, Stephan C, Erbersdobler A, et al. Areas suspicious for prostate cancer: MR-guided biopsy in patients with at least one transrectal US-guided biopsy with a negative finding--multiparametric MR imaging for detection and biopsy planning. Radiology. 2011;259(1):162–72.
75. Ogura K, Maekawa S, Okubo K, et al. Dynamic endorectal magnetic resonance imaging for local staging and detection of neurovascular bundle involvement of prostate cancer: correlation with histopathologic results. Urology. 2001;57(4):721–6.
76. Akin O, Gultekin DH, Vargas HA, et al. Incremental value of diffusion weighted and dynamic contrast enhanced MRI in the detection of locally recurrent prostate cancer after radiation treatment: preliminary results. Eur Radiol. 2011;21(9):1970–8.
77. Costello LC, Franklin RB. Concepts of citrate production and secretion by prostate. 1. Metabolic relationships. Prostate. 1991;18(1):25–46.
78. Kurhanewicz J, Swanson MG, Nelson SJ, et al. Combined magnetic resonance imaging and spectroscopic imaging approach to molecular imaging of prostate cancer. J Magn Reson Imaging. 2002;16(4):451–63.
79. Litjens GJ, Barentsz JO, Karssemeijer N, et al. Clinical evaluation of a computer-aided diagnosis system for determining cancer aggressiveness in prostate MRI. Eur Radiol. 2015;25(11):3187–99.
80. Hambrock T, Vos PC, Hulsbergen-van de Kaa CA, et al. Prostate cancer: computer-aided diagnosis with multiparametric 3-T MR imaging--effect on observer performance. Radiology. 2013;266(2):521–30.
81. Shiradkar R, Podder TK, Algohary A, et al. Radiomics based targeted radiotherapy planning (Rad-TRaP): a computational framework for prostate cancer treatment planning with MRI. Radiat Oncol. 2016;11(1):148.
82. Rosenkrantz AB, Ream JM, Nolan P, et al. Prostate cancer: utility of whole-lesion apparent diffusion coefficient metrics for prediction of biochemical recurrence after radical prostatectomy. AJR Am J Roentgenol. 2015;205(6):1208–14.
83. Tiwari P, Viswanath S, Kurhanewicz J, et al. Multimodal wavelet embedding representation for data combination (MaWERiC): integrating magnetic resonance imaging and spectroscopy for prostate cancer detection. NMR Biomed. 2012;25(4):607–19.
84. Viswanath SE, Bloch NB, Chappelow JC, et al. Central gland and peripheral zone prostate tumors have significantly different quantitative imaging signatures on 3 Tesla endorectal, in vivo T2-weighted MR imagery. J Magn Reson Imaging. 2012;36(1):213–24.
85. Moradi M, Salcudean SE, Chang SD, et al. Multiparametric MRI maps for detection and grading of dominant prostate tumors. J Magn Reson Imaging. 2012;35(6):1403–13.
86. Fehr D, Veeraraghavan H, Wibmer A, et al. Automatic classification of prostate cancer Gleason scores from multiparametric magnetic resonance images. Proc Natl Acad Sci U S A. 2015;112(46):E6265–73.
87. Nketiah G, Elschot M, Kim E, et al. T2-weighted MRI-derived textural features reflect prostate cancer aggressiveness: preliminary results. Eur Radiol. 2017;27(7):3050–9.
88. Lv D, Guo X, Wang X, et al. Computerized characterization of prostate cancer by fractal analysis in MR images. J Magn Reson Imaging. 2009;30(1):161–8.
89. Lopes R, Ayache A, Makni N, et al. Prostate cancer characterization on MR images using fractal features. Med Phys. 2011;38(1):83–95.
90. Ginsburg SB, Algohary A, Pahwa S, et al. Radiomic features for prostate cancer detection on MRI differ between the transition and peripheral zones: preliminary findings from a multi-institutional study. J Magn Reson Imaging. 2017;46(1):184–93.
91. Stoyanova R, Pollack A, Takhar M, et al. Association of multiparametric MRI quantitative imaging features with prostate cancer gene expression in MRI-targeted prostate biopsies. Oncotarget. 2016;7(33):53362–76.
92. McCann SM, Jiang Y, Fan X, et al. Quantitative multiparametric MRI features and PTEN expression of peripheral zone prostate cancer: a pilot study. AJR Am J Roentgenol. 2016;206(3):559–65.
93. Bellomo G, Marcocci F, Bianchini D, et al. MR spectroscopy in prostate cancer: new algorithms to optimize metabolite quantification. PLoS One. 2016;11(11):e0165730.

2 Anatomy of the Prostate

Oscar Laucirica, Violeta Catalá, and Joan C. Vilanova

Contents

O. Laucirica, M.D. (✉)
Department of Urology, Hospital Sant Joan Despí Moises Broggi, Jacinto Verdaguer 90, Sant Joan Despí, Barcelona, Spain
e-mail: olauciricag@hotmail.com

V. Catalá, M.D., Ph.D.
Department of Radiology, Fundació Puigvert, Cartagena 340, 08005 Barcelona, Spain
e-mail: violetacatala@yahoo.com.ar

J.C. Vilanova, M.D., Ph.D.
Department of Radiology, Clínica Girona, Institute Catalan of Health-IDI, University of Girona, Lorenzana 36, 17002 Girona, Spain
e-mail: kvilanova@comg.cat

2.1 Introduction

The McNeal anatomical model considers the prostate divided into four zones in relation to the different surrounding structures as described below [1, 2].

2.1.1 Urethra and Ejaculatory Ducts (Fig. 2.1)

The urethra is the anatomical landmark to describe the entire topographic anatomy of the prostate zone.

The urethra is made up of two segments, proximal and distal urethra, each one approximately 15 mm long, separated from each other by the verumontanum. There is a 35° angulation in the middle of the length of the prostatic urethra, immediately proximal to the verumontanum.

The urethral wall consists of longitudinally oriented smooth muscular fibres. Surrounding this internal longitudinal muscle layer, there is another layer in a circular position. Both smooth muscle layers constitute the so-called internal urethral sphincter (IUS), which extends from the bladder neck to the end of the membranous urethra. The IUS is of maximum thickness at the proximal level, in the bladder neck, and the thickness progressively reduces as it extends towards the membranous urethra. The IUS surrounds the membranous urethra along its entire circumference. On its anterior side, the intraprostatic IUS merges with the anterior fibromuscular stroma (AFMS).

The two ejaculatory ducts run in a plane parallel to the distal urethra. Their openings in the urethral lumen are in the *prostatic utricle*.

2.1.2 Transition Zone (TZ) (Fig. 2.2)

The TZ represents approximately 5% of the prostate gland tissue and comprises two lobes on either side of the proximal urethra. Its ductal system runs parallel to the urethral plane

J.C. Vilanova et al. (eds.), *Atlas of Multiparametric Prostate MRI*, DOI 10.1007/978-3-319-61786-2_2

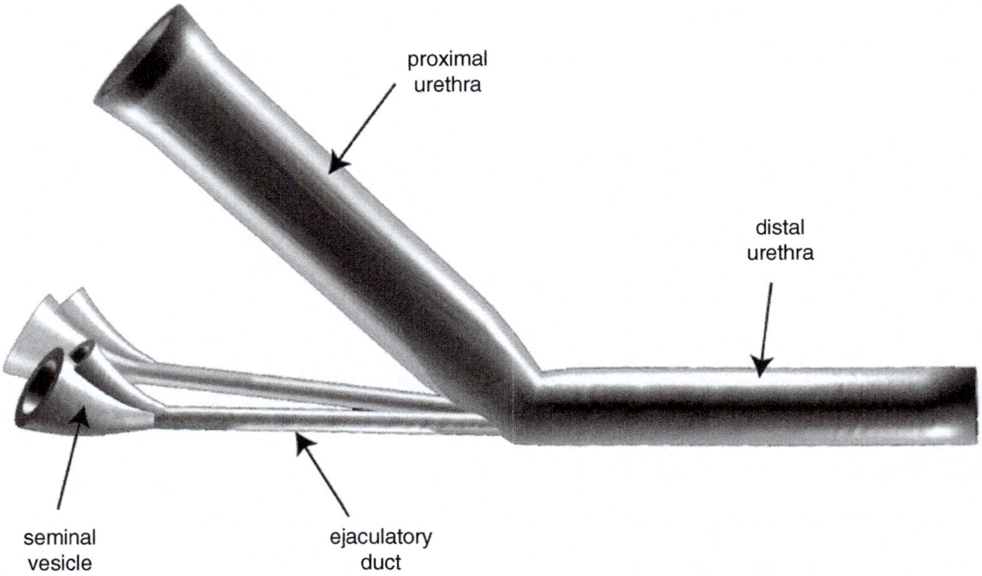

Fig. 2.1 Anatomical drawing sagittal view of urethra and ejaculatory ducts

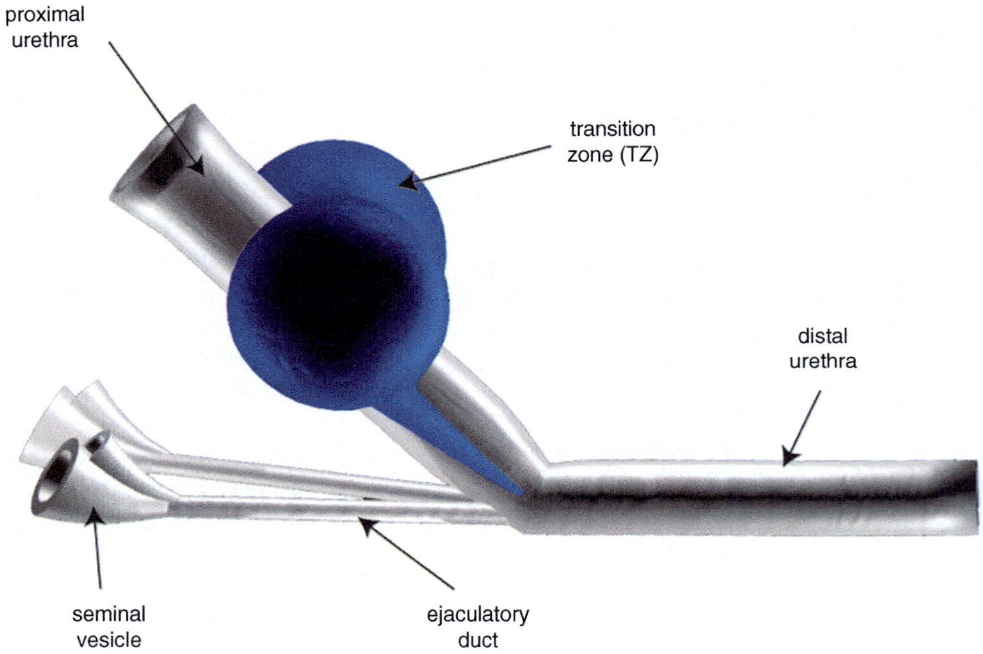

Fig. 2.2 Anatomical drawing sagittal view of transition zone (TZ)

and ends in the verumontanum, proximal to the opening of the ejaculatory ducts.

The TZ is adjacent to the peripheral zone, the central zone and the AFMS, which constitute the so-called surgical capsule, that is, they define the surgical cleavage plane for adenomectomy.

The TZ and the periurethral gland tissue are the seat of benign prostatic hyperplasia (BPH). The TZ is responsible for 10–20% of prostate cancers.

2.1.3 Central Zone (CZ) (Fig. 2.3)

The CZ represents approximately 25% of the prostate gland tissue. It forms a pyramidal or conical structure at the base of the prostate, narrowing to an apex at the level of the verumontanum. Its ducts run radially on both sides of the opening of the ejaculatory ducts.

The point at which the seminal vesicles and ductus deferens penetrate the CZ to form the ejaculatory ducts is called the "beak of the seminal vesicles". This represents an area of anatomical weakness due to the absence of prostatic capsule at this level.

The term *invaginated extraprostatic space* (IES) is used to denote the prolongation of the fascial and lymphovascular tissue inside the prostate, and more specifically in the CZ, that follows the path of the ejaculatory ducts. This represents another area of anatomical weakness due to the absence of any barrier to spread of a pathological process to this region from its seat in the CZ.

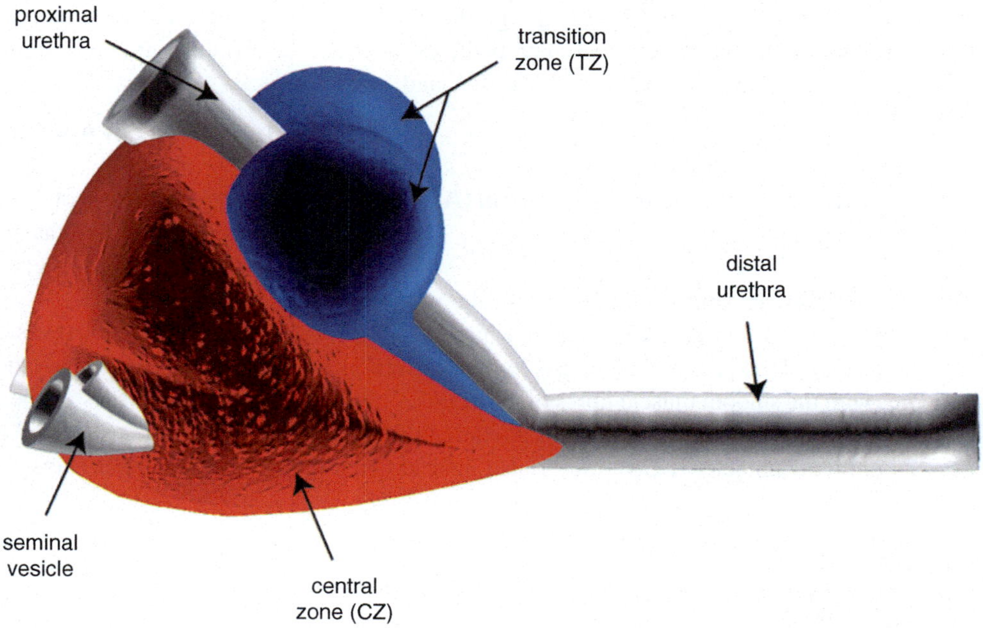

Fig. 2.3 Anatomical drawing sagittal view of central zone (CZ)

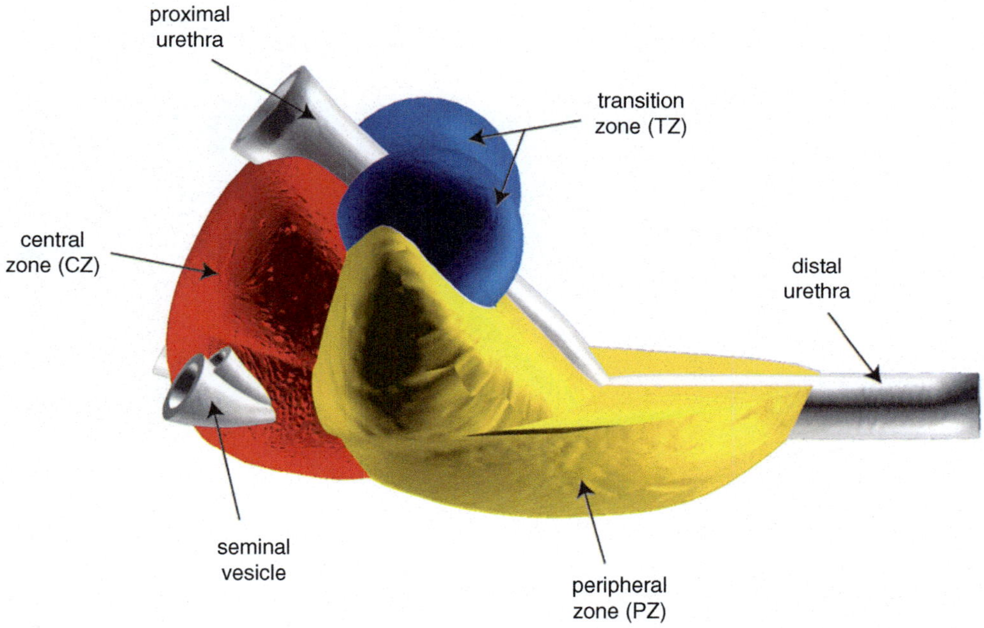

Fig. 2.4 Anatomical drawing sagittal view of peripheral zone (PZ)

The CZ is relatively resistant to development of pathology. It is considered that 5–10% of prostate cancers arise in this zone.

The absence of anatomical barriers between the peripheral and central zones, along with the IES, means that a tumour that arises in the prostatic apex can easily progress to the base of the prostate and give rise to early invasion of the structures of the extraprostatic space.

2.1.4 Peripheral Zone (PZ) (Fig. 2.4)

The PZ represents approximately 70% of the prostate gland tissue. It includes the lateral, dorsal and apical surfaces of the prostate, spreading ventrally in a variable way, where it maintains a relation of continuity with the AFMS.

The prostate does not contain a capsular structure "per se"; there is only a condensation of the glandular stroma, named "capsule". The prostatic "capsule" itself comprises the fibromuscular stroma, which forms a thin lamina around the gland. The prostatic apex lacks this stromal lamina, giving rise to an area of anatomical weakness named the *trapezoidal area.* This area is bordered ventrally by the membranous urethra, dorsally by the fascia of Denonvilliers and rectum, cranially by the prostatic apex (PZ) and caudally by the rectourethralis muscle.

The PZ is the seat of 70% of prostate cancers. When they arise close to the gland apex, they can invade the extraprostatic space at an early stage through the trapezoidal area. The dorsolateral neurovascular pedicles of the prostate also constitute tumour exteriorisation and invasion planes.

2.1.5 Anterior Fibromuscular Stroma (AFMS) (Fig. 2.5)

The AFMS represents approximately 33% of the volume of the prostate. It is a non-glandular region which forms the anterior surface of the prostate. In its most proximal section, it merges with the smooth muscle fibres of the detrusor muscle and of the IUS. Caudally, it maintains a relation with the external urethral sphincter (EUS); the striated muscle fibres of the EUS merge in this region, at the anterolateral side of the glandular apex, constituting the prostatic EUS apron.

2.1.6 Areas of Anatomical Weakness

In short, four areas of "anatomical weakness" are recognised, via which a prostate tumour can grow and invade adjacent structures. These are:

1. Beak of the seminal vesicles (Figs. 2.6 and 2.17)
2. Invaginated extraprostatic space (IES) (Fig. 2.6)
3. Perineural spaces of the prostatic dorsolateral neurovascular pedicles (Figs. 2.7 and 2.17)
4. Trapezoidal area (Figs. 2.8 and 2.17)

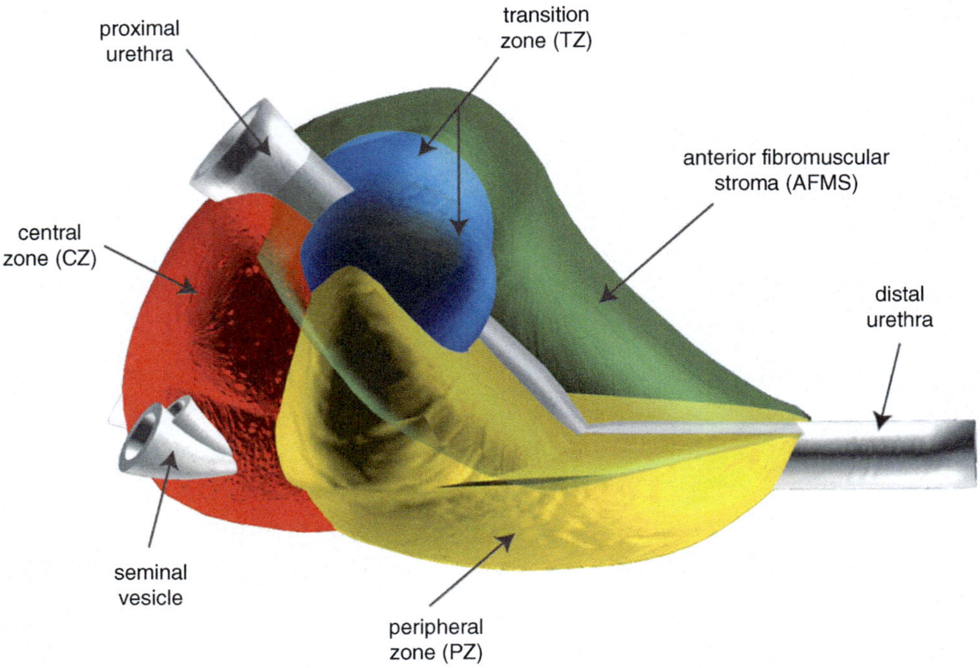

Fig. 2.5 Anatomical drawing sagittal view of anterior fibromuscular stroma (AFMS)

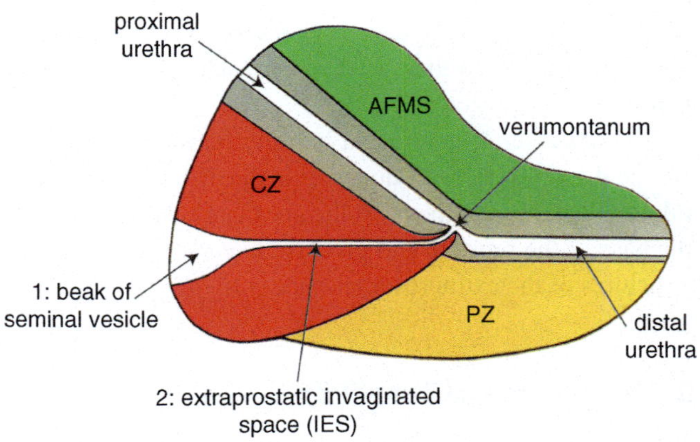

Fig. 2.6 Anatomical drawing of median section sagittal view of the McNeal prostate model showing the following elements: (*1*) beak of the seminal vesicles and (*2*) invaginated extraprostatic space (IES)

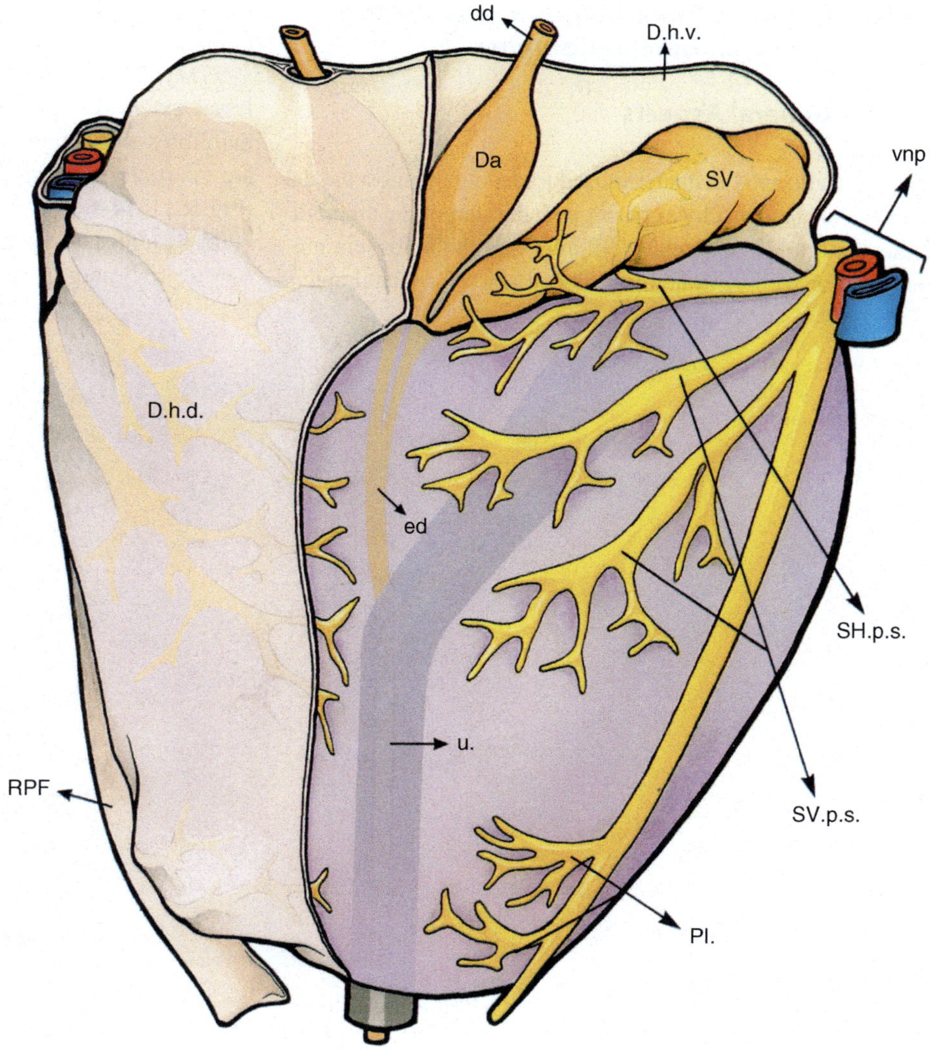

Fig. 2.7 Anatomical drawing of dorsal view of the prostate showing its dorsolateral neurovascular pedicles and the fascial complex that surround them. *RPF* Retzius periprostatic fascia; *SV* seminal vesicles; *PI* inferior pedicle; *Dhd* Denonvilliers fascia, dorsal sheath; *Dhv* Denonvilliers fascia, ventral sheath; *dd* ductus deferens; *Da* deferens ampulla; *HSsp* horizontal subdivision of the superior neurovascular pedicle; *VSsp* vertical subdivision of the superior neurovascular pedicle; *vnp* neurovascular pedicle; *ed* ejaculatory ducts; *u* urethra

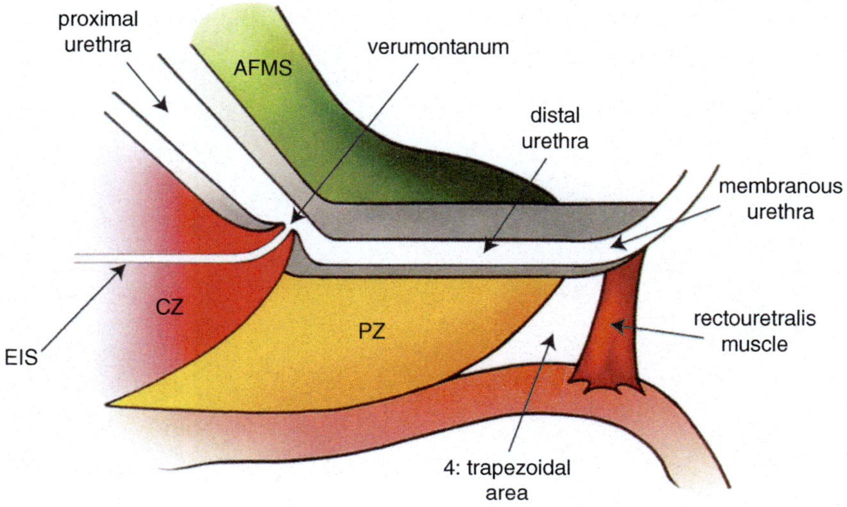

Fig. 2.8 Anatomical drawing of middle sagittal section of the McNeal prostate model showing the trapezoidal area (*4*). Invaginated extraprostatic space (IES)

2.2 Prostatic Apex, Membranous Urethra and Its Sphincter Complex

2.2.1 General Aspects

The prostatic apex is the term used to denote the most caudal part of the gland, in close contact with the start of the membranous urethra [3]. It displays different morphologies: circumferential or with ventral apical, dorsal apical or lateral apical lobes (Figs. 2.9 and 2.10) [3]. The importance of knowing the morphology of the prostatic apex lies mainly in two points:

First: The prostatic apex overlap (or cover) to a greater or lesser extent the most cranial portion of the EUS (rhabdomyofibres of the membranous urethra), such that these fibres are partially incorporated within the glandular apex (Fig. 2.11) [4–6].

In patients undergoing radical prostatectomy, it is necessary to apply surgical techniques capable of exteriorising and

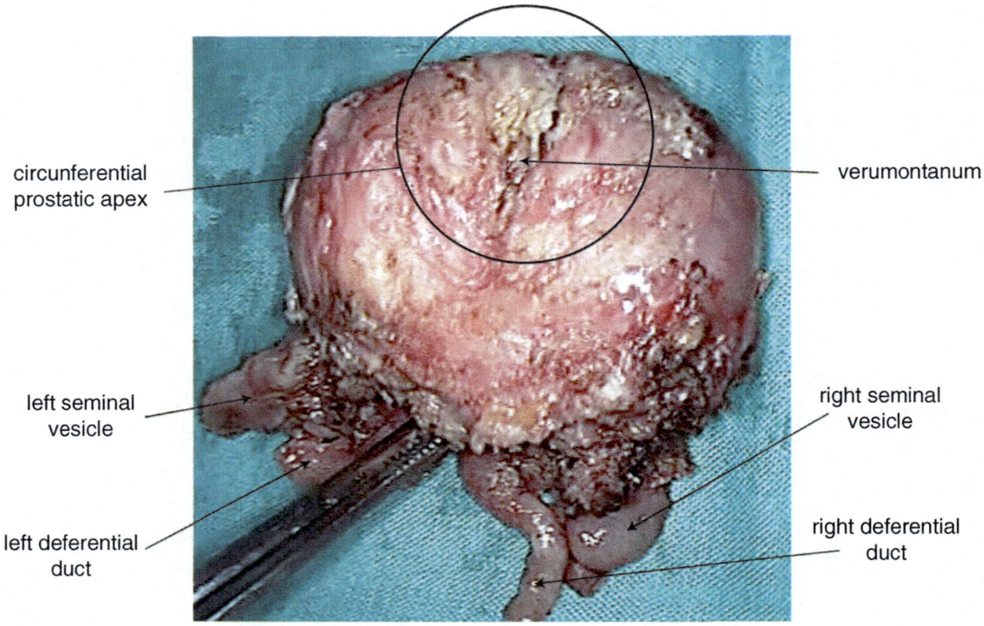

Fig. 2.9 Surgical specimen of the prostate, showing circumferential apex

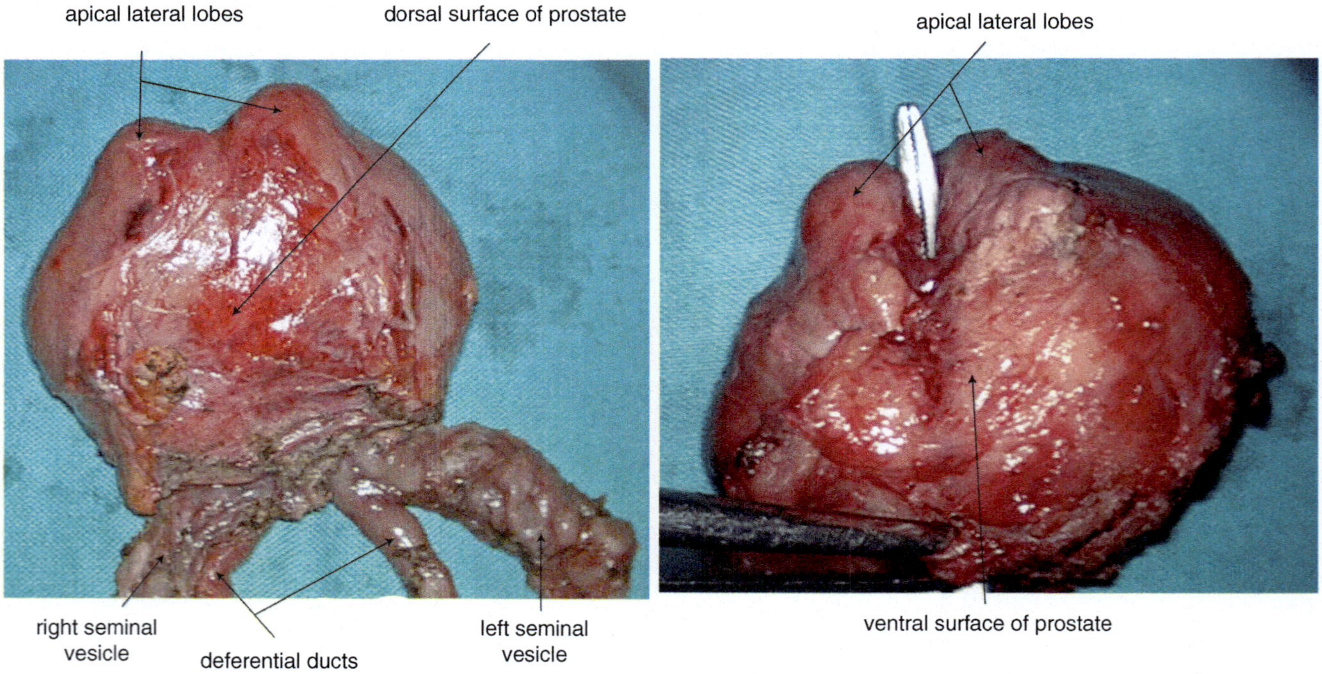

Fig. 2.10 Surgical specimen of the prostate, showing the apex with its lateral apical lobes

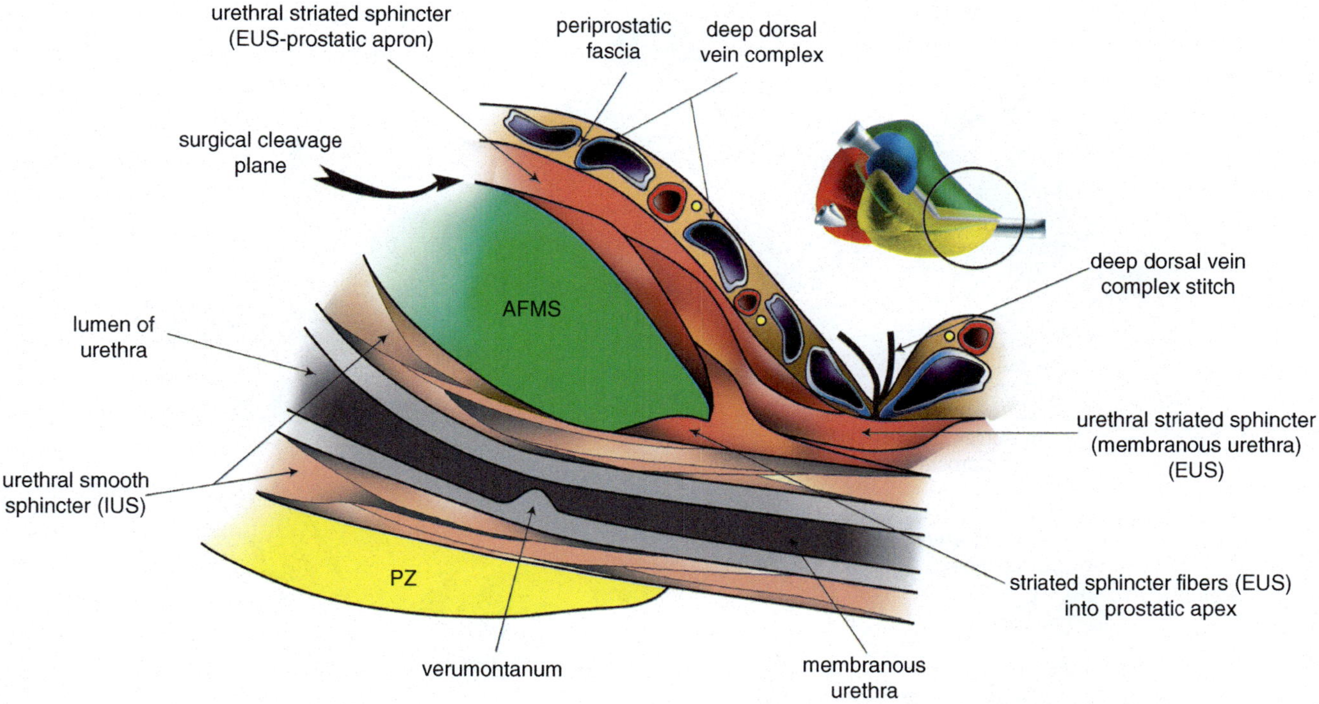

Fig. 2.11 Anatomical drawing of midline sagittal section of the prostatic apex. Showing the anterior fibromuscular stroma (AFMS) and the peripheral zone (PZ) of McNeal model, the urethra, the IUS and the EUS, along with the most cranial rhabdo-myofibres incorporated within the apex and the periprostatic fascial layers containing the deep dorsal venous plexus of the penis

dissecting this portion of rhabdo-myofibres, with the aim of preserving urinary continence (Fig. 2.12) [4, 6].

Second: Positive margins must be avoided during radical prostatectomy [4]. It is to be noted that at the apex level, the glandular tissue corresponds exclusively to the McNeal peripheral zone, except for a small anterior portion of the apex which comprises the AFMS of McNeal [7]. Moreover, the prostatic apex constitutes the roof of the so-called trapezoidal area, known to be an area of anatomical weakness, where progression of cancer to the extraprostatic space can occur more easily (Fig. 2.8) [1, 2].

On its anterolateral sides, the prostatic apex is covered by the EUS apron, merging with the AFMS and the apron of detrusor smooth muscle extending from the vesical neck (Fig. 2.13) [3–5, 7–11].

The prostatic apex continues caudally with the start of the membranous urethra. The membranous urethra in males is considered to be the portion of the urethra which is located between the prostatic apex and the urethral bulb, with an approximate length of 1 cm [3, 4]. It contains both the internal urethral sphincter (IUS) and the EUS [3, 7–9, 12].

The IUS extends from the vesical neck, where it acquires its maximum thickness, to the bulbar urethra, progressively reducing in thickness in the caudal direction. It surrounds the membranous urethra in all its circumference and is composed of a double layer of smooth muscular fibres (leio-myofibres), one longitudinal interior and one circular (Figs. 2.13 and 2.14) [3, 7–9, 12].

The innervation of the IUS is received from the autonomic, sympathetic and parasympathetic nervous systems [3, 9, 12–21].

The inferior hypogastric plexus is responsible for all the autonomic innervation to the prostate, the glandular apex and the membranous urethra. Its terminal fibres run medially to the puboperinealis muscle and laterally to the EUS of the membranous urethra, ventrally constituting the so-called cavernous nerves (responsible for the erection mechanism) and dorsally the corpus spongiosum nerves (responsible for the autonomic afferent innervation of the mucosa of the membranous urethra, directly involved in the mechanism of continence [14]) (Figs. 2.13 and 2.14) [3, 12–21].

The EUS constitutes a striated muscular plane (rhabdomyofibres) that surrounds the IUS at the level of the membranous urethra, spreading cranially over the anterolateral sides of the prostatic apex and constituting at this level the so-called EUS apron (Fig. 2.13). Its muscular fibres are mainly of type I, that is, without muscle spindles, being specialised for prolonged contractions, although of low intensity. The function of the EUS consists in maintaining a constant tone which collapses the urethral lumen in intermicturitional periods, thus preventing involuntary urine leakage [3–5, 7, 8, 12, 22].

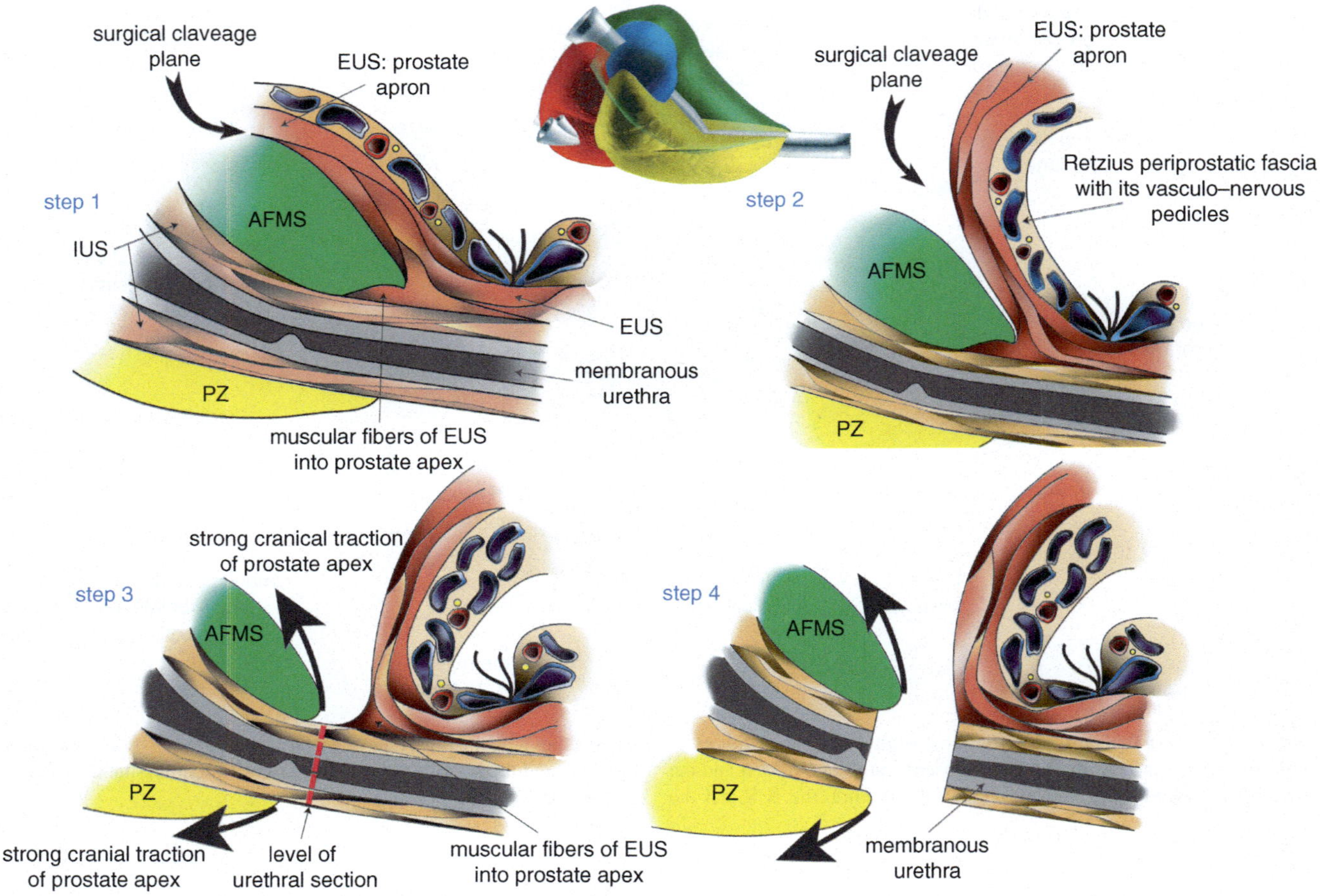

Fig. 2.12 Anatomical drawing of midline midsagittal sections of the prostatic apex showing the different stages in correct preservation of the EUS during radical prostatectomy

The EUS is at its maximum thickness at the level of the membranous urethra, and the thickness progressively reduces as it progresses cranially until it forms the prostatic apron. Its omega-shaped arrangement surrounds the body of the membranous urethra except in its middorsal position, constituting the "middorsal raphe" (Figs. 2.13 and 2.14) [3–5, 7, 8, 12, 22]. Moreover, some of the rhabdo-myofibres of the EUS are incorporated in the interior of the glandular apex, under the verumontanum and in variable amounts depending on the morphology of the glandular apex (Fig. 2.11) [4–6].

The innervation and the arterial supply of the EUS are from the internal pudendal nerve and artery. The innervation is somatic, and the EUS is therefore under voluntary control [3, 12, 14, 19]. The internal pudendal nerve and artery both run cranially to the transverse deep muscle of the perineum, emitting branches that reach the most caudal portion of the EUS, and then become the dorsal nerve and dorsal artery of the penis. There is a distance of 3–13 mm between the prostatic apex and the branches of the internal pudendal nerve that innervate the EUS (Fig. 2.13) [3, 12, 19, 23, 24].

The IUS and EUS constitute the so-called *passive or intrinsic factor of urinary continence.* Their function basically consists in "collapsing" the urethral lumen against the middorsal raphe, thus preventing the involuntary "leakage" of intermicturitional urine (Figs. 2.11 and 2.13) [3].

The cavernous nerves run within both the dorsolateral and anterolateral sides of the periprostatic fascia. Preservation of these lateral branches during the surgical procedure is highly important in order to ensure recovery of erectile function after radical prostatectomy [3, 12].

2.2.2 Perineal Body or Central Perineum Tendon

The perineal body is a fibromuscular structure that is difficult to evaluate anatomically and has the function of supporting all the musculo-aponeurotic structures that make up

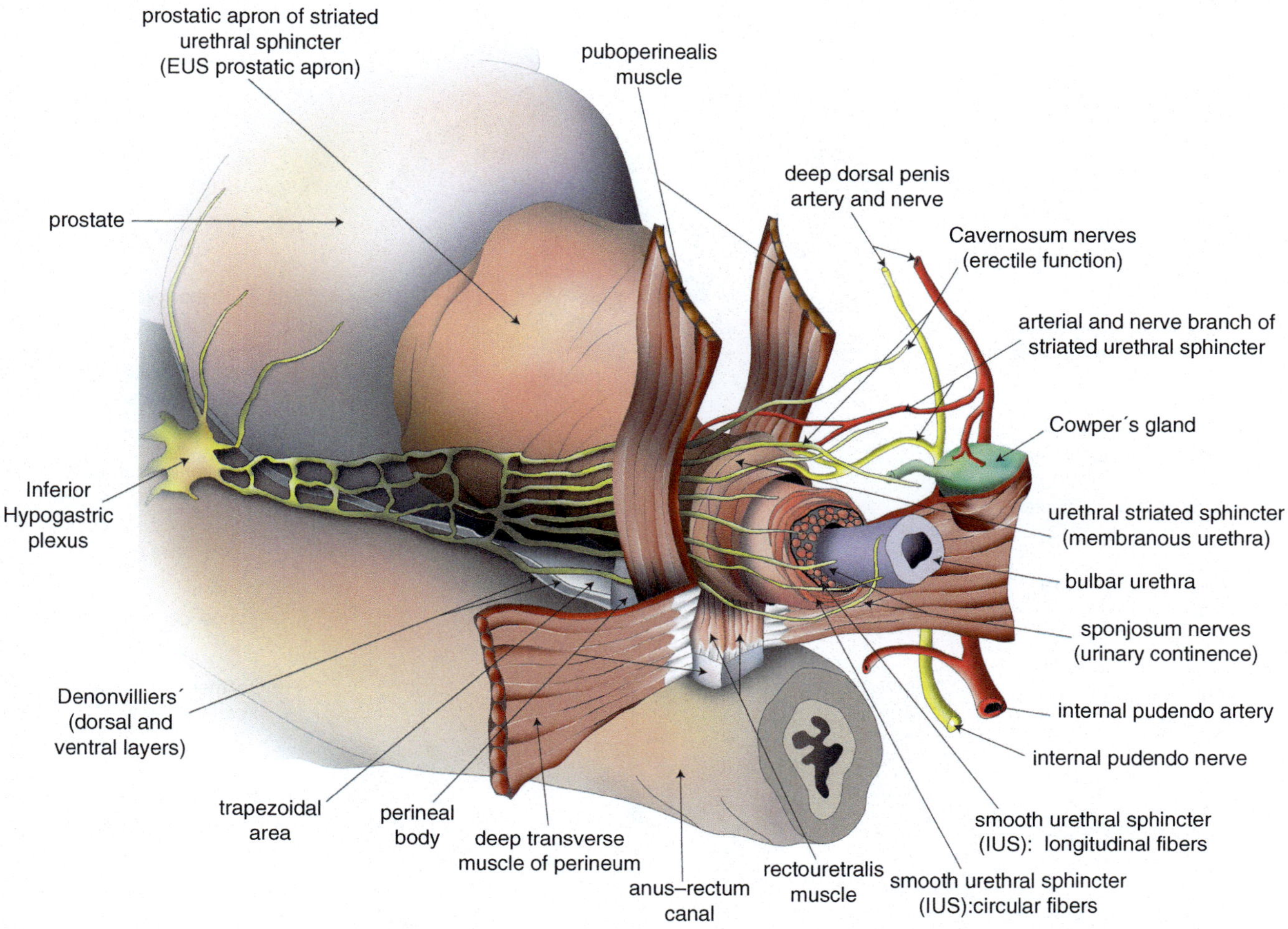

Fig. 2.13 Anatomical drawing of caudal view of the prostatic apex and membranous urethra along with its sphincter systems. The extension of the EUS apron on the anterolateral sides of the gland and the arrangement of the most ventromedial muscle fibres of the puboperinealis muscle are seen. The cavernous and corpus spongiosum nerves run medially to the puboperineal muscle plane, within of the multiple sheaths of fibre conjunctive tissue, elastic fibres and smooth muscle fibres that make up the periurethral fascial plane. In this figure, the pubic symphysis and puboprostatic ligaments have been eliminated in order to correctly identify the described anatomical elements

the perineal floor and support the pelvic viscera [3, 5, 6, 8, 22]. Regarding urinary continence, it provides a fixing basal plate which enables the EUS to perform correctly by means of the "impaction" of the striated muscle plane of the EUS against this basal plate, thus achieving correct collapse of the urethral lumen during intermicturitional periods [3, 5, 6, 8, 22].

The perineal body is made up of the following elements (Figs. 2.13 and 2.14) [3, 23, 25]:

- Medial insertion of the deep transverse muscles of the perineum
- Medial insertion of the puboperinealis muscle
- Terminal portion (more caudal) of Denonvilliers fascia with its ventral and dorsal sheaths merged
- Middorsal raphe of the membranous urethra
- Rectourethralis muscle

2.2.3 **Puboperinealis Muscle** (Figs. 2.13 and 2.14) [3, 23, 25]

The levator muscle of the anus constitutes the so-called active or extrinsic factor of urinary continence. It is made up of two muscular planes, the pubococcygeus and iliococcygeus muscles.

The pubococcygeus muscle originates in the mid-branches of the pubis and inserts dorsally at the level of the anococcygeal ligament and coccyx. Medial fibres of the pubococcygeus muscle move medially, configuring a loop behind the external anal sphincter at the level of the anorectal canal, causing an inflexion at this level that contributes to the anal pressure and closing mechanism. This is the puborectalis muscle.

At the same time, the medial fibres of the puborectalis muscle displace mid-caudally, running laterally to the

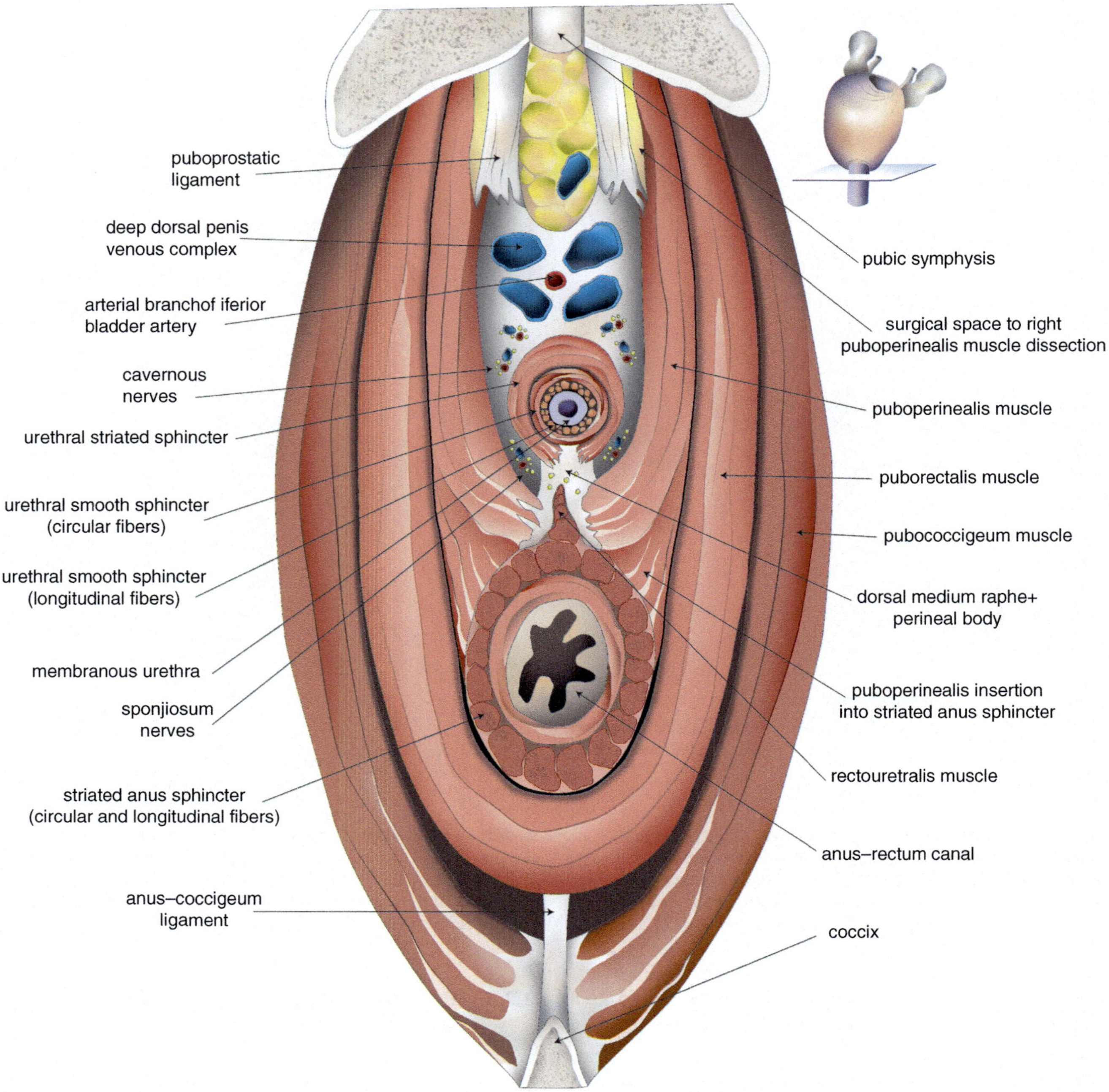

Fig. 2.14 Anatomical drawing of transverse section at the level of the membranous urethra. The urethral sphincter and external anal system are shown, as are the muscle fascicles that make up the pubococcygeus muscle and the deep dorsal venous plexus of the penis. Laterally to the puboprostatic ligaments, one can see the cleavage plane for dissection of the puboperinealis muscle

membranous urethra and prostatic apex along with their sphincter systems, and insert at the level of the perineal body, the deepest section of the external anal sphincter and the urethral bulb. These muscle fibres are referred to as the puboperinealis muscle (also named the pubourethral or the levator prostatae muscle). The puboperinealis muscle configures the most ventromedial section of the perineal floor and can end up covering the lateral surface of the puboprostatic ligaments, so that its more distal fibres follow a path parallel to the axis of the membranous urethra. The preservation “ad integrum” of this muscular plane in most cases demands the partial section of the puboprostatic ligaments, with the aim of locating the correct cleavage plane for its surgical dissection (Fig. 2.15).

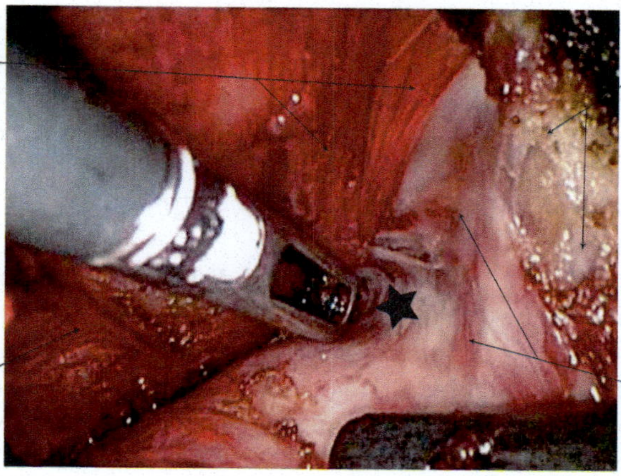

Fig. 2.15 Surgical photograph showing the lateral fascial surface of the puboprostatic ligament once dissection of the most ventromedial fibres of the puboperinealis muscle has been completed. Note the central "invagination" (*star* in the image); this corresponds to the point at which the needle should be passed in the ligation of the deep dorsal venous complex of the penis, thus preventing decapitation of the EUS at this level as well as ensuring correct preservation of the puboperinealis muscle

2.3 The Role of MRI in Evaluation of the Prostatic Apex, Membranous Urethra and Urethral Sphincter Complex

Radical prostate surgery has two main objectives: complete removal of the tumour and satisfactory postsurgical functional results, that is, recovery of urinary continence and penile erectile function [4, 6]. In order to achieve early urinary continence after radical prostatectomy, complete preservation of the urethral sphincter system is required, together with "ad integrum" preservation of the puborectalis and puboperinealis muscles (the latter being more important) [4, 6, 25].

The preservation of the EUS starts with a thorough dissection of the EUS apron on the anterolateral sides of the glandular apex, moving in the caudal direction. The EUS of the membranous urethra is correctly identified and dissected, respecting the periurethral fascia, which is the site of the nerve endings of the cavernous and corpus spongiosum nerves (Figs. 2.12, 2.13 and 2.14) [3, 4, 6, 7, 10, 11, 21, 26–28].

MRI evaluation of the AFMS and prostatic apex may reveal the presence of a tumour in these areas, either as a primary growth or, more frequently, as a result of local spread of a tumour that has originally arisen in other anatomical areas of the gland and has invaded the anterior side of the prostate and/or anterior glandular apex. In these cases, sphincter preservation surgery is contraindicated due to the high risk of obtaining positive margins at this level.

2.4 Pelvic and Prostate Fascias

Between the musculoskeletal walls of the lateral and inferior walls of the pelvic cavity and the anterior parietal peritoneal recess on its cranial side lies the "pelvisubperitoneal space", which houses the pelvic viscera in their middle line and their neurovascular pedicles in their lateral sides. This space also contains abundant celluloadipose tissue, which continues cranially with the retroperitoneal adipose tissue and laterally, through the sciatic notches, with the adipose tissue of the gluteal and perineal region [23].

The pelvisubperitoneal space is septated, although not completely, by different cellular-fibrous sheaths, which arise in the vascular sheaths of the pelvic vessels and accompany the latter in their path from the lateral walls where they originate to their respective irrigation viscera. It is also known as "vascular septa", they are composed of fibrous conjunctive tissue, elastic fibres, adipose tissue and smooth muscle fibres in. It is important to know the distribution of these fascias which, located in the interior of the pelvic cavity, transport all the vascularisation and innervation of the pelvic viscera, throughout the thickness of their multiple sheaths, and will constitute the different surgical cleavage planes employed in radical prostatectomy.

Schematically five fascias are distinguished (Figs. 2.16 and 2.17) [23]:

Two sagittal fascias:

- Farabeuf sacro-recto-genito-vesical-pubic sheaths

Three transverse fascias:

- Umbilicoprevesical aponeurosis
- Genital artery septa
- Septum of the mid-haemorrhoidal artery

In the prostate, these sheaths are also called "Retzius periprostatic fascias", "periprostatic fascias", "prostate lateral bands" or, more recently, "visceral covering of the endopelvic fascia". They cover the lateral and ventral sides of the gland, merging at the level of the ventral side with the AFMS of McNeal. The entire vascularisation and innervation run within these sheaths. These sheaths, on both lateral sides of the prostate, constitute the surgical cleavage planes once the prostatic posterior or prerectal plane has been dissected [3, 4, 7, 11, 28].

The prostate does not contain a capsular structure "per se"; there is only a condensation of the glandular stroma, which shows high interindividual variability and is absent at certain points, constituting an area of anatomical weakness as described by McNeal [1, 2].

So, from a practical point of view, we consider that although the prostate does not have its own capsular structure, it does have three "pseudocapsules", as described below [3, 4, 7]:

- *Retzius periprostatic capsule*, more recently named visceral covering of the endopelvic fascia, made up by the set of multiple fibre conjunctive tissue sheaths, elastic fibres, smooth muscle fibres, vessels and nerves which merge with the AFMS on its ventral side
- *False "capsule"*, referring only to the condensation of the glandular stroma
- *Surgical capsule*, referring to the external compression that the AFMS, CZ and PZ undergo when BPH develops, forming the surgical cleavage plane for correct exeresis of the adenomatous tissue

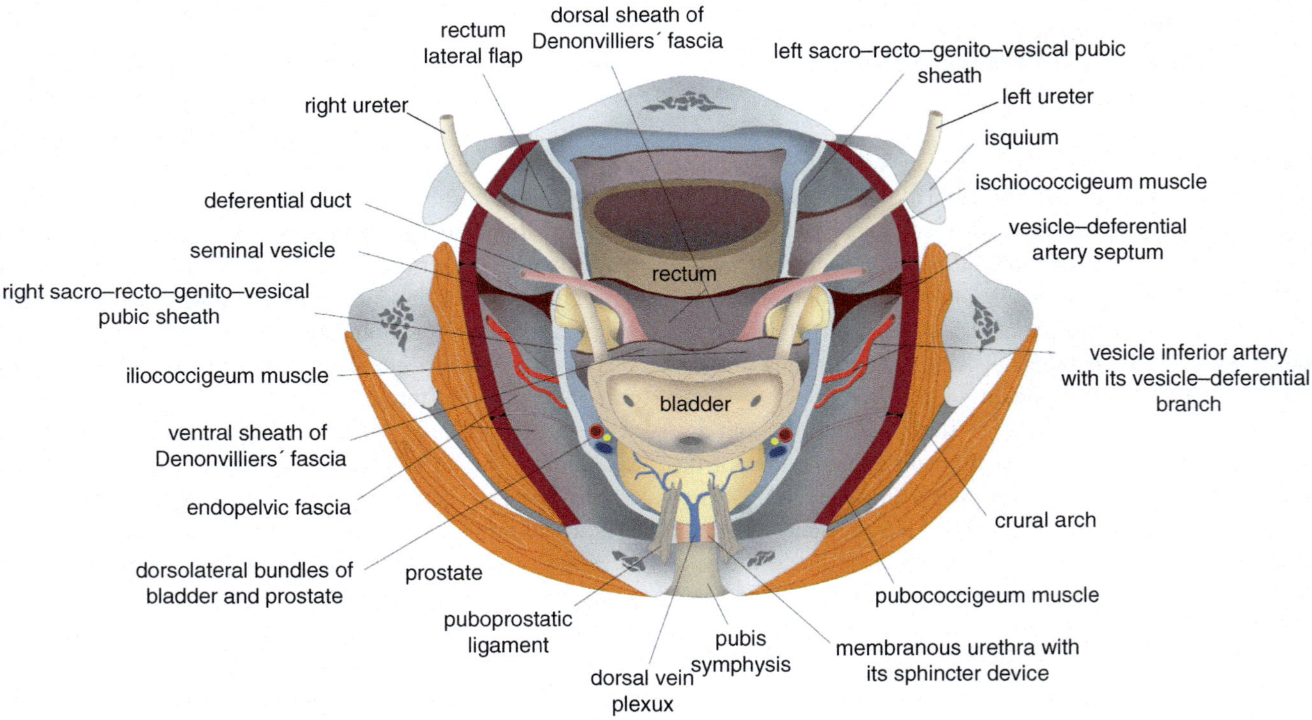

Fig. 2.16 Anatomical drawing of cranial view of the pelvis in a male. See the location of the two sagittal sheaths and the three transverse sheaths that make up the vascular septa of the pelvis

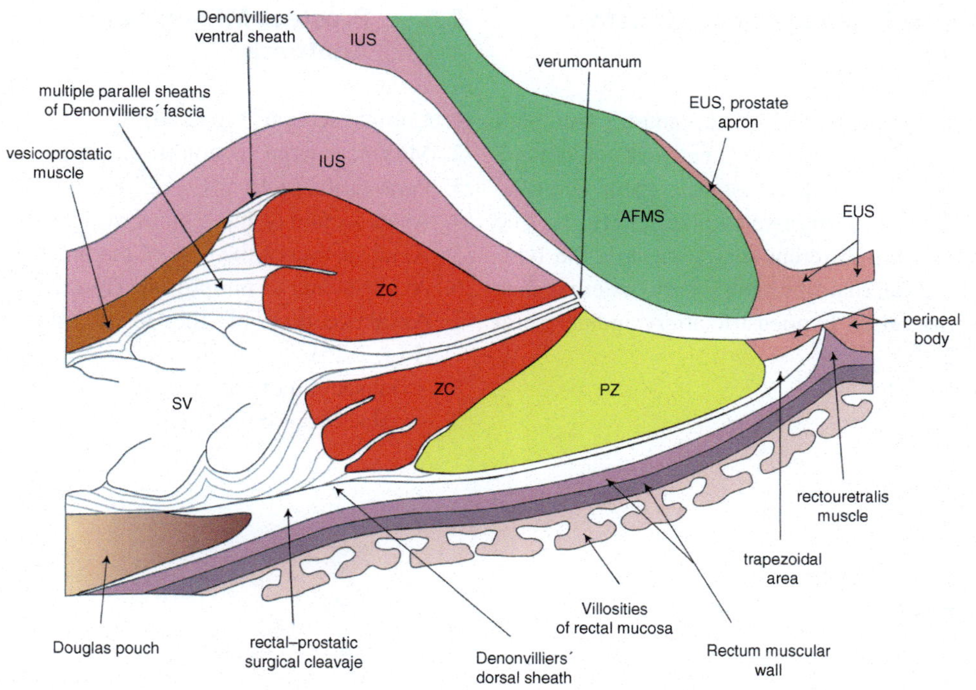

Fig. 2.17 Anatomical drawing of midline midsagittal section of the prostate showing the central zones (CZ), peripheral zone (PZ) and the anterior fibromuscular stroma (AFMS). Note the scarce capsular delimitation at the level of the seminal vesical beak, at the base of the CZ. The Denonvilliers fascia is made up of multiple parallel sheaths and has a craniocaudal arrangement. Histologically it shows fibroelastic connective tissue with smooth muscle fibres, vessels and nerves. At its lateral margins, it merges with the lateral sheaths of the Farabeuf sacro-recto-genito-vesical-pubic fascia and the transverse septa of the vesico-deferential artery. The rectal-prostatic surgical cleavage runs dorsally to the sheath complex that makes up the Denonvilliers fascia. It shows a lax areolar tissue. *AFMZ* anterior fibromuscular zone; *CZ* central zone; *PZ* peripheral zone; *VVSS* seminal vesicles; *IUS* internal urethral sphincter; *EUS* external urethral sphincter

2.5 Lymphatic Drainage of the Prostate (Fig. 2.18)

Small interlobular lymphatic capillaries anastomose with each other, forming lymphatic drainage networks of increasing diameter until they cross the prostatic capsule and configure a dense periprostatic lymphatic drainage network. The latter finally spreads via different routes towards the lymphatic chains of the internal obturator artery, external iliac artery, common iliac artery, hypogastric artery and presacral lymph nodes [23].

2.6 Prostate MRI and Cross-sectional Anatomy

1. Coronal section (Fig. 2.19)
2. Midline sagittal section (Fig. 2.20)
3. Parasagittal section (Fig. 2.21)
4. Axial section of the seminal vesicles (Fig. 2.22)
5. Axial section of the base of the prostate (Fig. 2.23)
6. Axial section of midprostate (Fig. 2.24)
7. Axial section of the lower part of the prostate (Fig. 2.25)
8. Axial section of the prostate apex (Fig. 2.26)
9. Axial section of the membranous urethra (Fig. 2.27)

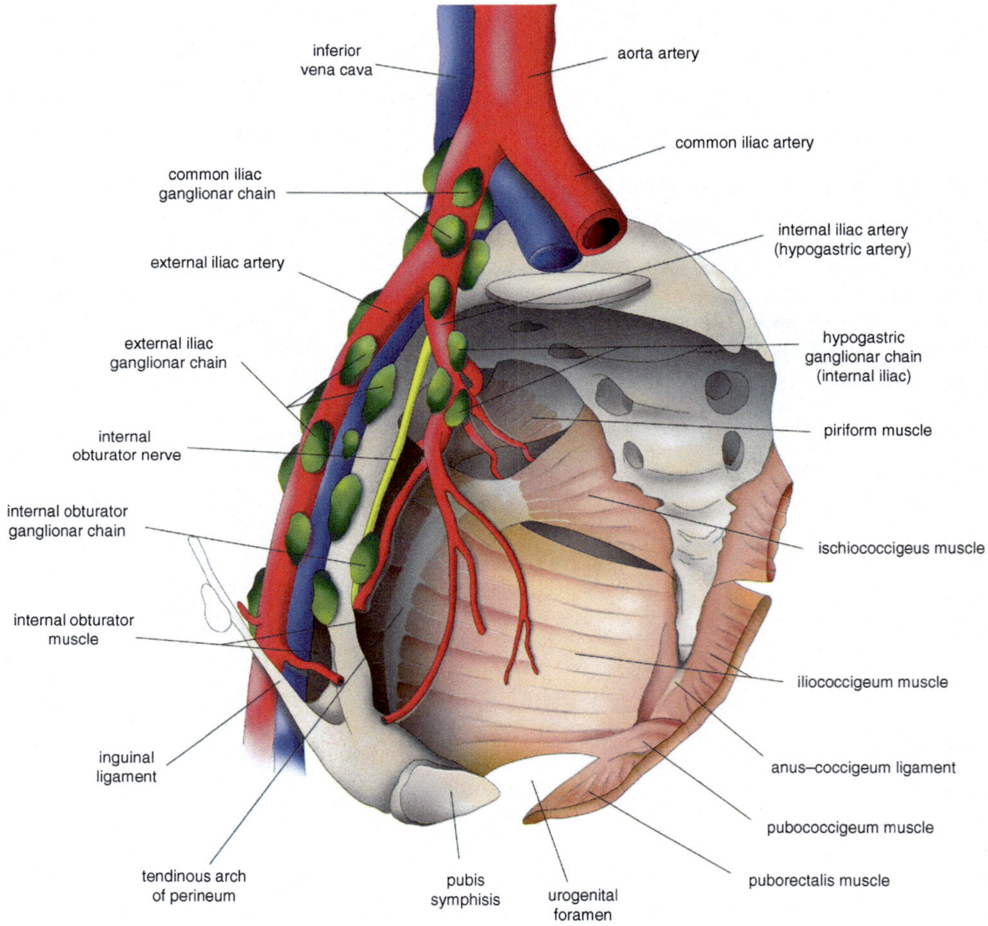

Fig. 2.18 Anatomical drawing of schematic overview of the lymphatic drainage chains of the prostate

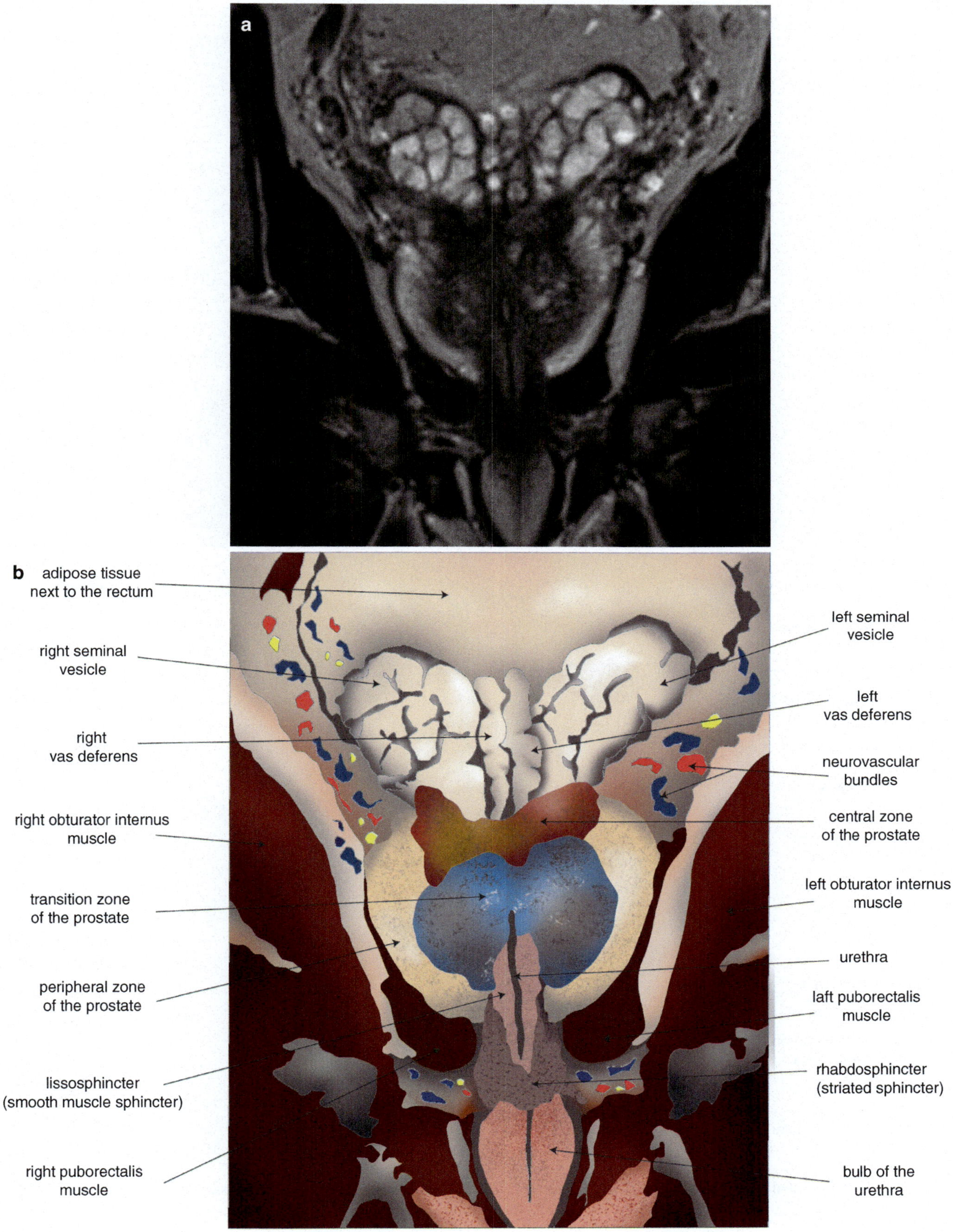

Fig. 2.19 Coronal section of prostate. (**a**) Appearance on T2 WI MRI. (**b**) Anatomical drawing of the same location as shown in "**a**"

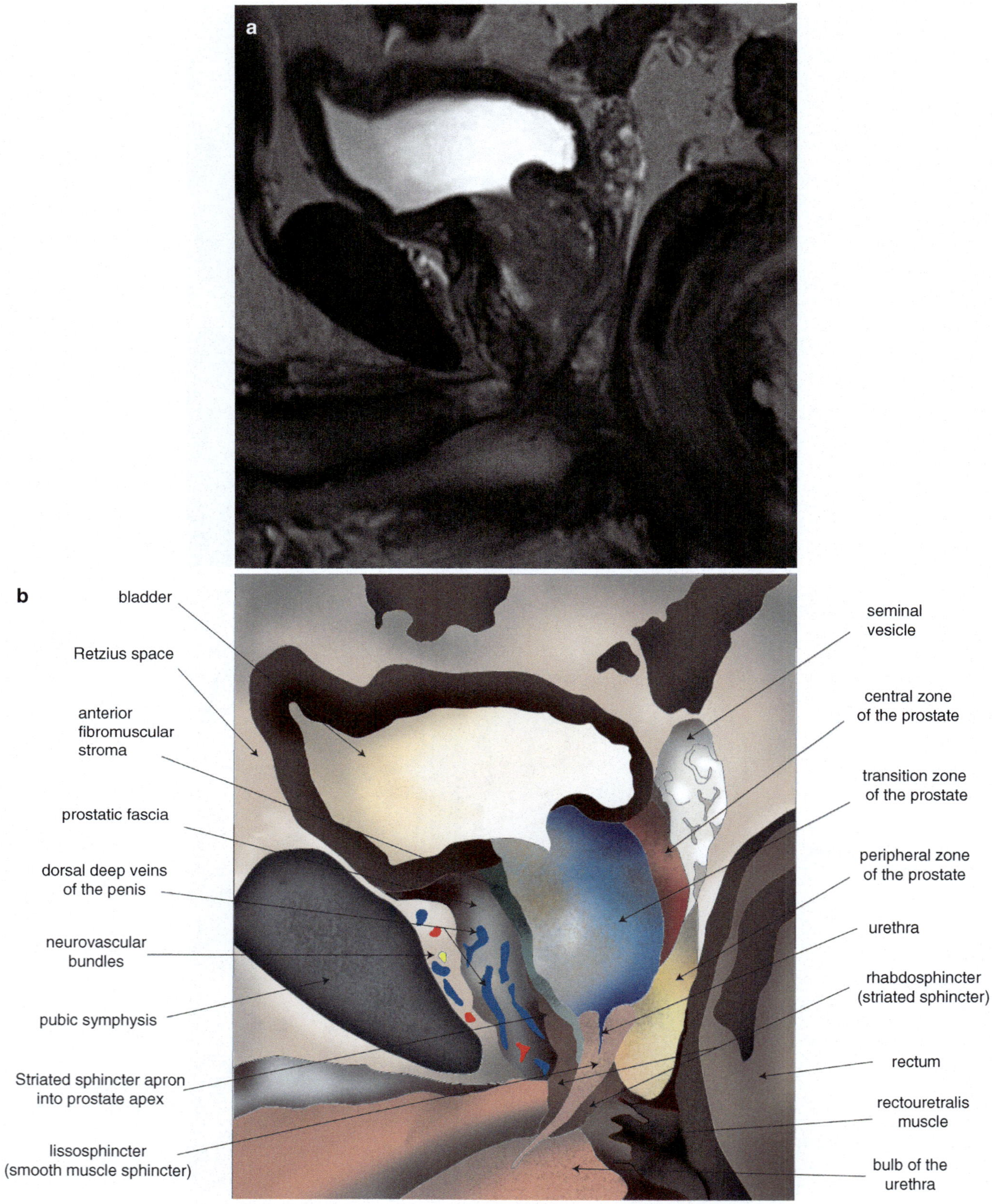

Fig. 2.20 Midline sagittal section of prostate. (**a**) Appearance on T2 WI MRI. (**b**) Anatomical drawing of the same location as shown in "**a**"

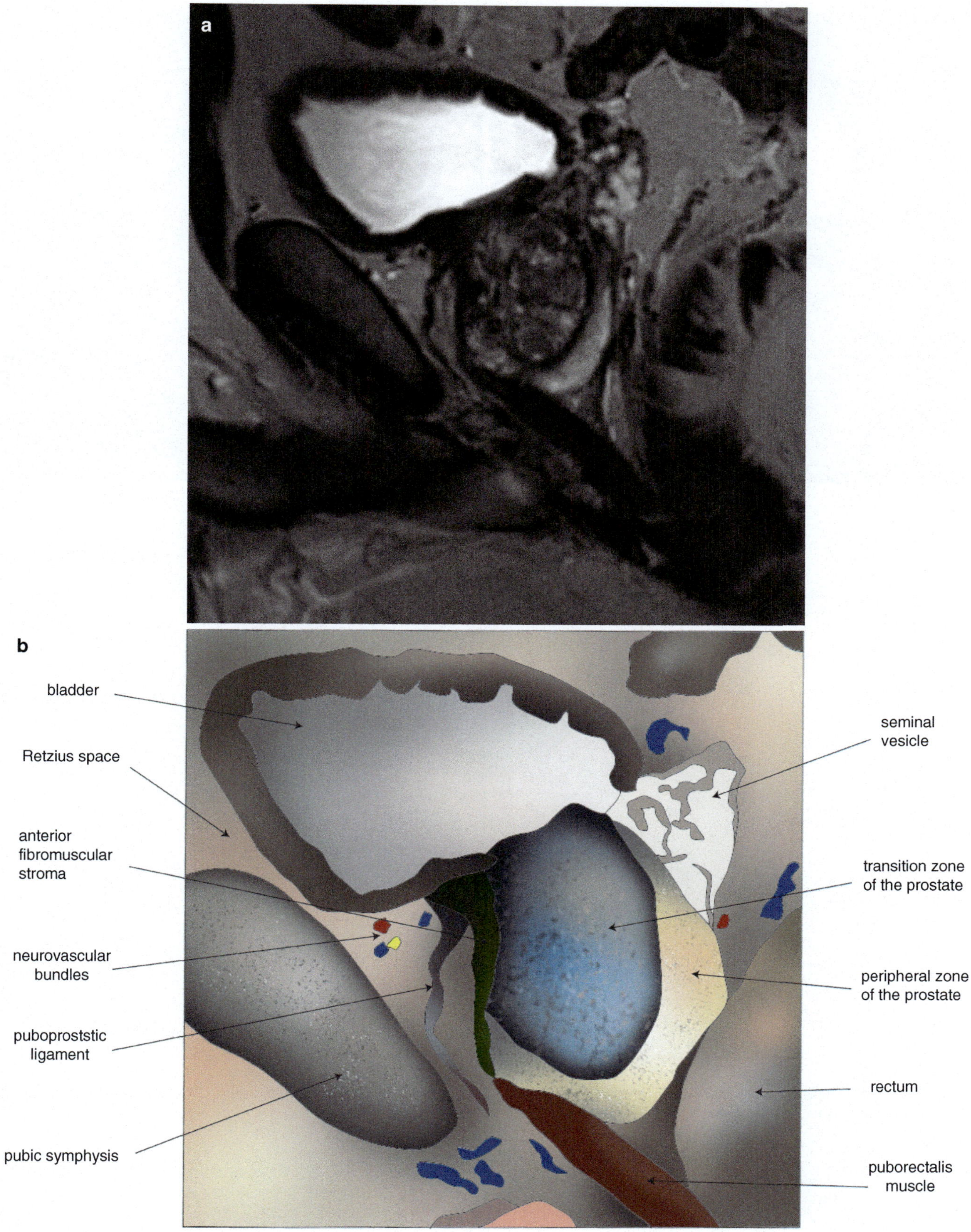

Fig. 2.21 Parasagittal section of the prostate. (**a**) Appearance on T2 WI MRI. (**b**) Anatomical drawing of the same location as shown in "**a**"

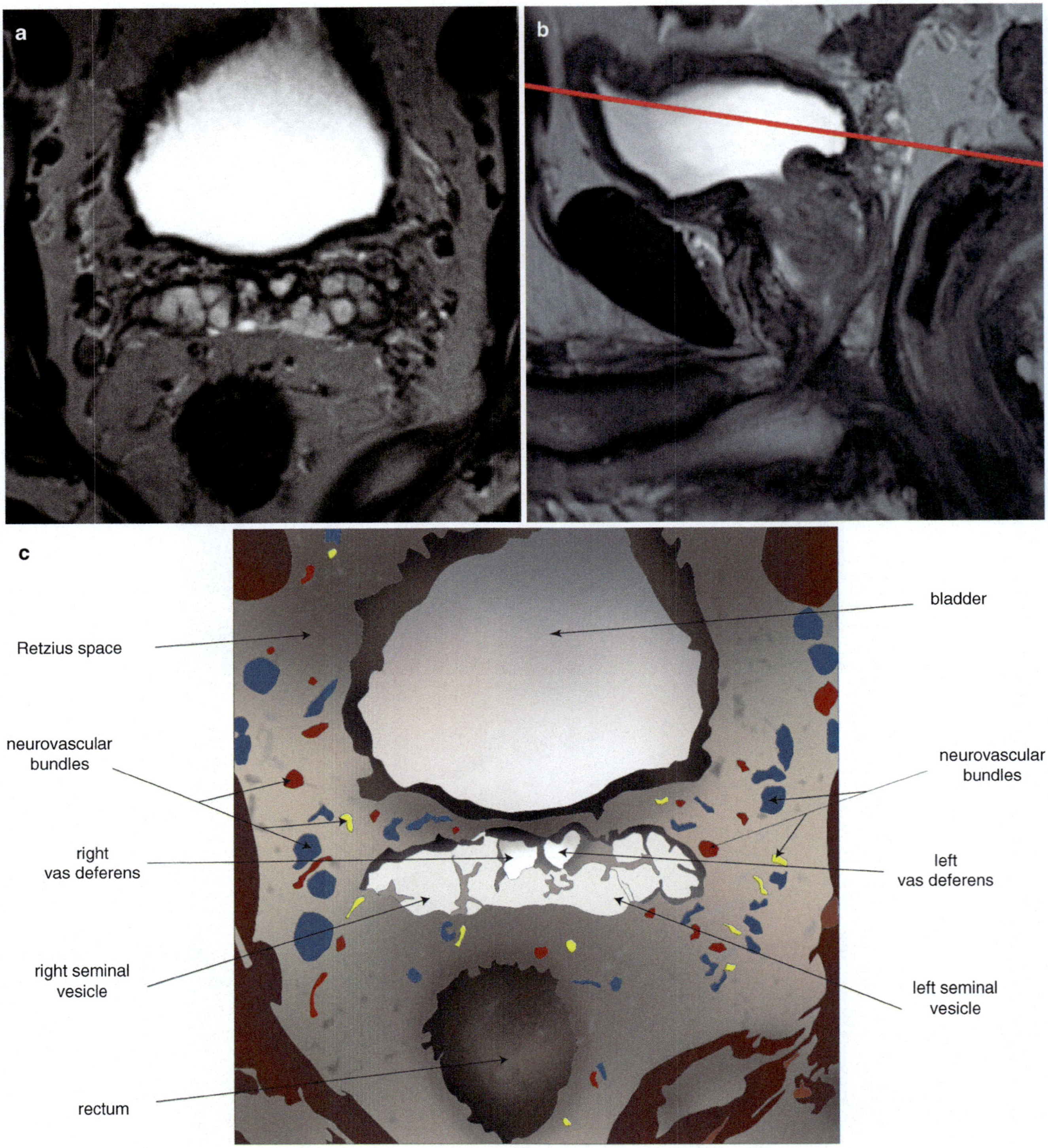

Fig. 2.22 (**a**) Axial section of the seminal vesicles on T2 WI MRI. (**b**) Midline sagittal section of the prostate on T2 WI MRI. Red line shows the level of section (**c**) Anatomical drawing of the same location as shown in "**a**"

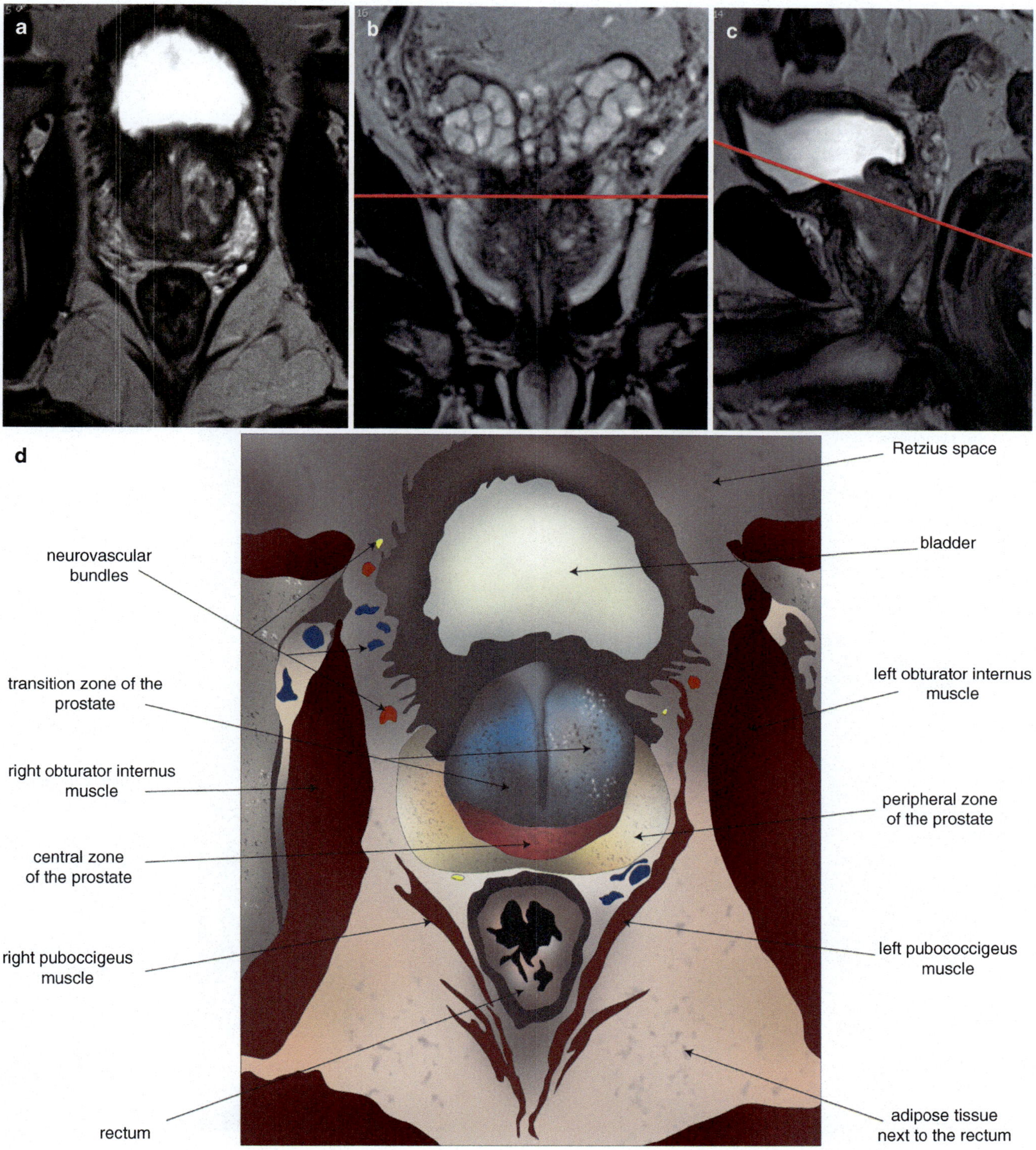

Fig. 2.23 (**a**) Axial section of the base of the prostate on T2 WI. (**b**) Coronal section of the prostate on T2 WI MRI. *Red line* shows the level of section. (**c**) Midline sagittal section of the prostate on T2 WI MRI. *Red line* shows the level of section. (**d**) Anatomical drawing of the same location as shown in "**a**"

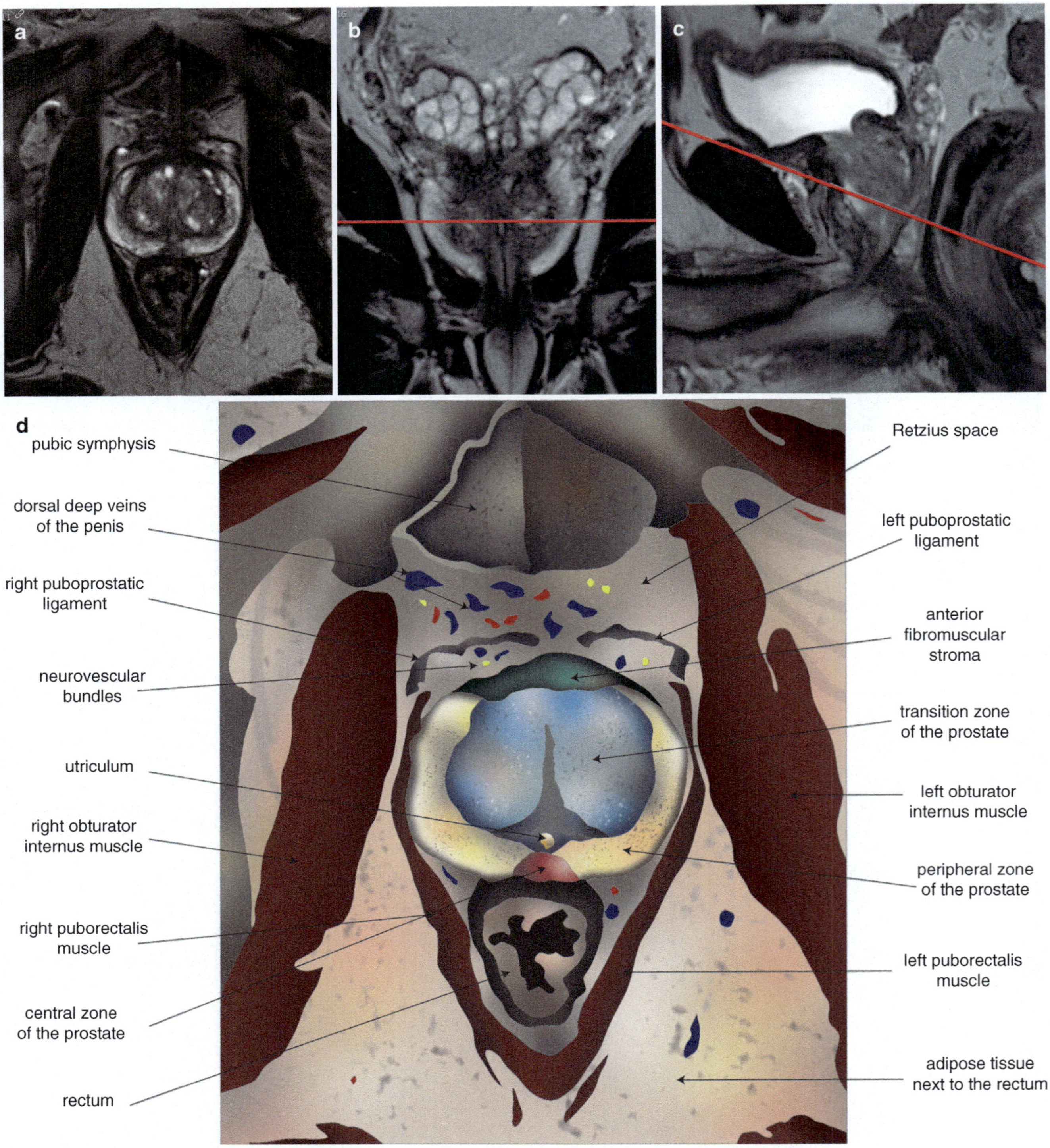

Fig. 2.24 (**a**) Axial section of the midprostate on T2 WI MRI. (**b**) Coronal section of the prostate on T2 WI MRI. *Red line* shows the level of section. (**c**) Midline sagittal section of the prostate on T2 WI MRI. *Red line* shows the level of section. (**d**) Anatomical drawing of the same location as shown in "**a**"

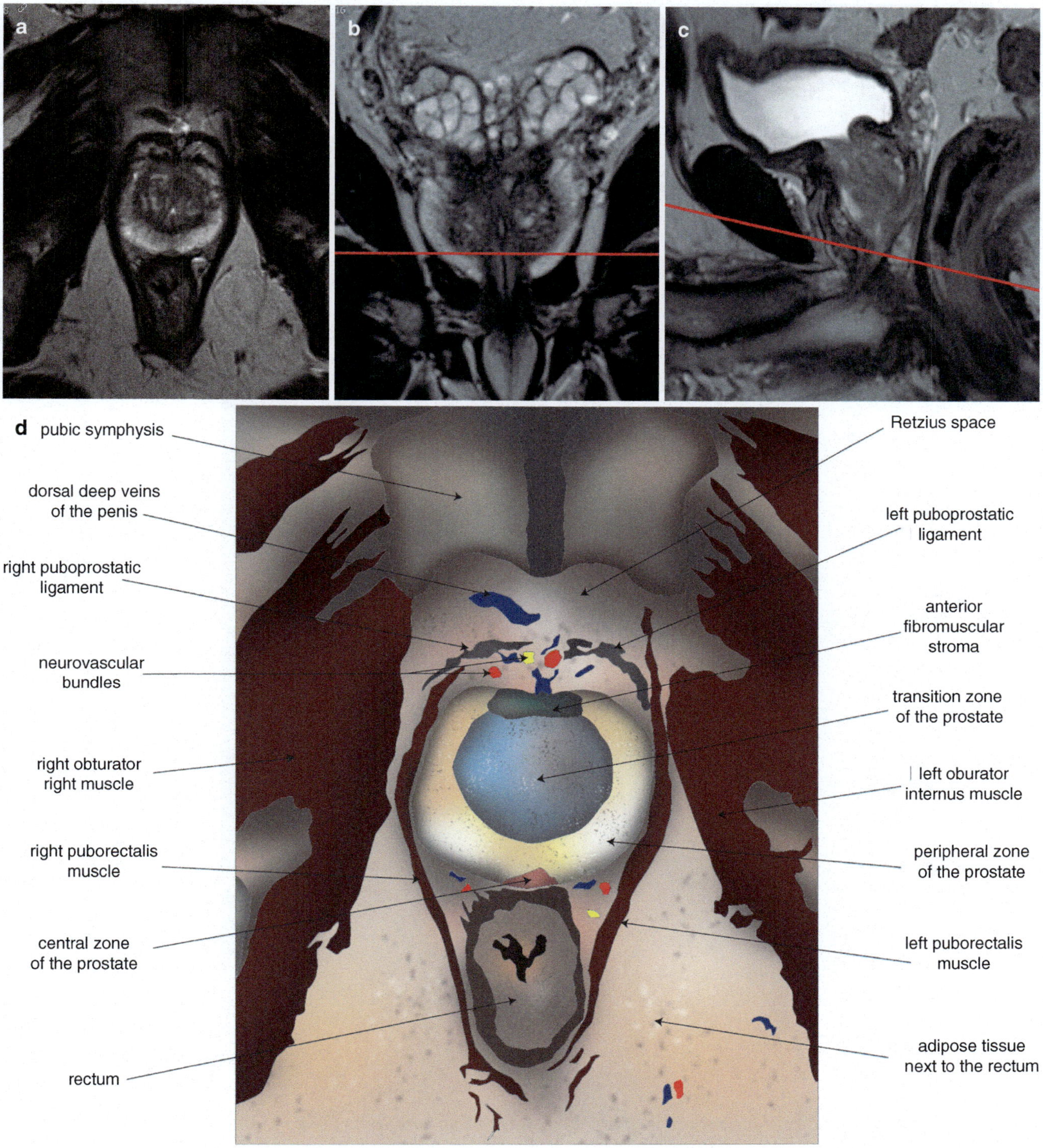

Fig. 2.25 (**a**) Axial section of the lower part of prostate on T2 WI MRI. (**b**) Coronal section of the prostate on T2 WI MRI. *Red line* shows level of section. (**c**) Midline sagittal section of the prostate on T2 WI MRI. *Red line* shows level of section. (**d**) Anatomical drawing of the same location as shown in "**a**"

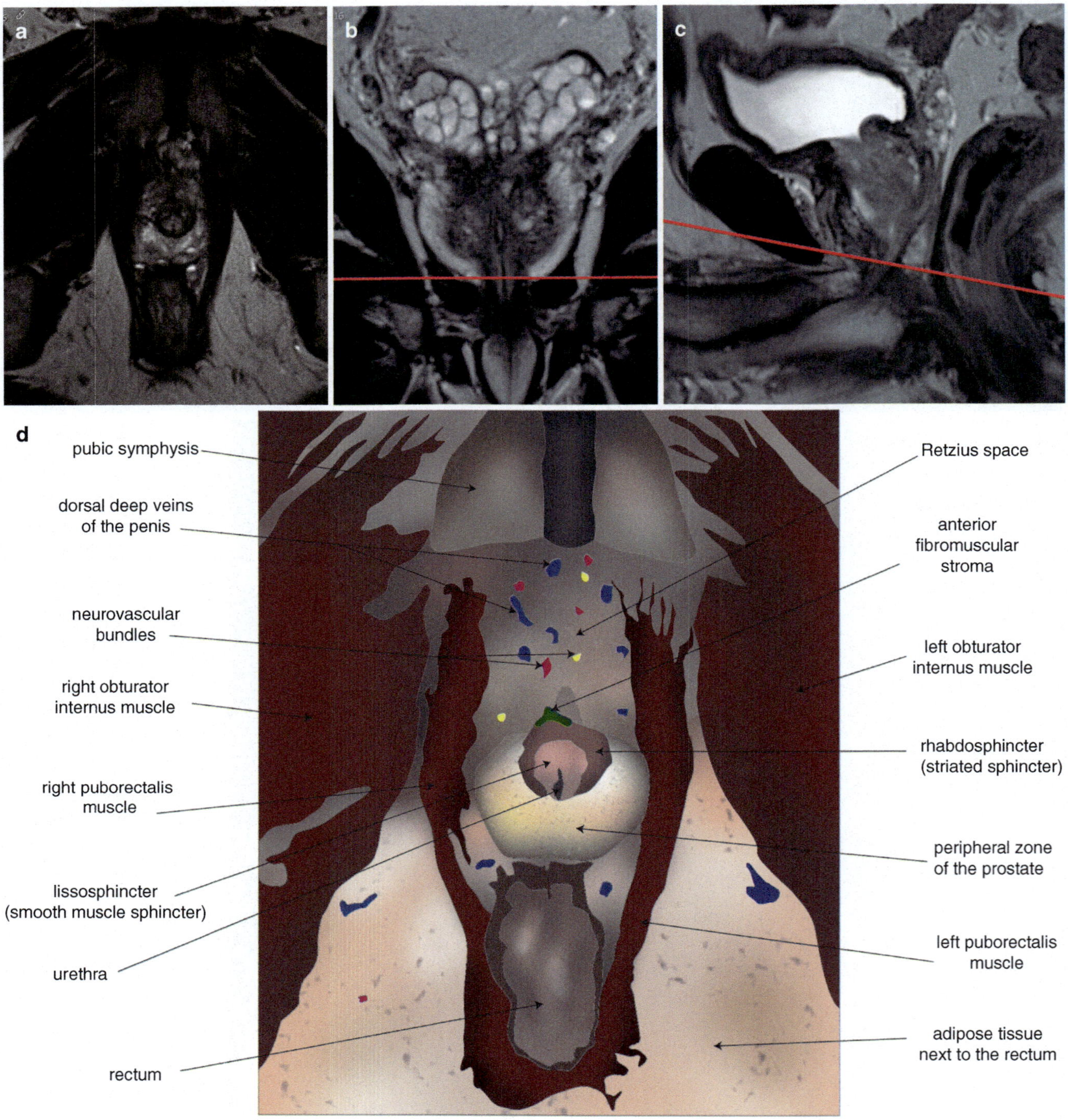

Fig. 2.26 (**a**) Axial section of the prostate apex on T2 WI MRI. (**b**) Coronal section of the prostate on T2 WI MRI. *Red line* shows the level of section. (**c**) Midline sagittal section of the prostate on T2 WI MRI. *Red line* shows level of section. (**d**) Anatomical drawing of the same location as shown in "**a**"

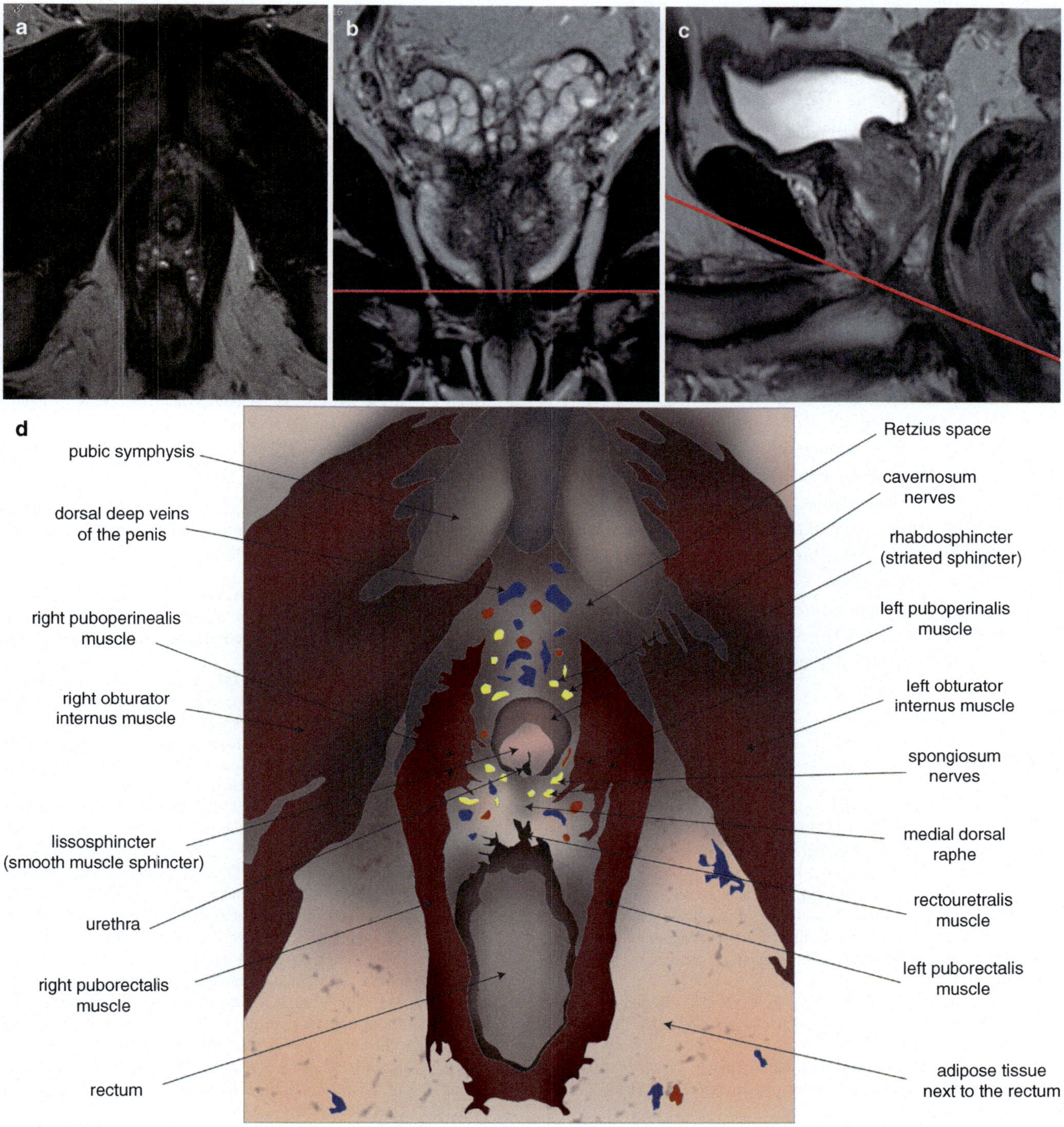

Fig. 2.27 (**a**) Axial section of the membranous urethra on T2 WI MRI. (**b**) Coronal section of the prostate on T2 WI MRI. *Red line* shows level of section. (**c**) Midline sagittal section of the prostate on T2 WI MRI. *Red line* shows level of section. (**d**) Anatomical drawing of the same location as shown in "**a**"

Key Points

- The prostate is divided into four zones: transition zone, central zone (CZ), peripheral zone (PZ) and anterior fibromuscular stromal zone (AFMS).
- Anatomical weakness areas can be recognised: (1) beak of the seminal vesicles, (2) invaginated extraprostatic space (IES), (3) perineural spaces of the prostatic dorsolateral neurovascular pedicles and (4) trapezoidal area.
- Prostatic apex is an important part of gland due to the following points: (1) its glandular tissue correspond to the Mc Neal peripheral zone; (2) its proximity with the trapezoidal area; and (3) cover a variable portion of EUS.
- Precise MRI evaluation of Prostatic Apex will allow us to achieve a complete removal of the tumour during the surgical procedure and satisfactory postsurgical functional results, that is, recovery of early urinary continence and penile erectile function.
- The prostate has three "pseudocapsules": (1) *Retzius periprostatic capsule,* merging with the AFMS; (2) *True capsule*, condensation of the glandular stroma; and (3) *Surgical capsule*, compression of the AFMS, CZ and PZ from BPH.

References

1. McNeal JE. The prostate gland: morphology and pathology. Monogr Urol. 1988;9(3):36–54.
2. Laucirica O. Anatomía topográfica zonal de la próstata. Madrid: Laboratorios Elfar-Drag S.A.; 1993.
3. Walz J, Burnett AL, Costello AJ, Eastham JA, et al. A critical analysis of the current knowledge of surgical anatomy related to optimization of cancer control and preservation of continence and erection in candidates for radical prostatectomy. Eur Urol. 2010;57:179–92.
4. Stolzenburg J-U, Schwalenberg T, Horn L-C, Neuhaus J, et al. Anatomical landmarks of radical prostatectomy. Eur Urol. 2007;51:629–39.
5. Koraitim M. The male urethral sphincter complex revisited: an anatomical concept and its physiological correlate. J Urol. 2008;179:1683–9.
6. Schlomm T, Heinzer H, Steuber T, et al. Full functional-length urethral sphincter preservation during radical prostatectomy. Eur Urol. 2011;60:320–9.
7. Myers RP. Detrusor apron, associated vascular plexus and avascular plane: relevance to radical retropubic prostatectomy; anatomical and surgical commentary. Urology. 2002;59:472–9.
8. Burnett AL, Mostwin JL. In situ anatomical study of the male urethral sphincteric complex: relevance to continence preservation following major pelvic surgery. J Urol. 1998;160:1301–6.
9. Wallner C, Dabhoiwala NF, DeRutier MC, et al. The anatomical components of urinary continence. Eur Urol. 2009;55:932–44.
10. Daouacher G, Waldén M. A simple reconstruction of the posterior aspect of rhabdosphincter and sparing of puboprostatic collar reduces the time to early continence after laparoscopic radical prostatectomy. J Endourol. 2014;28:1–6.
11. Tewari AK, Bigelow K, Rao S, et al. Anatomical restoration technique of continence mechanism and preservation of puboprostatic collar: a novel modification to achieve early urinary continence in men undergoing robotic prostatectomy. Urology. 2007;69:726–31.
12. Alsaid B, Bessede T, Diallo D, et al. Division of autonomic nerves within neurovascular bundles distally into corpora cavernosa and corpus spongiosum components: immunohistochemical confirmation with three-dimensional reconstruction. Eur Urol. 2011;59:902–9.
13. Burkhard FC, Kessler TM, Fleischmann A, et al. Nerve sparing open radical retropubic prostatectomy - does it have an impact on urinary continence? J Urol. 2006;176:189–95.
14. Guarnieri Catarin MV, Mastrocola MG, Nobrega JAM, et al. The role of membranous urethral afferent autonomic innervations in the continence mechanism after nerve sparing radical prostatectomy: a clinical and prospective study. J Urol. 2008;180:2527–31.
15. Hyun PY, Wook JC, Lee SE. A comprehensive review of neuroanatomy of the prostate. Prostate Int. 2013;1(4):139–45.
16. Nandipati KC, Raina R, Agarwal A, et al. Nerve-sparing surgery significantly affects long-term continence after radical prostatectomy. Urology. 2007;70:1127–30.
17. Srivastava A, Chopra S, Pham A, et al. Effect of a risk-stratified grade of nerve-sparing technique on early return of continence after robot-assisted laparoscopic radical prostatectomy. Eur Urol. 2013;63:438–44.
18. Suardi N, Moschini M, Gallina A, et al. Nerve-sparing approach during radical prostatectomy is strongly associated with the rate of postoperative urinary continence recovery. BJU Int. 2012;111:717–22.
19. Arango TO, Domenech Mateu JM. Evidencias anatomicalas y clinicas sobre el pudendo intrapelvico y su relación con el esfinter estriado de la uretra. Actas Urol Esp. 2000;24(3):248–54.
20. Ahmad E, Schenk Eric A. A new theory of the innervations of bladder musculature. Part 4. Innervation of the vesicourethral junction and external urethral sphincter. J Urol. 1974;111:613–5.
21. Kaiho Y, Nakagawa H, Ikeda Y, et al. Intraoperative electrophysiological confirmation of urinary continence after radical prostatectomy. J Urol. 2005;173:1139–42.
22. Soga H, Takenaka A, Murakami G, et al. Topographical relationship between urethral rhabdosphincter and rectourethralis muscle: a better understanding of the apical dissection and the posterior stitches in radical prostatectomy. Int J Urol. 2008;15:729–32.
23. Bouchet A, Cuilleret J. Anatomía descriptiva, topográfica y funcional. Pamplona: Ed Médica Panamericana; 1980.
24. Gil-Vernet JM, Arango O, Alvarez-Vijande R. Topographic anatomy and its development in urology in the 20th century. The work of Salvador Gil-Vernet. Eur J Anat. 2016;20(3):231–47.
25. Myers RP, Cahill DR, Kay PA, et al. Puboperineales: muscular boundaries of the male urogenital hiatus in 3D magnetic resonance imaging. J Urol. 2000;164:1421–15.
26. Rocco B, Gregori A, Stener S, et al. Posterior reconstruction of the rhabdosphincter allows a rapid recovery of continence after transperitoneal videolaparoscopic radical prostatectomy. Eur Urol. 2007;51:996–1003.
27. Kojima Y, Takahashi N, Haga N, et al. Urinary incontinence after robot-assisted radical prostatectomy: pathophysiology and intraoperative techniques to improve surgical outcome. Urology. 2013;20:1052–63.
28. Asimakopoulos AD, Annino F, D'Orazio A, et al. Complete periprostatic preservation during robot-assisted laparoscopic radical prostatectomy (RALP): the new pubovesical complex-sparing technique. Eur Urol. 2010;58:407–17.

Pathology of Prostate Cancer

3

Ferran Algaba

Contents

F. Algaba, M.D., Ph.D.
Pathology Department, Universitat Autònoma de Barcelona, Fundació Puigvert, Carrer Cartagena, 340-350, 08025 Barcelona, Spain
e-mail: falgaba@fundacio-puigvert.es

3.1 Introduction

Prostate carcinoma is the most frequent neoplasm and the sixth leading cause of cancer death in men. Although the risk of prostate cancer is higher in men with relatives who have had prostate cancer, the majority of cases are sporadic. The incidence of prostate cancer is closely related to age, geographical area (higher prevalence in Western countries than in Asia), and race (higher prevalence in the black race). These differences may be due to genetic factors, dietary factors, and diagnostic practices.

It is already known that some prostate carcinomas are not life-threatening [1, 2]. However, the widespread use of PSA determination has led to a large increase in the number of prostate biopsies, which in turn has resulted in the detection of such carcinomas. One of the great challenges today is to be able to distinguish between carcinomas at risk of progression and carcinomas which are clinically insignificant.

Because PSA is not a specific marker of prostate cancer an increase in its level motivates a search for the neoplasm by means of needle biopsy; if no neoplasm is found patients tend to undergo repeated needle biopsies. Until recently, the methods of imaging diagnosis have not been sufficiently accurate to locate the areas to be biopsied, but the introduction of multiparametric magnetic resonance imaging (mpMRI) appears to allow better recognition of tumor foci, especially the more aggressive ones [3].

The basis of Gleason grading for evaluation of the aggressiveness of prostate carcinoma lies in the variability of the tumor architecture, so there may be a relationship between the image seen by the pathologist and the image seen by the radiologist. Exchange of information between the pathologist and the radiologist will permit optimal interpretation of radiological images, and therefore it is very useful to know the morphological characteristics of the normal prostate and prostate cancer.

J.C. Vilanova et al. (eds.), *Atlas of Multiparametric Prostate MRI*, DOI 10.1007/978-3-319-61786-2_3

3.2 Prostate Microanatomy

The prostate comprises a number of tubuloalveolar glands (30–50) which drain directly into the urethra through 16–32 ducts, surrounded by a stromal component with abundant smooth muscle. The distribution of these glands was debated for a long time until the introduction of McNeal's model. McNeal divided the prostate into four zones [4], of which one is mainly stromal and three are chiefly glandular:

- The *anterior fibromuscular zone* is composed of collagen and spindle-shaped smooth muscle cells that are proximally contiguous with the detrusor fibers of the anterior bladder wall.
- The *central zone*, the base of which is at the bladder neck and the vertex toward the urethra, surrounding part of the proximal urethra; it is crossed by the ejaculatory ducts. The acini are large with irregular contours, and branching is very elaborate, with a homogeneous texture.
- The *transition zone* is located around the proximal urethra and has small, simple, round glands with a stroma similar to that in the central zone, with a low stroma/glandular index (Fig. 3.1).
- The *peripheral zone* constitutes the mid and the apex of the prostate and is therefore the area most accessible for digital rectal examination. The acini are either small and round or triangular, and the muscle bundles are multidirectional and loose (Fig. 3.2).

The histological structure of the acini and ducts is identical. The cells that form the gland are arranged in two layers, basal and luminal or secretory cells.

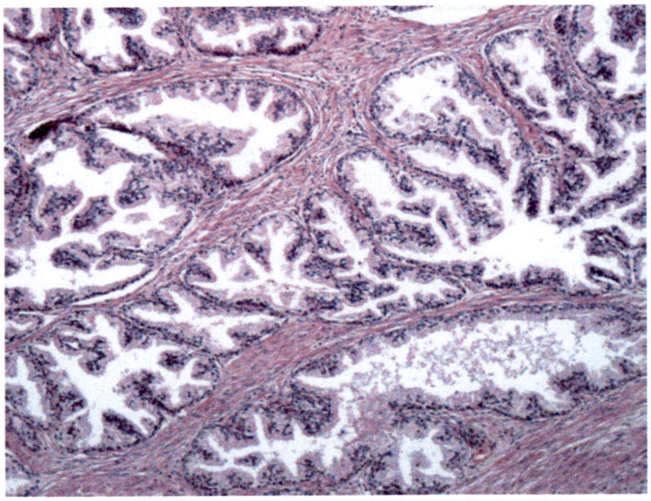

Fig. 3.1 Normal prostate transition zone

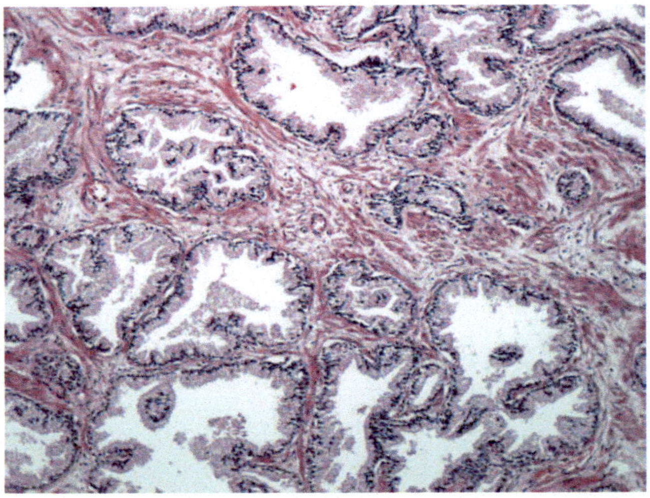

Fig. 3.2 Normal prostate peripheral zone

3.3 Morphology of Prostate Cancer

Prostate cancer is a glandular malignant neoplasia (adenocarcinoma), mostly of secretory or luminal phenotype with only a minimal percentage of cases having another histological morphology. The typical morphological features are microglandular monolayer proliferation with absence of basal cells and irregular nuclei with large nucleoli, which are multiple in some cases.

Using McNeal's model, around 70% of prostate carcinomas are in the peripheral zone (90% in the posterior or posterolateral area and 10% in the anterior horns) [5, 6], 7% are exclusively in the transition zone, and the remainder are in both zones or of indeterminate location [7]. Tumors with a smaller volume tend to be located in the apical portion, but as their volume increases, the subvesical portion also becomes involved [8]. Multifocality is present in approximately 80% of patients, half of whom have more than two nodules with frequent heterogeneous features [9].

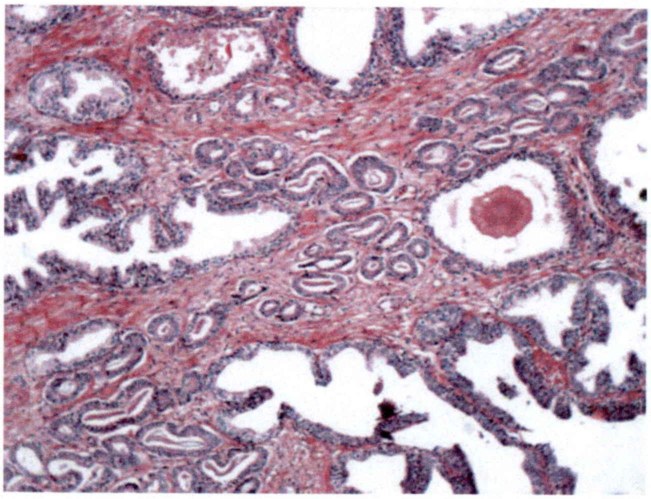

Fig. 3.3 Prostate adenocarcinoma pattern Gleason 3. Notice the tumoral growth among normal prostate glands

3.4 Morphological Variability of Acinar Prostate Cancer

The aggressiveness of cancer is related to the increase in genetic (chromosomal) changes. The nuclear changes produce cytoplasmic and intercellular adhesion molecule lesions expressed by changes in the architectural arrangement of the neoplastic cells.

For prostate cancer grading, WHO recommends the Gleason score with the 2014 International Society of Urological Pathology (ISUP) criteria and grade groups. The Gleason system only evaluates the architectural changes [10]. The ISUP guidelines claimed to be more precise in the criteria for every pattern.

Patterns 1, 2, and 3 consist in discrete glandular proliferation with marked variation in size and shape, with infiltration among nonneoplastic prostate acini and with different quantities of interglandular stroma (Fig. 3.3).

Pattern 4 has four different subtypes:

- *Fused glands* composed of a group of glands that are no longer completely separated by stroma (Fig. 3.4).
- *Cribriform glands* representing a glandular proliferation with multiple punched-out lumina (Fig. 3.5).
- *Poorly defined glands* with ill-formed or absent glandular lumina (Fig. 3.6). Classification for this subtype requires the presence of a cluster of such glands, to exclude the possibility of tangentially sectioned glands for Gleason pattern 3.
- *Glomeruloid glands*. These are dilated glands containing a cribriform proliferation attached to only one edge of the

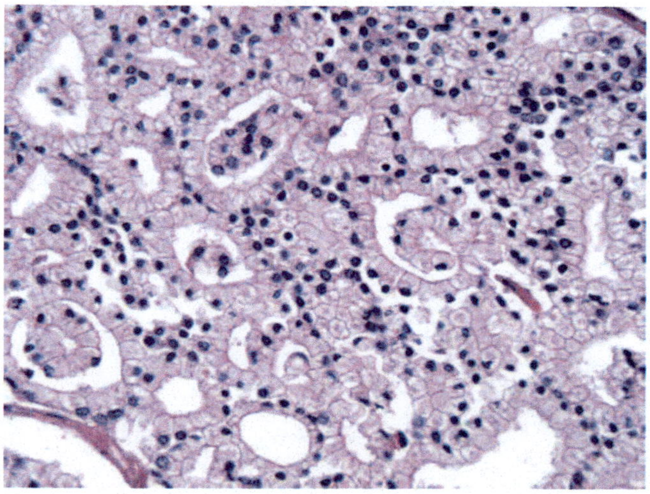

Fig. 3.4 Prostate adenocarcinoma, Gleason pattern 4, fused type

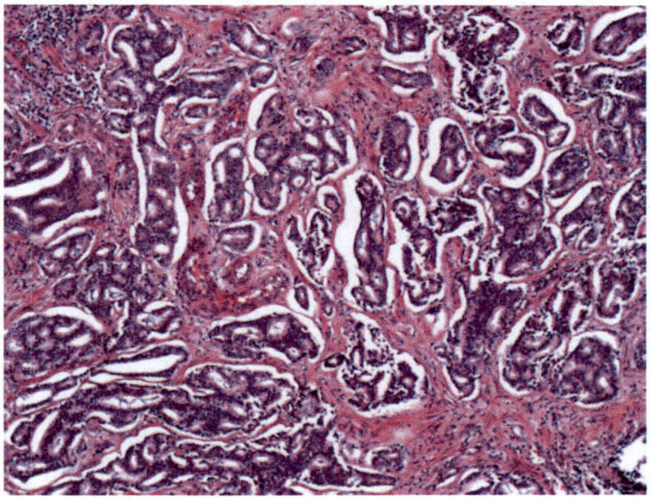

Fig. 3.5 Prostate adenocarcinoma, Gleason pattern 4, cribriform type

gland, resulting in the structure resembling a glomerulus (Fig. 3.7).

Pattern 5 is essentially no glandular differentiation with or without necrosis (Fig. 3.8).

The grade groups proposed by ISUP correspond to various combinations of these different patterns (Table 3.1). These grade groups show a good correlation with prognosis in prostate carcinoma in biopsy and radical prostatectomy [11] and with the number of genetic changes [12].

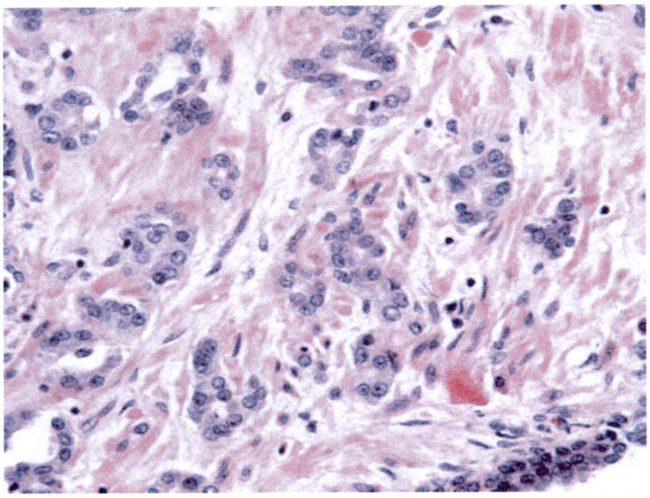

Fig. 3.6 Prostate adenocarcinoma, Gleason pattern 4, poorly or ill-defined gland type

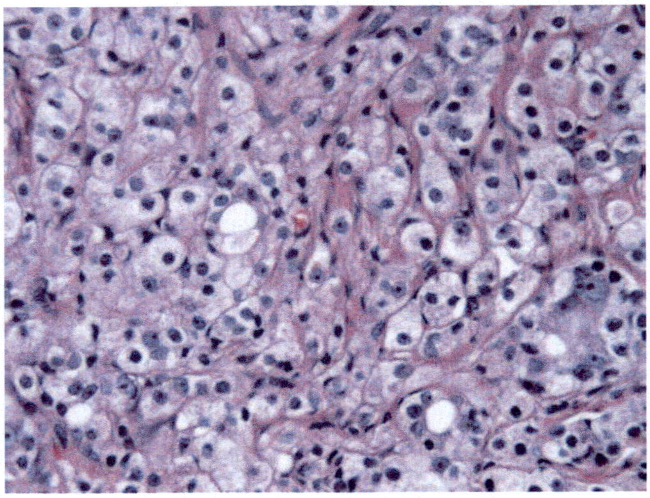

Fig. 3.8 Prostate adenocarcinoma, Gleason pattern 5

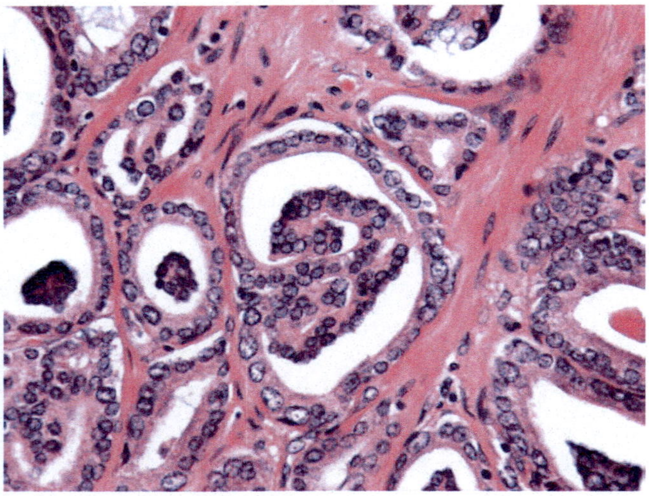

Fig. 3.7 Prostate adenocarcinoma, Gleason pattern 4, glomeruloid type

Table 3.1 Different combinations of Gleason patterns in the different grade groups proposed by ISUP

Group	Gleason	Description
1	≤6	Only individual discrete well-formed glands
2	3 + 4 = 7	Predominantly well-formed glands with a lesser component of poorly formed/fused/cribriform glands
3	4 + 3 = 7	Predominantly poorly formed/fused/cribriform glands with lesser component of well-formed glands
4	8	Only poorly formed/fused/cribriform glands or predominantly well-formed glands and lesser component lacking glands or predominantly lacking glands and lesser component of well-formed glands
5	9–10	Lack of gland formation (or with necrosis) with or without poorly formed/fused/cribriform glands

3.5 Prostate Cancer Morphology and Imaging Diagnosis

Diagnostic imaging methods are used with the aim of distinguishing foci of carcinoma from normal prostate tissue, and the criteria employed for this purpose may vary depending on whether one is considering the peripheral zone or the central portion (comprising the central and transitional zones) of the organ. Taking this fact into account, it is very important to re-read the normal and pathological morphology according to the distribution of the glands in the stroma and the possible amount of water molecules in the tissue since the mpMRI appearances correlate with them [13].

The peripheral zone is characterized by a loose stromal tissue interstitium which is distributed in a multidirectional manner with a high water content (Fig. 3.9) [14].

In the central portion of the prostate, the stroma is compact and has thick muscular bundles with less water content than in the peripheral zone (Fig. 3.10).

Looking at the different patterns of prostate carcinoma, it can be seen that variations in the size of the lumens and nuclei correlate with Gleason patterns and prognosis [15]: thus,

Group 1 prostate carcinomas (Gleason 3+ 3) are formed by glands similar to each other, with a regular stroma that infiltrates between normal glands, so that the amount of water can be variable and similar to peripheral zone normal tissue. Tumors with Gleason pattern 4 may have very different areas. The fused subtype of pattern 4 is characterized by tightly packed cells (fused and poorly formed glands) with little intercellular water (Fig. 3.4) and therefore with little mobility of molecules. On the other hand, the cribriform and glomeruloid subtypes are characterized by loose glands with abundant water (Fig. 3.5) and greater mobility of molecules, resembling normal tissue of the peripheral zone.

Gleason pattern 5 may range from compact accumulations of neoplastic cells with little intercellular fluid to cell strands between areas of thick connective tissue or solid masses with central necrosis.

On mpMRI, tumors smaller than 0.5 cm are not visible. When correlating the histology of prostate carcinomas above this size with the appearances on mpMRI, all of the abovementioned characteristics must be taken into account. In the case of tumor foci that are predominantly Gleason pattern 4, the detection rate on mpMRI varies from 36% for the cribriform subtype to more than 75% for the other subtypes. Consequently, in order to be visible on mpMRI, tumors of the cribriform subtype must be larger (1.25 cm) compared with tumors having other architectures (0.75–0.95 cm) [16]. In this study by Truong et al., among tumor foci containing Gleason pattern 4, the only independent predictors of tumor detection were accordingly increasing tumor size and noncribriform predominant architecture ($p = 0.003$ and $p = 0.013$, respectively).

Because the mpMRI image is dependent upon the cellular distribution and the mobility of the water molecules, it can be easily understood that certain nonneoplastic pathologies may be confused for a tumor lesion when they are characterized by sufficiently large accumulations of isolated cells in a liquid medium or by necrosis, as occurs in inflammatory processes or cystic glandular atrophy.

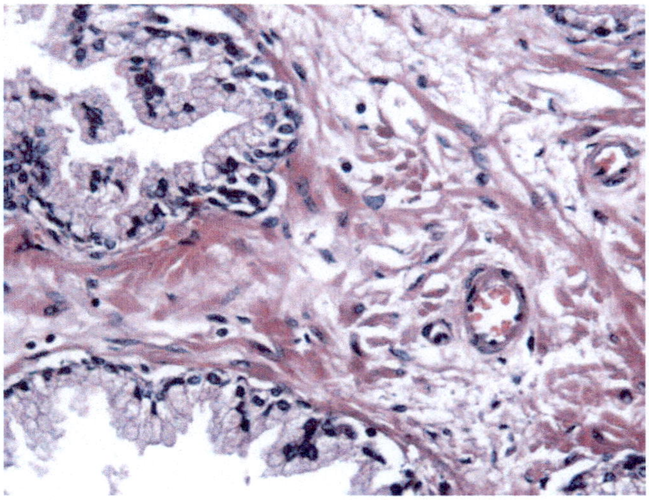

Fig. 3.9 Peripheral zone with a loose stroma

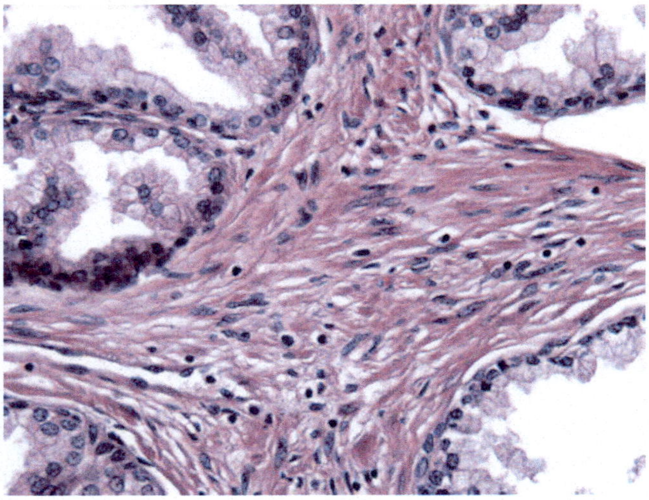

Fig. 3.10 Transition zone with a compact stroma

Key Points

- Prostate cancer grade is performed with the Gleason score according to the tumor architecture, from a pattern 1 (differentiated) to pattern 5 (undifferentiated).
- A new grading system uses modified Gleason score groups: Group 1 = Gleason score $\leq$ 6, Group 2 = Gleason score 3 + 4 = 7, Group 3 = Gleason score 4 + 3 = 7, Group 4 = Gleason score 8, Group 5 = Gleason scores 9 and 10.
- mpMRI appearance correlates with the distribution of the glands in the stroma and the possible amount of water molecules in the tissue.
- The peripheral zone is characterized with a high water content, and the central and transition zones have compacted stroma and thicker muscular bundles.
- Tumors of the pattern 4 cribriform subtype must be larger compared with tumors pattern 4 having other architectures for mpMRI detection.

References

1. Sakr WA, Haas GP, Cassin BF, et al. The frequency of carcinoma and intraepithelial neoplasia of the prostate in young male patients. J Urol. 1993;150:379–85.
2. Alsinnawi M, Loftus B, Flynn R, et al. The incidence and relevance of prostate cancer in radical cystoprostatectomy specimens. Int Urol Nephrol. 2012;44:1705–10.
3. Roethke M, Anastasiadis AG, Lichy M, et al. MRI-guided prostate biopsy detects clinically significant cancer: analysis of a cohort of 100 patients after previous negative TRUS biopsy. World J Urol. 2012;30(2):213–8.
4. McNeal JE. Regional morphology and pathology of the prostate. Am J Clin Pathol. 1968;49:347–57.
5. McNeal JE, Redwine EA, Freiha FS, et al. Zonal distribution of prostatic adenocarcinoma. Correlation with histologic pattern and direction of spread. Am J Surg Pathol. 1988;12:897–906.
6. Abdelsayed GA, Danial T, Kaswick JA, et al. Tumors of the anterior prostate: implications for diagnosis and treatment. Urology. 2015;85:1224–8.
7. Erbersdobler H, Augustin T, Schlomm T, et al. Prostate cancers in the transition zone: part 1; pathological aspects. BJU Int. 2004;94:1221–5.
8. Egawa S, Takashima R, Matsumoto K, et al. Infrequent involvement of the anterior base in low-risk patients with clinically localized prostate cancer and its possible significance in definitive radiation therapy. Jpn J Clin Oncol. 2000;30:126–30.
9. Arora R, Koch MO, Eble JN, et al. Heterogeneity of Gleason grade in multifocal adenocarcinoma of the prostate. Cancer. 2004;100:2362–6.
10. Epstein JI, Egevad L, Amin MB, et al.; Grading Committee. The 2014 International Society of Urological Pathology (ISUP) Consensus Conference on Gleason Grading of Prostatic Carcinoma: definition of grading patterns and proposal for a new grading system. Am J Surg Pathol. 2016;40:244–52.
11. Epstein JI, Zelefsky MJ, Sjoberg DD, et al. A contemporary prostate cancer grading system: a validated alternative to the Gleason score. Eur Urol. 2016;69:428–35.
12. Rubin MA, Girelli G, Demichelis F. Genomic correlates to the newly proposed grading prognostic groups for prostate cancer. Eur Urol. 2016;69:557–60.
13. Langer DL, van der Kwast TH, Evans AJ, et al. Prostate tissue composition and MR measurements: investigating the relationships between ADC, T2, K(trans), v(e), and corresponding histologic features. Radiology. 2010;255:485–94.
14. McNeal JE. Prostate. In: Sternberg SS, editor. Histology for pathologists. Chapter 40. New York: Raven Press; 1992. p. 749–63.
15. Venkataraman G, Rycyna K, Rabanser A, et al. Morphometric signature differences in nuclei of Gleason pattern 4 areas in Gleason 7 prostate cancer with differing primary grades on needle biopsy. J Urol. 2009;181:88–93.
16. Truong M, Hollenberg G, Weinberg E, et al. Impact of Gleason subtype on prostate cancer detection using multiparametric MRI: correlation with final histopathology. J Urol. 2017. doi:10.1016/j.juro.2017.01.077, pii: S0022-5347(17)30197-0.

4 PI-RADS v2: Reading Model

Joan C. Vilanova, Violeta Catalá, Roberto García-Figueiras, and Maria Boada

Contents

J.C. Vilanova, M.D., Ph.D. (✉)
Department of Radiology, Clínica Girona, Institute Catalan of Health-IDI, University of Girona, Lorenzana 36, 17002 Girona, Spain
e-mail: kvilanova@comg.cat

V. Catalá, M.D., Ph.D.
Department of Radiology, Fundació Puigvert, Cartagena 340, 08005 Barcelona, Spain
e-mail: violetacatala@yahoo.com.ar

R. García-Figueiras, M.D., Ph.D.
Department of Radiology, Hospital Clínico Universitario de Santiago de Compostela (CHUS), 15706 Santiago de Compostela, A Coruña, Spain
e-mail: elhabibi.xray@gmail.com

M. Boada, M.D.
Department of Radiology, Clínica Girona, Lorenzana 36, 17002 Girona, Spain
e-mail: mariaboada@comg.cat

4.1 Introduction

Multiparametric MRI (mpMRI) is the method of choice to evaluate the prostate for clinically significant adenocarcinoma. The widespread implementation and acceptance of mpMRI requires a standardization of image acquisition, interpretation, and reporting to achieve an optimal test for daily practice on the work-up of prostate cancer (PCa).

For this purpose, Prostate Imaging Reporting and Data System (PI-RADS) guidelines for mpMRI have been provided with the specific goals [1]: (a) to establish minimum technical parameters for prostate MRI; (b) to standardize radiology reports to reduce variability in imaging interpretation; (c) to develop assessment categories that summarize levels of suspicion or risk for clinically significant prostate cancer, to be used to triage patients for appropriate management; and (d) to promote research and quality assurance to improve patient's outcome.

The current PI-RADS v2 guidelines should be followed considering the information provided on clinical considerations, technical specifications for mpMRI (see Chap. 1), normal anatomy and benign findings to perform appropriate assessment criteria for detection, and diagnosis of significant PCa [2]. The PI-RADS v2 guidelines are intended for diagnostic evaluation and risk assessment of patients with suspected PCa prior to or after transrectal ultrasound (TRUS) biopsy but not for detecting suspected recurrence following PCa therapy.

A major objective of the PI-RADS reporting is to identify clinically significant PCa. Clinically significant cancer is defined on pathology/histology as Gleason score $\geq$ 7, and/or volume $\geq$ 0.5 cc, and/or extra prostatic extension (EPE) [3].

PI-RADS v2 assessment uses a final 5-point scale based on the likelihood (probability) that a combination of mpMRI

J.C. Vilanova et al. (eds.), *Atlas of Multiparametric Prostate MRI*, DOI 10.1007/978-3-319-61786-2_4

Table 4.1 PI-RADS v2 assessment categories (Typical examples on Fig. 4.22)

PI-RADS 1—very low (clinically significant cancer is highly unlikely to be present)
PI-RADS 2—low (clinically significant cancer is unlikely to be present)
PI-RADS 3—intermediate (the presence of clinically significant cancer is equivocal)
PI-RADS 4—high (clinically significant cancer is likely to be present)
PI-RADS 5—very high (clinically significant cancer is highly likely to be present)

findings on T2W, DWI, and DCE correlates with the presence of a clinically significant cancer for each lesion in the prostate gland (Table 4.1).

This chapter illustrates a comprehensive overview to perform an appropriate interpretation of mpMRI following the PI-RADS v2 guidelines approach providing an imaging atlas algorithm in order to decide a final PI-RADS score.

4.2 Systematic Reading Method

It is mandatory to evaluate the MRI examination displaying the relevant sequences at the same time, correlated and synchronized when viewing, using a single or additional monitors. A standardized layout displaying the morphological (with different planes) and multiparametric sequences (DWI and/or DCE), including the ADC map, should be configured (Fig. 4.21a). The T1 WI should be analyzed to rule out the presence of hemorrhage post-biopsy, before the initial evaluation of the different sequences.

The reasonable approach to read a mpMRI should use a lesion-based location score. PI-RADS v2 uses an algorithm to arrive at the overall score based on the zonal location of the lesion, related to the peripheral (PZ) or transition-central zone (TZ).

DWI with corresponding ADC map is the dominant sequence in the peripheral zone that will determine the overall suspicious score (Fig. 4.1). For a detected PZ lesion, if the DWI score is 4 and the T2WI score (Fig. 4.2) is 3, the PI-RADS assessment category should be 4. Dynamic contrast enhancement (DCE) sequence has secondary role in equivocal cases (PI-RADS 3), where a positive DCE (fast and early focal uptake corresponding to suspicious findings on T2WI and/or DWI) score can upgrade the lesion to a PI-RADS 4 (Fig. 4.1) (Table 4.2). The criteria for a negative DCE are as follows: no early enhancement or diffuse enhancement not corresponding to a focal finding on T2WI

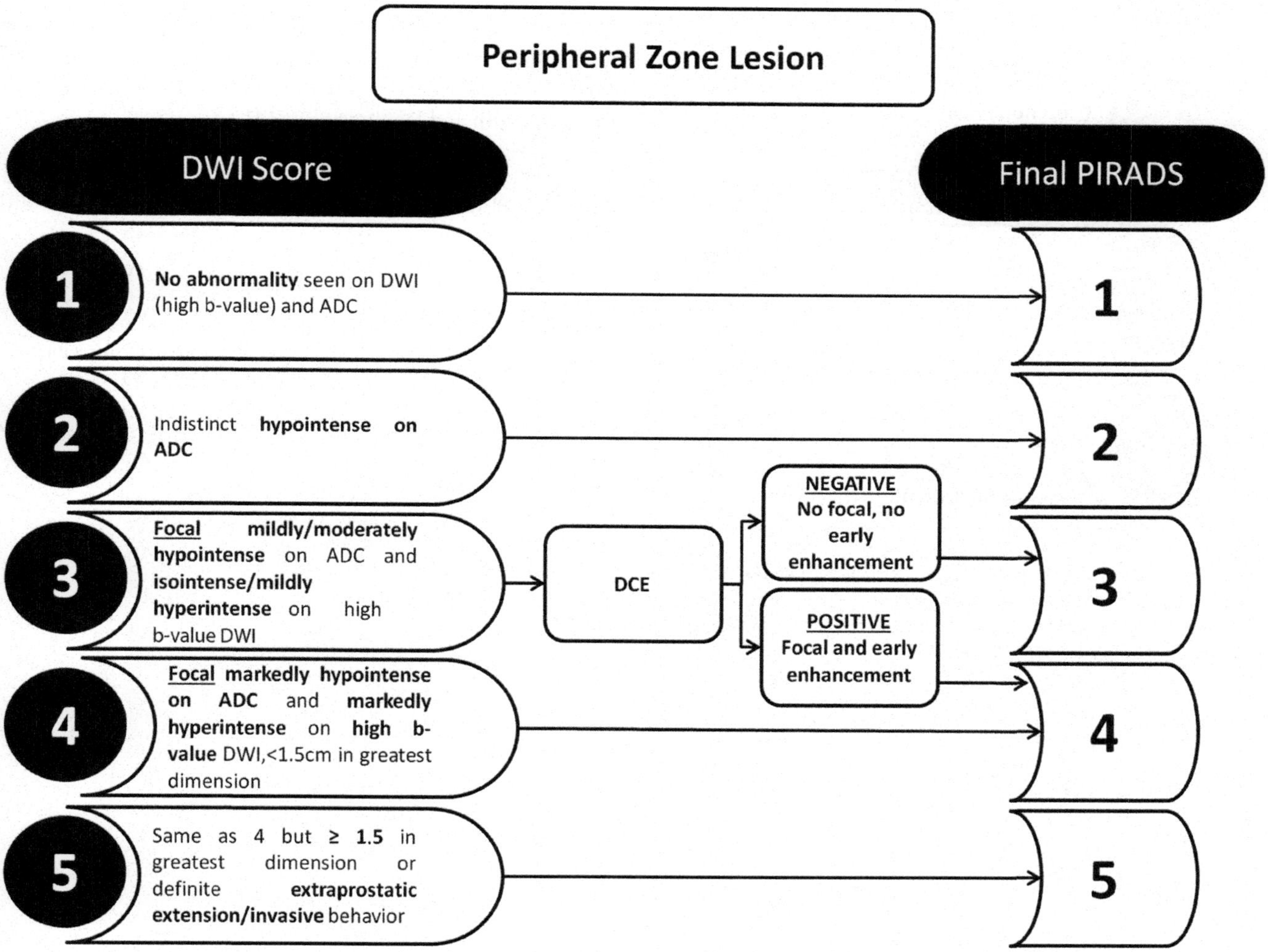

Fig. 4.1 Stepwise approach to assign and overall PI-RADS v2 score for the peripheral zone (see Fig. 4.22 for corresponding typical examples). *ADC* apparent diffusion coefficient, *DWI* diffusion-weighted imaging, *DCE* dynamic contrast enhancement

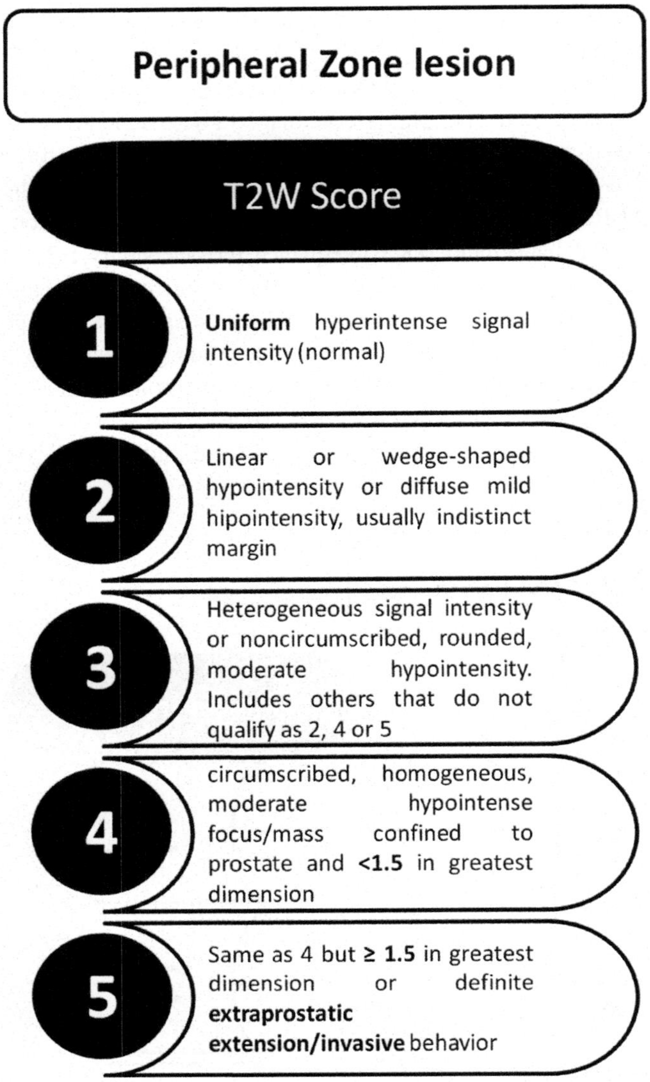

Fig. 4.2 PI-RADS scoring system for peripheral zone on T2WI. The final PI-RADS assessment for the peripheral zone is the DWI score (Fig. 4.1), as is the determining sequence. See Fig. 4.22 for corresponding typical examples

and/or DWI or focal enhancement corresponding to a lesion demonstrating features of benign prostatic hypertrophy (BPH) on T2WI (Table 4.2).

T2W imaging is the dominant sequence in the transition-central zone that will determine the overall suspicion score (Fig. 4.3). DWI has a secondary role in the transition zone for equivocal cases (PI-RADS 3), where a large corresponding abnormality (PI-RADS 5, >1.5 cm) can upgrade the lesion to an overall PI-RADS 4 (Fig. 4.3).

A lesion within the central zone or fibromuscular stroma should be scored using the transition zone scoring algorithm (Fig. 4.3), that is, T2W imaging is the dominant sequence.

Lesion should be localized using the PI-RADS v2 39-sector map (Fig. 4.4) and provide the corresponding measurement in greatest dimension (Fig. 4.5).

It is recommended that ADC maps from a particular MR equipment are set for clinically significant prostate cancers so that they appear markedly hypointense on ADC maps, and they should be consistently viewed with the same contrast (window with and level) settings [4].

Table 4.2 PI-RADS assessment for dynamic contrast enhanced MRI (DCE)

Negative DCE (example on Fig. 4.12)	Positive DCE (example on Fig. 4.13)
– No early enhancement	– Fast and early focal uptake corresponding to suspicious findings on T2WI and/or DWI
– Diffuse enhancement not corresponding to a focal finding on T2WI and/or DWI	
– Focal enhancement corresponding to a lesion demonstrating features of benign prostatic hypertrophy (BPH) on T2WI	

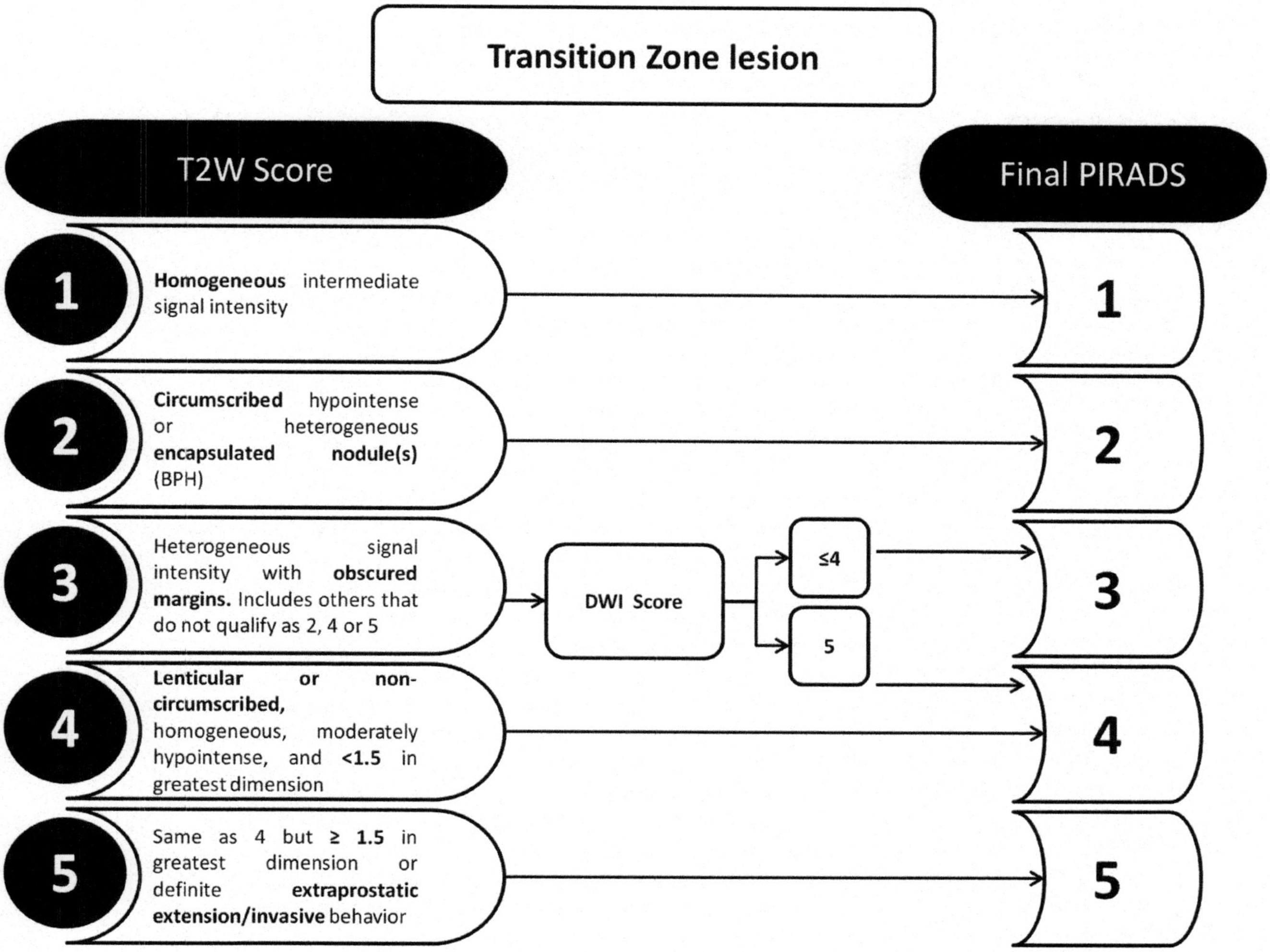

Fig. 4.3 Stepwise approach to assign and overall PI-RADS v2 score for the transition zone. See Fig. 4.22 for corresponding typical examples. *DWI* diffusion-weighted imaging, *BPH* benign prostatic hyperplasia

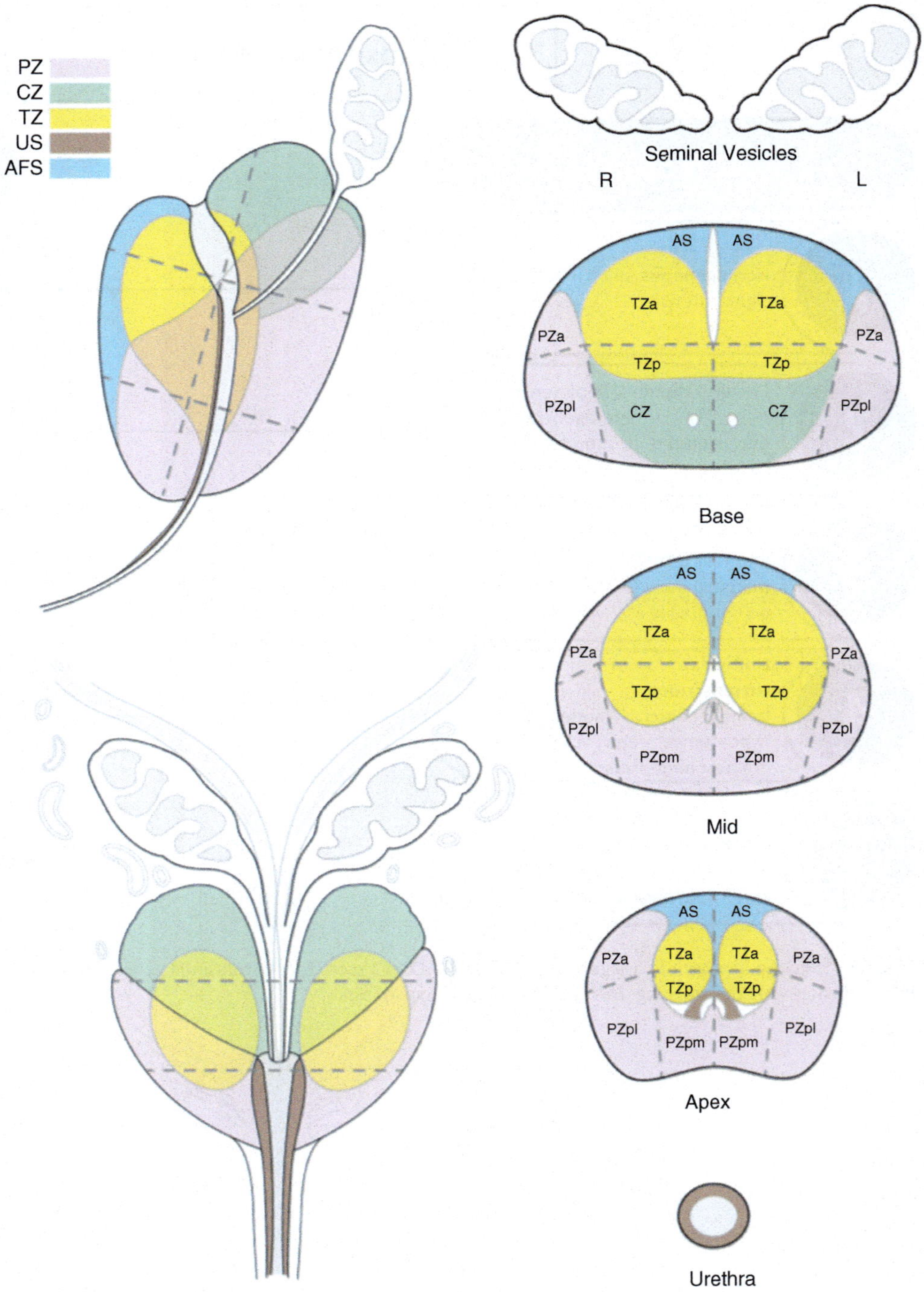

Fig. 4.4 Sector map used in PI-RADS v2. *AFS* (AS) anterior fibromuscular stroma, *CZ* central zone, *TZ* transition zone, *PZ* peripheral zone, *US* urethral sphincter. *a* anterior, *p* posterior, *m* medial, *l* lateral. From European Society of Urogenital Radiology. MR Prostate Imaging Reporting and Data System version 2.0. Accessed January 2017, from http://www.esur.org/fileadmin/content/user_upload/PI-RADS_v2_20141223.pdf

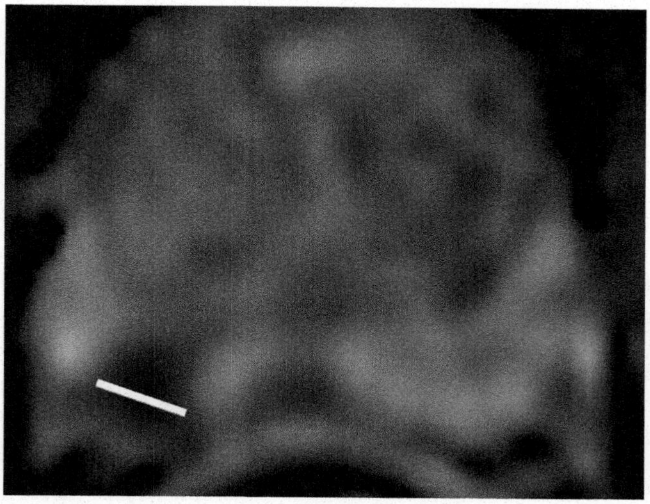

Fig. 4.5 Axial ADC map image showing a right focal nodular lesion in the peripheral zone with the maximum diameter of 12 mm, which is key feature to discriminate between an overall PI-RADS suspicion score of 4 or 5. A lesion in the transition zone should be measured on T2WI. If a lesion is difficult to measure in the recommended sequence, measurement should be performed using the sequence or plane with the best lesion conspicuity

4.3 PI-RADS 1

Clinically significant cancer is highly unlikely to be present.

No abnormality in the peripheral zone on DWI and no lesion on T2WI in the transition zone, homogeneous intermediate signal intensity (Fig. 4.6).

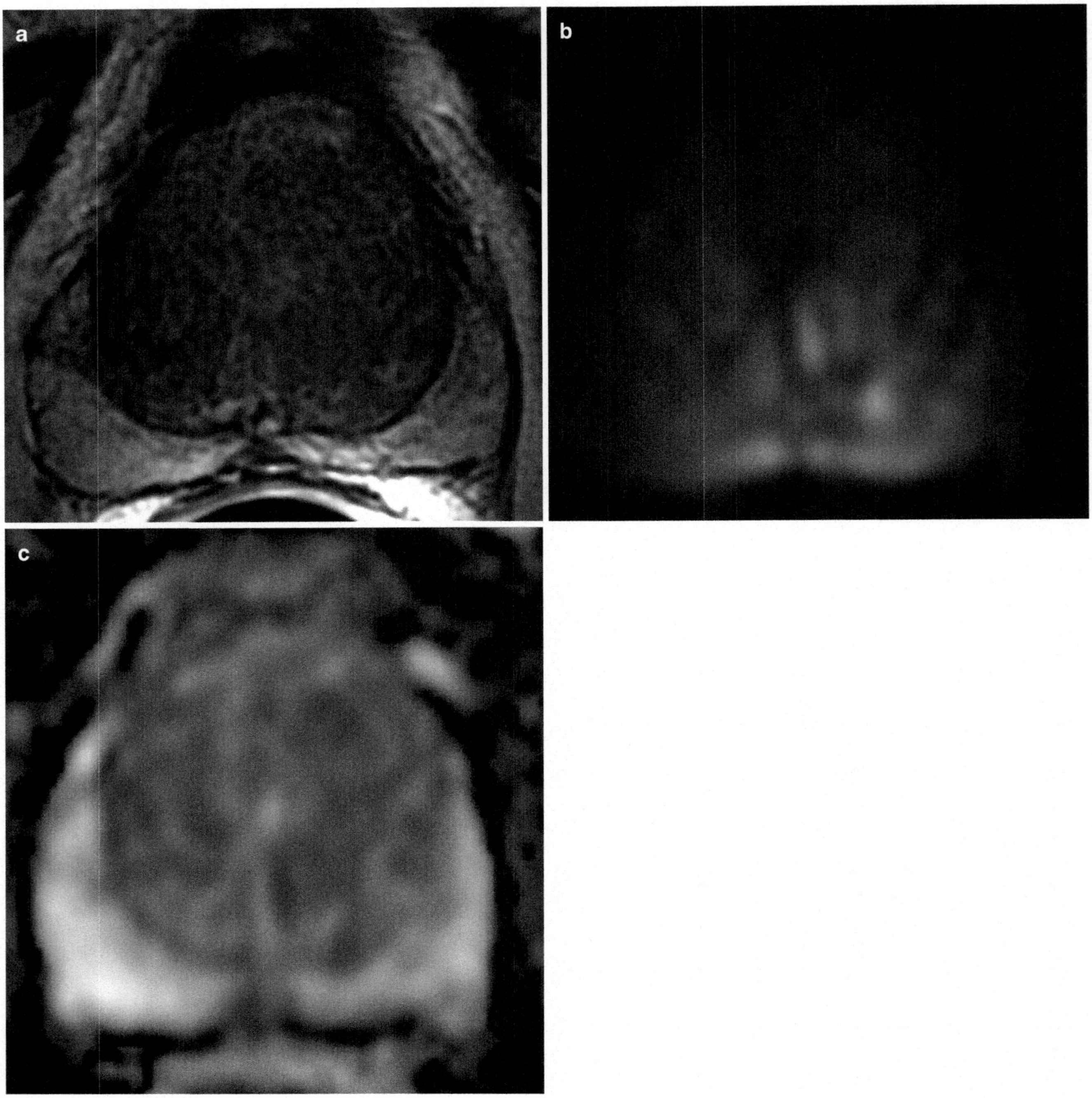

Fig. 4.6 PI-RADS 1. (**a**) Axial T2WI, (**b**) b1400 DWI, and (**c**) ADC map, without any abnormality on DWI/ADC in the peripheral zone and homogeneous intermediate signal intensity of the transition zone on T2WI; assigning a PI-RADS 1

4.4 PI-RADS 2: Peripheral Zone

Clinically significant cancer is unlikely to be present.

No peripheral focal restriction on DWI. Indistinct hypointense on ADC (Fig. 4.7). An area of low signal in the peripheral zone on T2WI but no focal restriction on DWI imaging would correspond to a PI-RADS score 2. Be aware that in any lesion seen on the peripheral zone on T2WI or in DWI without focal shape, the maximum PI-RADS score would be 2 (Figs. 4.8 and 4.9), as the dominant sequence for PI-RADS assessment in the peripheral zone is DWI (Fig. 4.1).

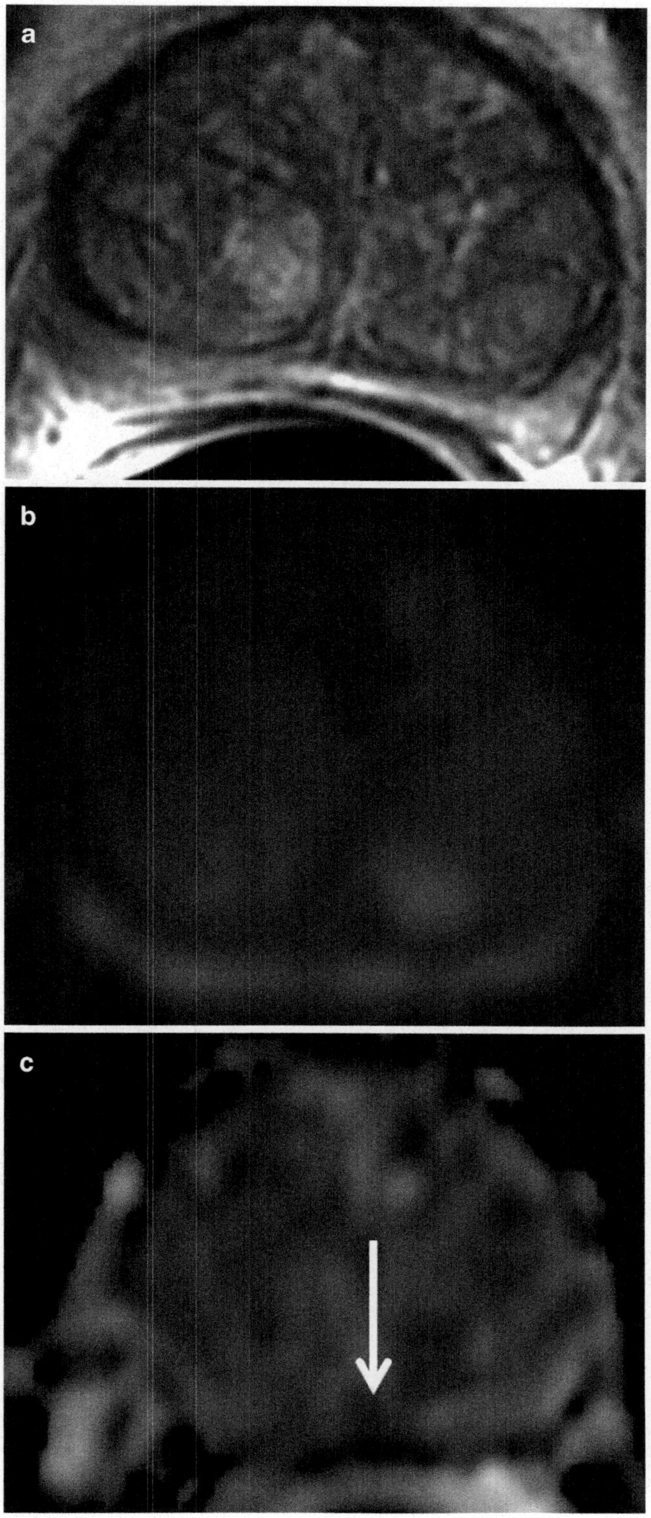

Fig. 4.7 PI-RADS 2. Peripheral zone. (**a**) Axial T2WI, (**b**) b1400 DWI, and (**c**) ADC map, without any focal lesion on DWI and a mild low signal intensity on ADC map (*arrow*) in the peripheral zone; assigning a final PI-RADS of 2

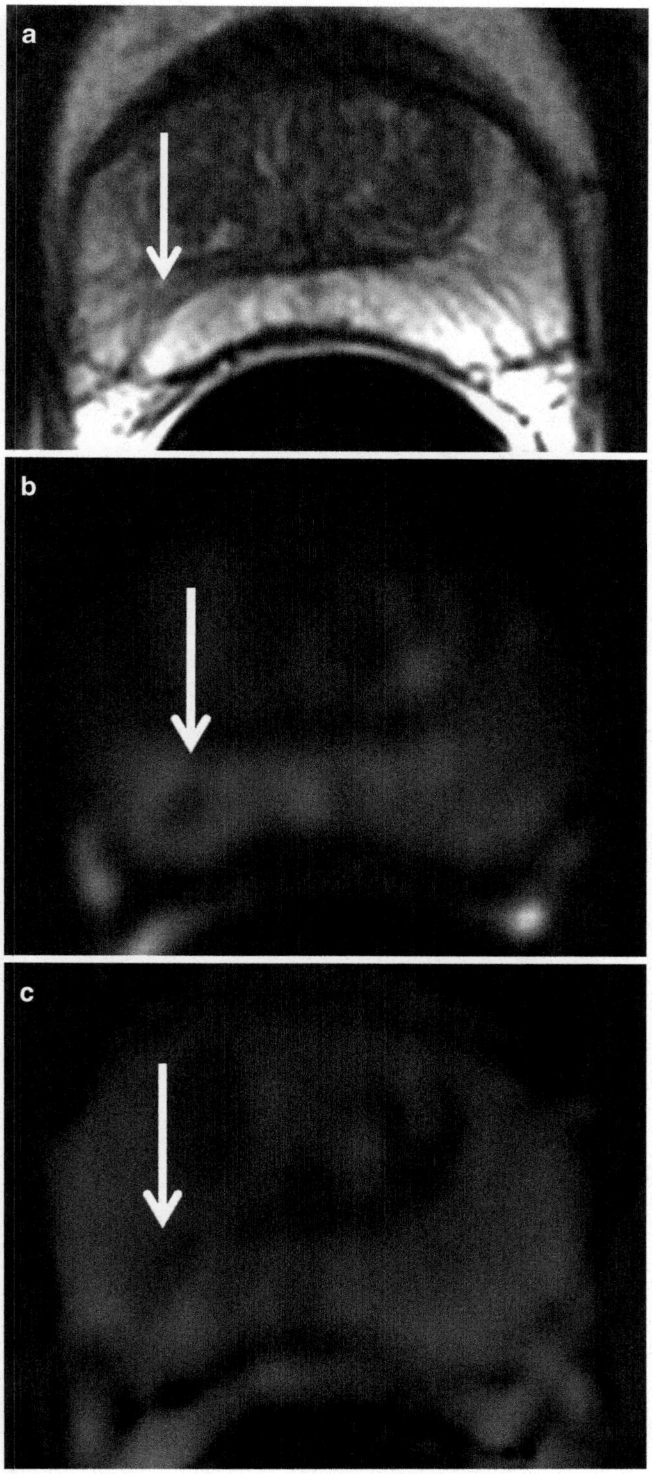

Fig. 4.8 PI-RADS 2. Peripheral zone. (**a**) Axial T2WI, (**b**) b1400 DWI, and (**c**) ADC map, showing linear, heterogeneous hypointensity in the right peripheral zone, without hyperintense signal on DWI and hypointense on ADC map (*arrows*), assigning a final PI-RADS of 2

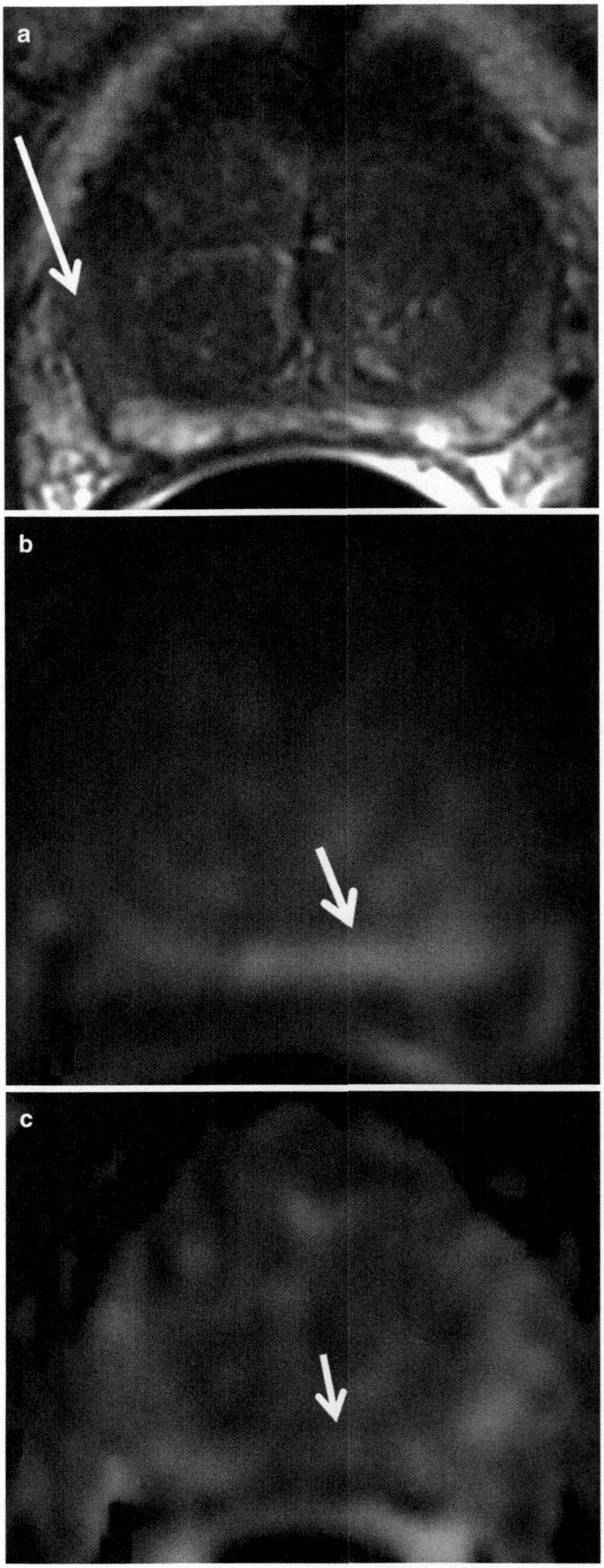

Fig. 4.9 PI-RADS 2. Peripheral zone. (**a**) Axial T2WI, (**b**) b1400 DWI, and (**c**) ADC map, showing homogeneous hypointensity in the right peripheral zone (*long arrow*), without hyperintense signal on DWI. The peripheral assessment should be decided on the DWI/ADC images; thus, no concern should be on this location. On DWI there is mild hyperintense signal on the left peripheral zone, but not focal; with mild indistinct hypointensity (*short arrows*), assigning a final PI-RADS score of 2

4.5 PI-RADS 2 Transition Zone

Clinically significant cancer is unlikely to be present.

Encapsulated, circumscribed, round hypointense, or heterogeneous encapsulated nodule(s) (BPH) (Fig. 4.10). It is important to evaluate the lesion in different planes to realize the encapsulated margins overall the BPH nodule (Fig. 4.11); in order to avoid false interpretation of pseudo ill-defined nodules corresponding to a encapsulated heterogeneous BPH nodule.

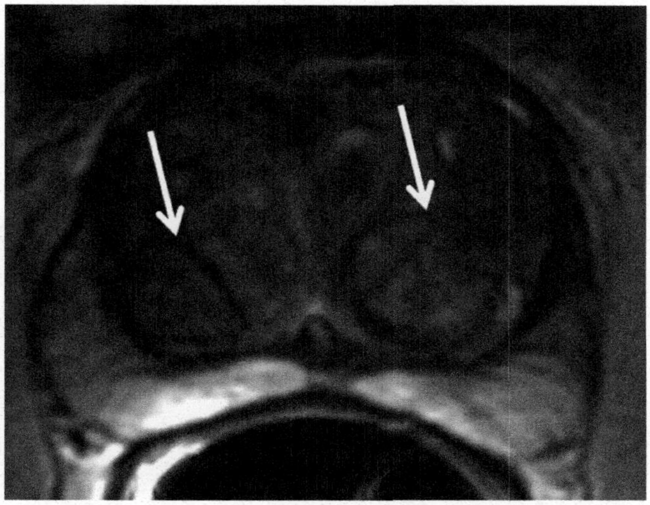

Fig. 4.10 PI-RADS 2. Transition zone. Axial T2WI showing different encapsulated and round nodules in the transition zone, assigning a final PI-RADS score of 2

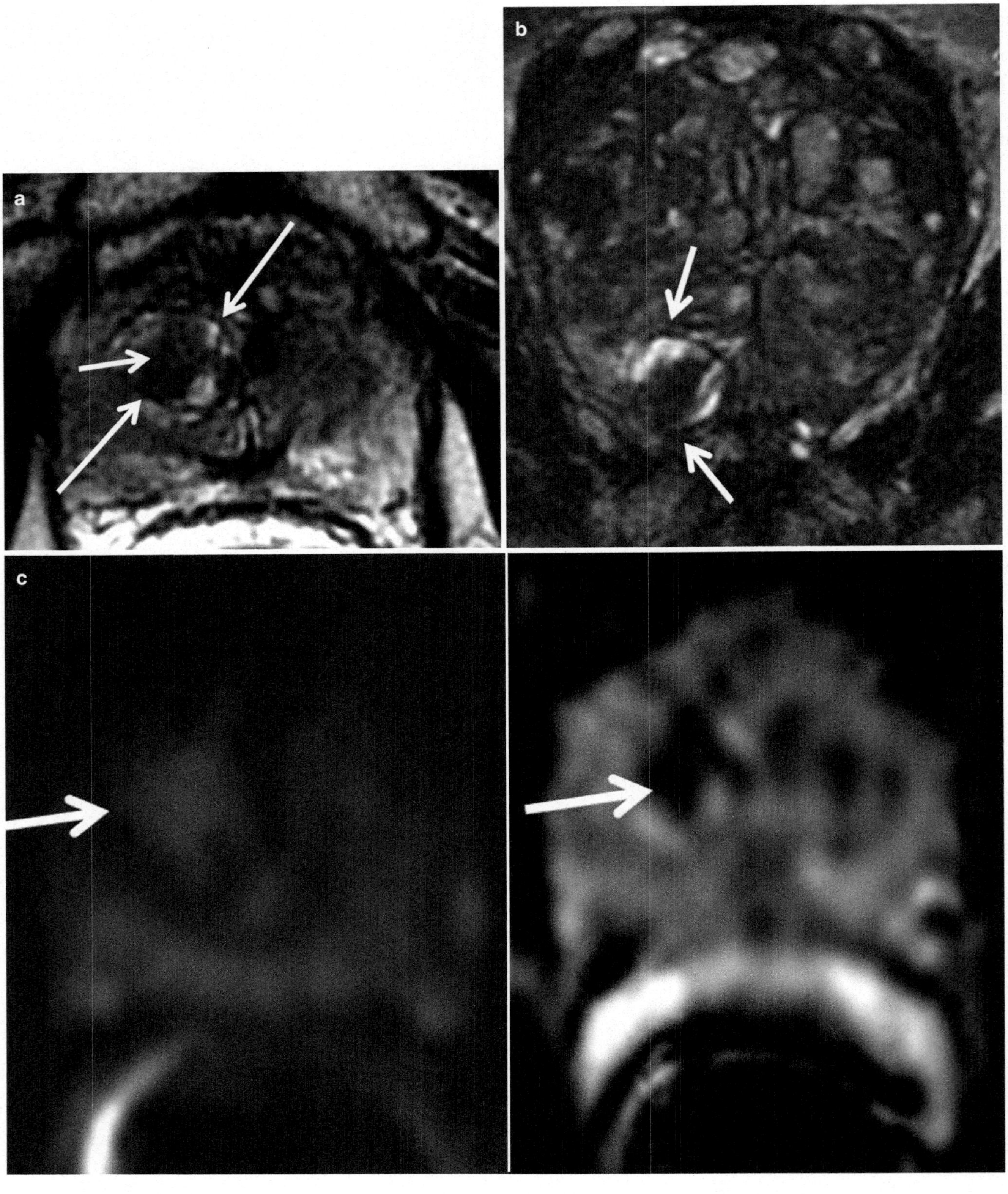

Fig. 4.11 PI-RADS 2. Transition zone. (**a**) Axial T2WI shows a low signal intensity nodule (*short arrow*) with obscured margins; but it should be evaluated the outer margin, encapsulated (*long arrows*) on a heterogeneous mixed BPH with peripheral high signal due to glandular tissue. The coronal plane (**b**) confirms the encapsulated margin of the BPH (**b**) (*arrows*), with a final assessment of PI-RADS 2, as the nodule is circumscribed within a typical BPH. The false interpretation of an obscured margins nodule (*short arrow* in **a**) would have scored a PI-RADS 3; and the axial DWI and corresponding ADC images (**c**), showing restriction, would upgraded to a PI-RADS 4

4.6 PI-RADS 3 Peripheral Zone

The presence of clinically significant cancer is equivocal.

Minimal focal restriction. Focal mildly/moderately hypointense on ADC and isointense/mildly hyperintense on high b-value DWI. Dynamic contrast enhancement (DCE) differentiates lesions into PI-RADS 3 (negative contrast) or upgrades to PI-RADS 4 (positive contrast) (Table 4.2) (Figs. 4.1, 4.12, and 4.13).

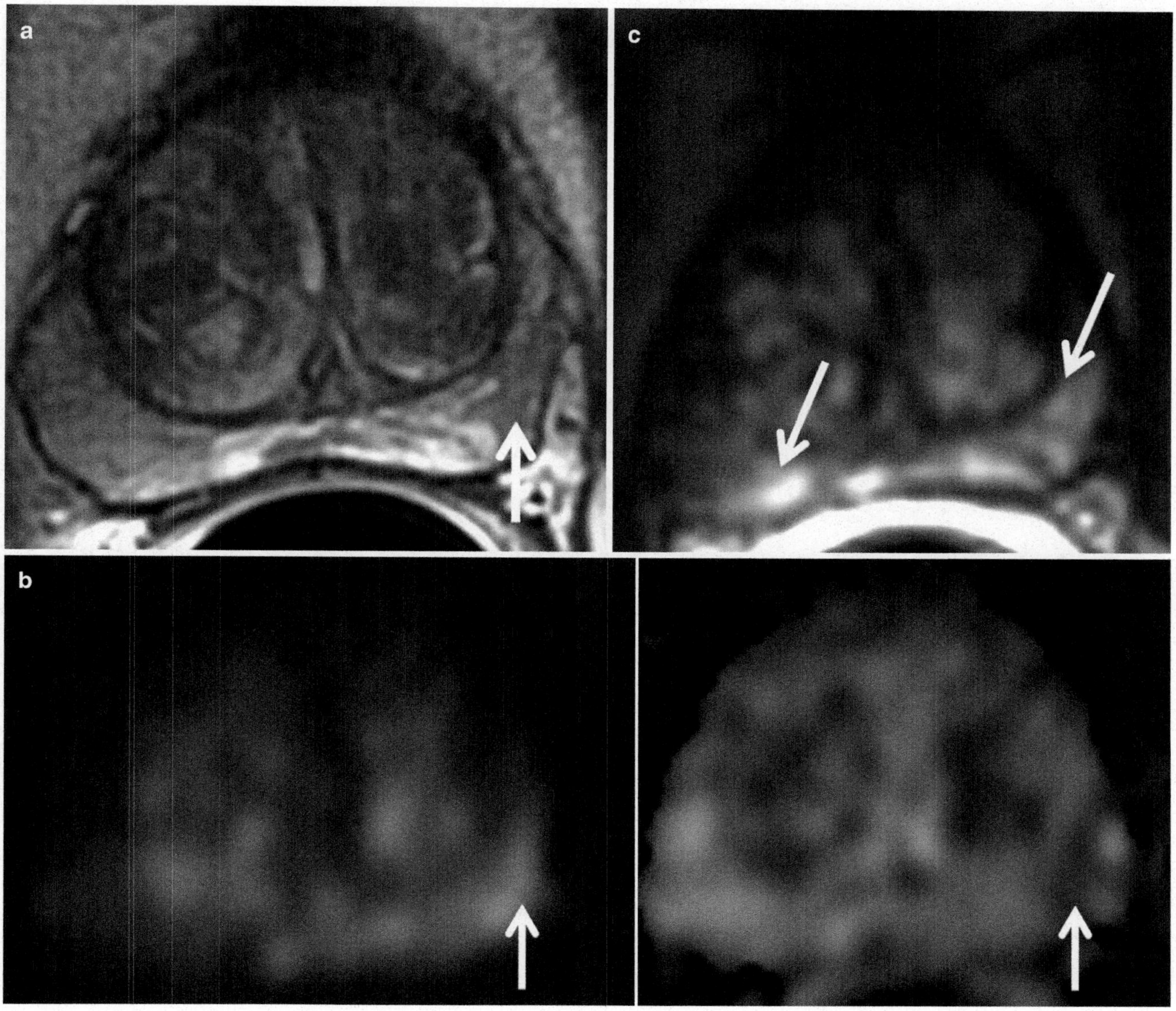

Fig. 4.12 PI-RADS 3. Peripheral zone. (**a**) Axial T2WI, (**b**) b1400DWI and ADC map, and (**c**) dynamic contrast imaging at 10s; shows a mildly focal high signal area on DWI and mildly hypointense on ADC (*arrows*) in the left peripheral zone, corresponding to an intermediate signal intensity on T2WI. These findings correspond to a PI-RADS score of 3. Dynamic contrast imaging (**c**) shows early diffuse uptake of the peripheral zone bilateral (*arrows*), indicating negative contrast assessment and making a final PI-RADS score of 3. The clinical management and work-up of the patient should rely on the clinical factors and whether there is low or high clinical suspicion of prostate cancer to perform a biopsy or clinical follow-up. The target biopsy was negative for prostate cancer

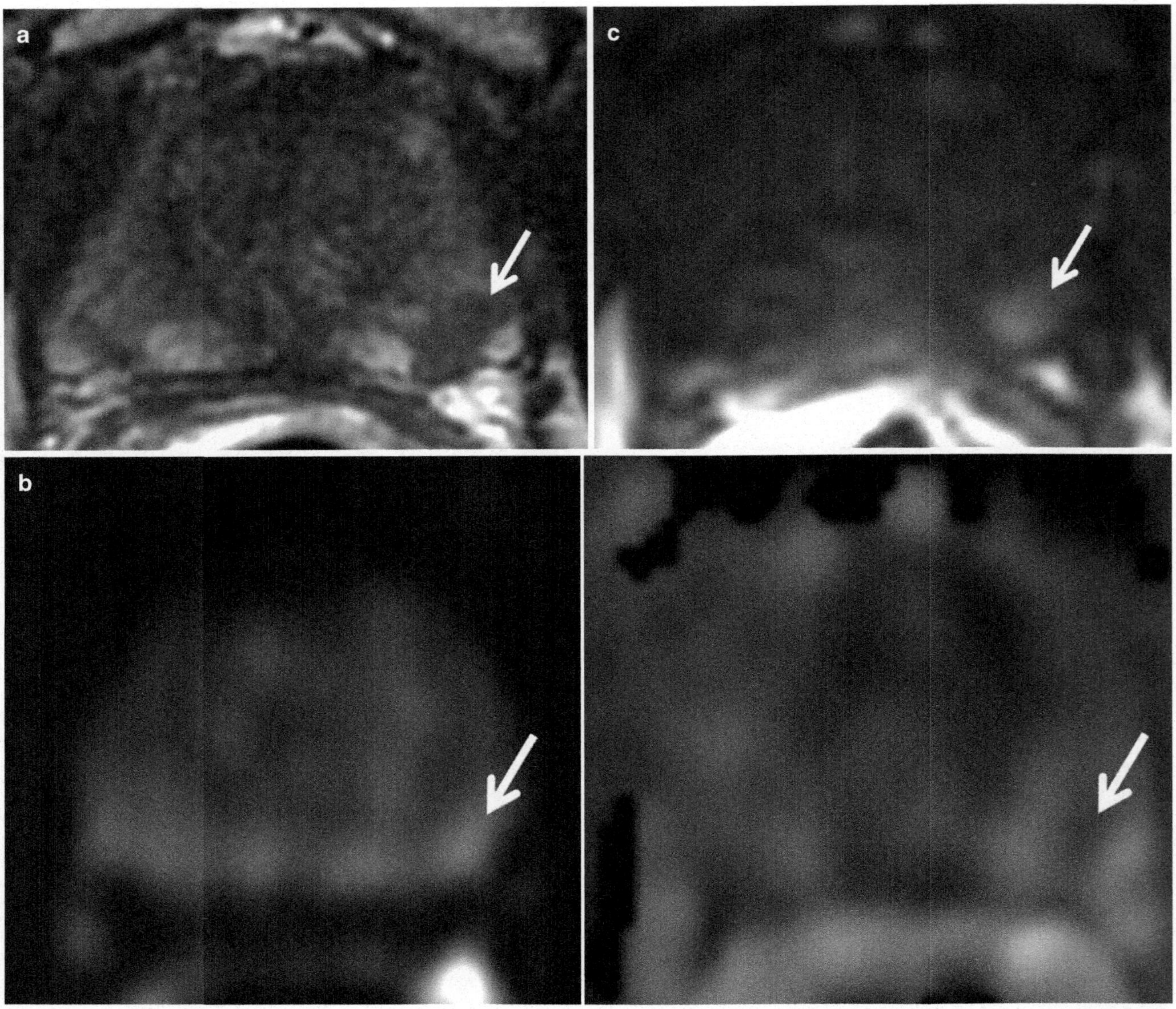

Fig. 4.13 PI-RADS 3. Peripheral zone. (**a**) Axial T2WI, (**b**) b1400DWI and ADC, and (**c**) dynamic contrast imaging at 10 s; shows a mildly focal high signal area on DWI and mildly hypointense on ADC (*arrows*), corresponding to a low signal intensity on T2WI (*arrows*). These findings correspond to a PI-RADS score of 3. Dynamic contrast imaging (**c**) shows early focal uptake at the same location (*arrow*), indicating positive contrast assessment; upgrading a final PI-RADS score of 4. The target biopsy showed inflammatory tissue and negative for prostate cancer

4.7 PI-RADS 3 Transition Zone

The presence of clinically significant cancer is equivocal.

Heterogeneous lesion with obscured margins. Includes others that do not qualify as 2, 4, or 5 (Fig. 4.14). Diffusion restriction plays a role in upgrading what would be a PI-RADS 3 lesion to a PI-RADS 4 lesion in the transition zone whether the DWI score is 5, restricted diffusion >1.5 cm (Fig. 4.1, 4.3, and 4.15).

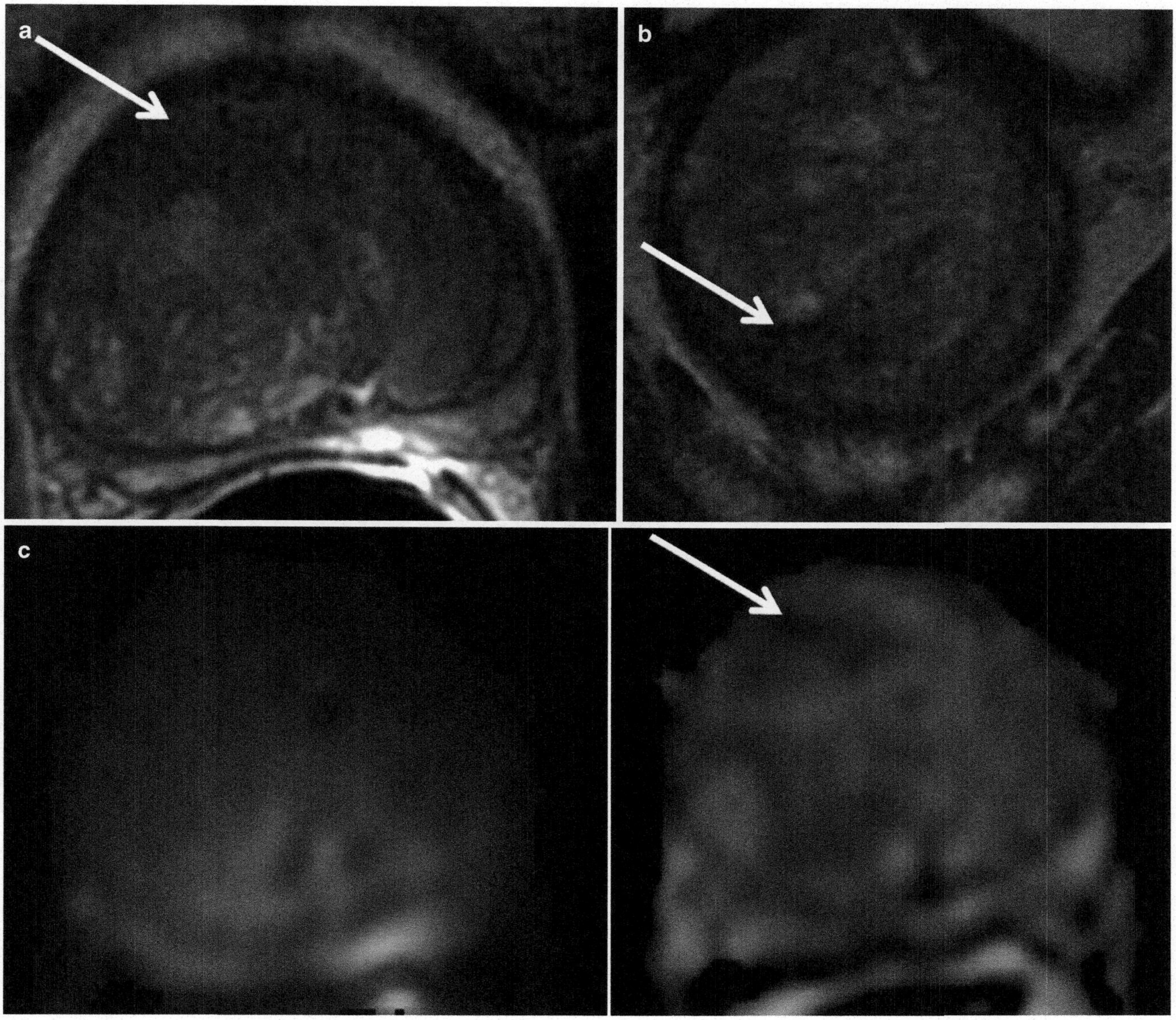

Fig. 4.14 PI-RADS 3. Transition zone. (**a**) Axial, (**b**) coronal T2WI, and (**c**) b1400 DWI and ADC map. There is a heterogeneous low signal intensity area in the right TZ with obscured margins without restriction assigning a PI-RADS score of 3. The DWI score is <4 which assigns a final PI-RADS score of 3. The clinical management and work-up of the patient should rely on the clinical factors and whether there is low or high clinical suspicion of prostate cancer to perform a biopsy or clinical follow-up. The target biopsy was negative for prostate cancer

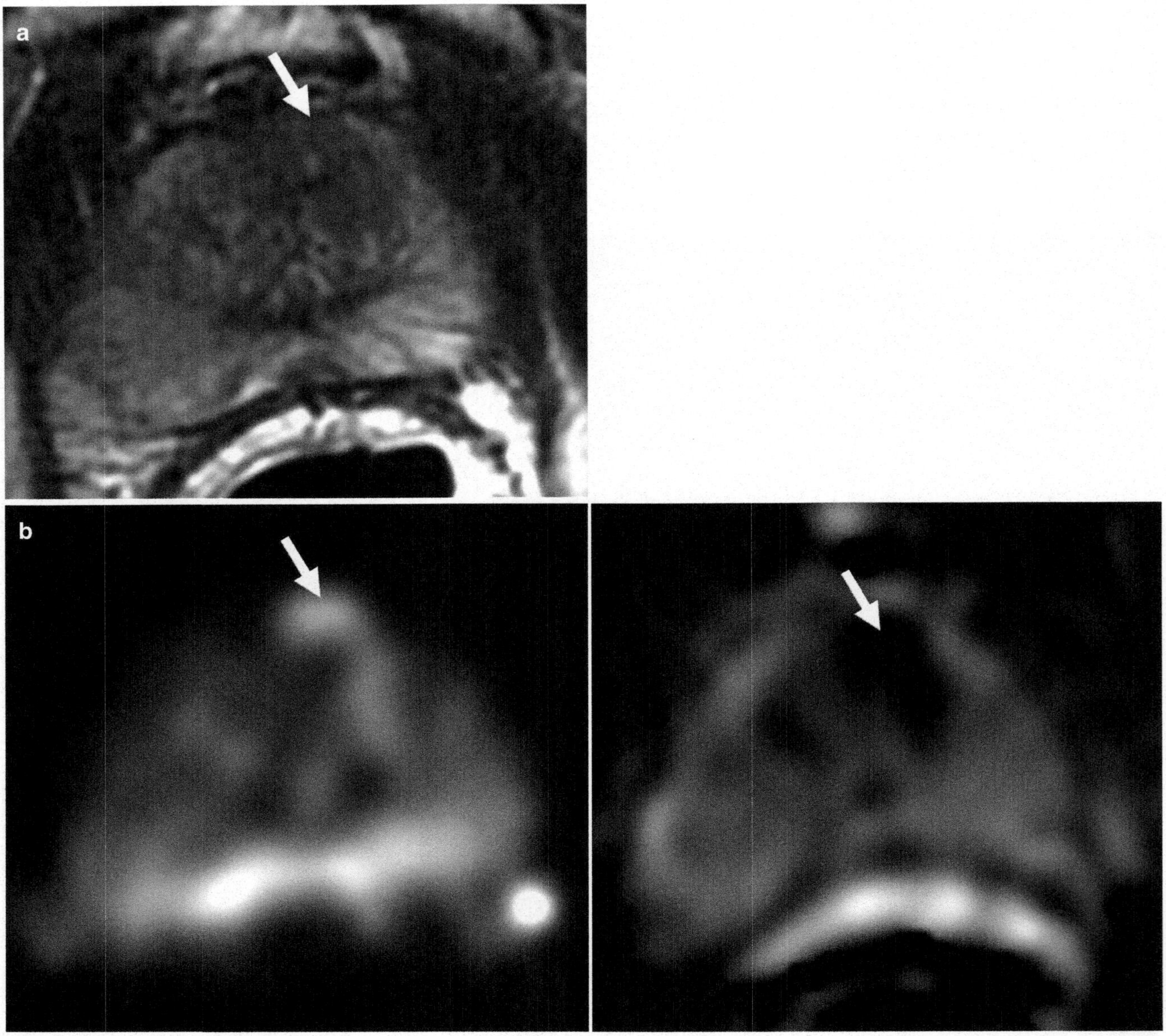

Fig. 4.15 PI-RADS 3. Transition zone. (**a**) Axial T2 WI, (**b**) axial b1400 DWI, and ADC map. There is a heterogeneous signal intensity area in the left anterior TZ with obscured margins (*arrow*) assigning a PI-RADS score of 3. The focal lesion shows high signal on DWI and low signal in ADC with longest diameter of 16 mm consistent with a DWI component score of 5, upgrading the final PI-RADS assessment of 4. A target biopsy was positive for adenocarcinoma Gleason 3 + 4

4.8 PI-RADS 4 Peripheral Zone

Clinically significant cancer is likely to be present.

Marked focal restriction (Fig. 4.16) on high b-value DWI, <1.5 cm in greatest dimension.

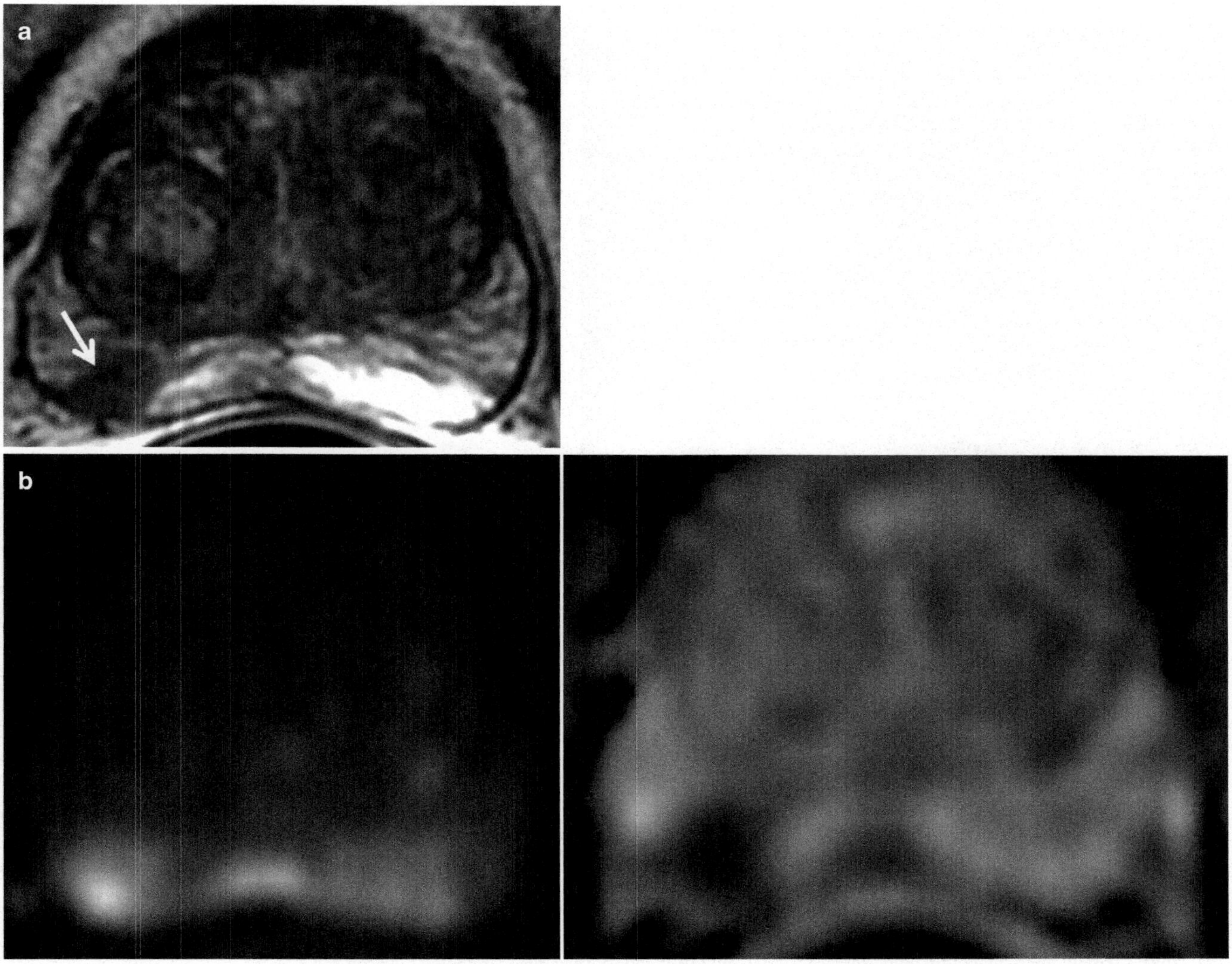

Fig. 4.16 PI-RADS 4. Peripheral zone. (**a**) Axial T2WI and (**b**) b1400 DWI and ADC map, shows focal low signal lesion in the right peripheral zone (*arrow*) on T2WI, with markedly hyperintense signal on DWI and markedly hypointense signal on ADC, < 1.5 cm, assigning a final PI-RADS score of 4. Pathologic diagnosis was adenocarcinoma Gleason 3 + 4

4.9 PI-RADS 5 Peripheral Zone

Clinically significant cancer is highly likely to be present.

Same as PI-RADS 4 but ≥1.5 cm in greatest dimension or definitive extraprostatic extension (Fig. 4.17).

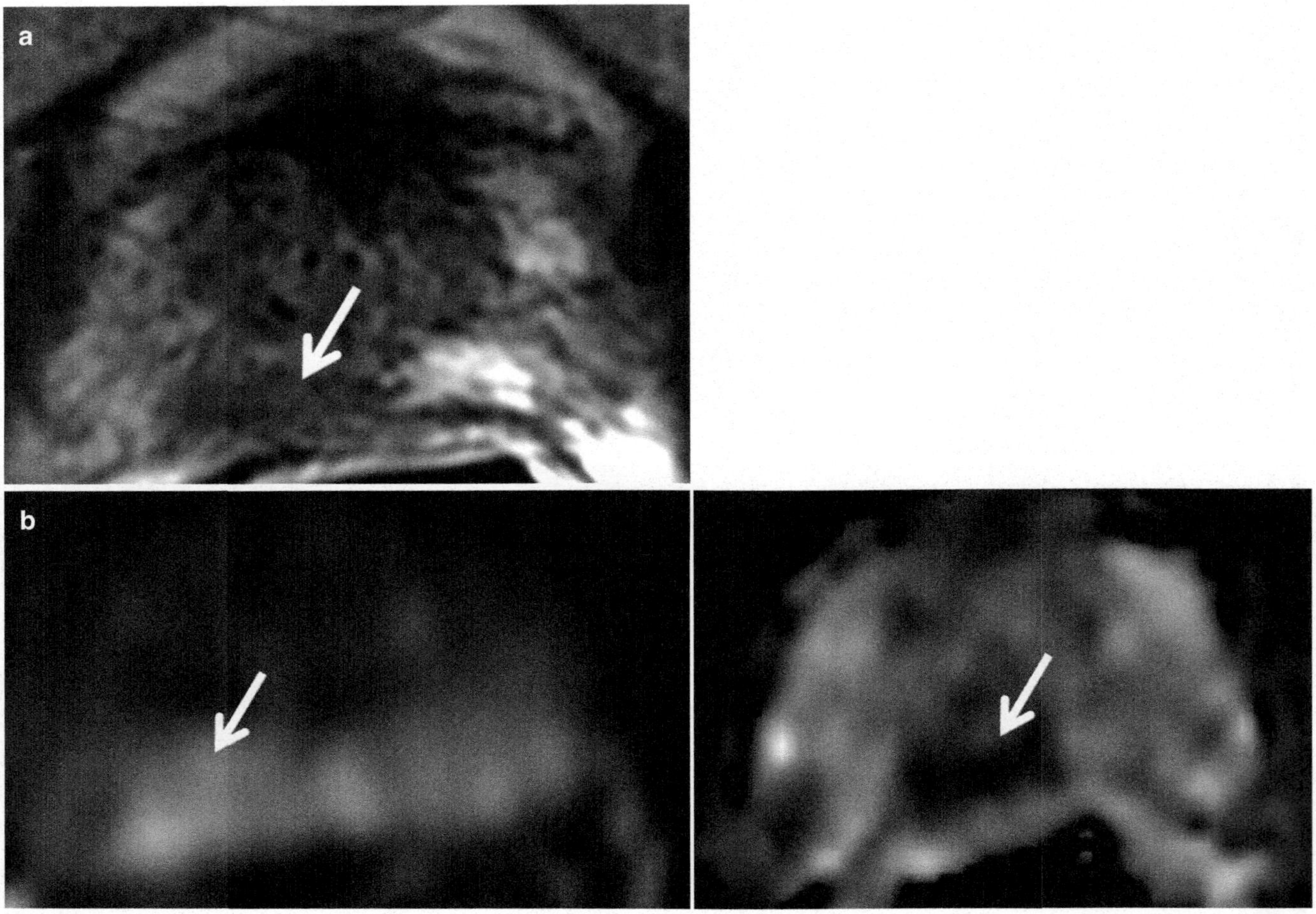

Fig. 4.17 PI-RADS 5. Peripheral zone. (**a**) Axial T2WI and (**b**) b1400 DWI and ADC map, shows focal low signal lesion in the right peripheral zone (*arrow*), with markedly hyperintense signal on DWI and marked hypointense signal on ADC, with features of extraprostatic extension, assigning a final PI-RADS score of 5. Pathologic diagnosis was adenocarcinoma Gleason 4 + 4

4.10 PI-RADS 4 Transition Zone

Clinically significant cancer is likely to be present.

Lenticular or non-circumscribed homogeneous hypointense lesion, and <1.5 cm in greatest dimension (Fig. 4.18).

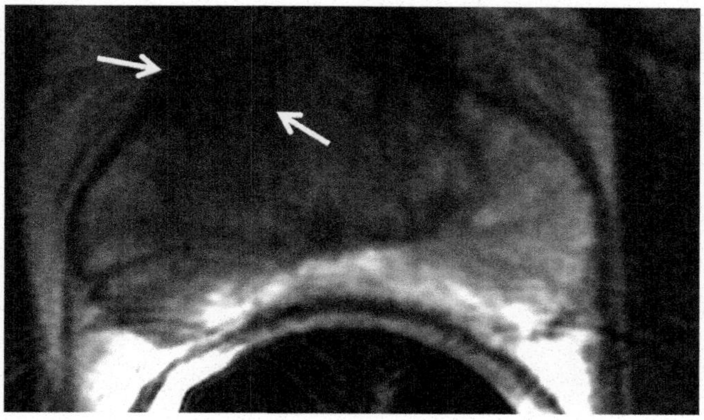

Fig. 4.18 PI-RADS 4. Transition zone. Axial T2WI showing a non-circumscribed homogeneous lesion (*arrows*) on the anterior right TZ <1.5 cm assigning a final PI-RADS score of 4. Pathologic diagnosis was adenocarcinoma Gleason 3 + 4

4.11 PI-RADS 5 Transition Zone

Clinically significant cancer is highly likely to be present.

Same as PI-RADS 4 but ≥1.5 cm in greatest dimension or definitive extraprostatic extension (Fig. 4.19).

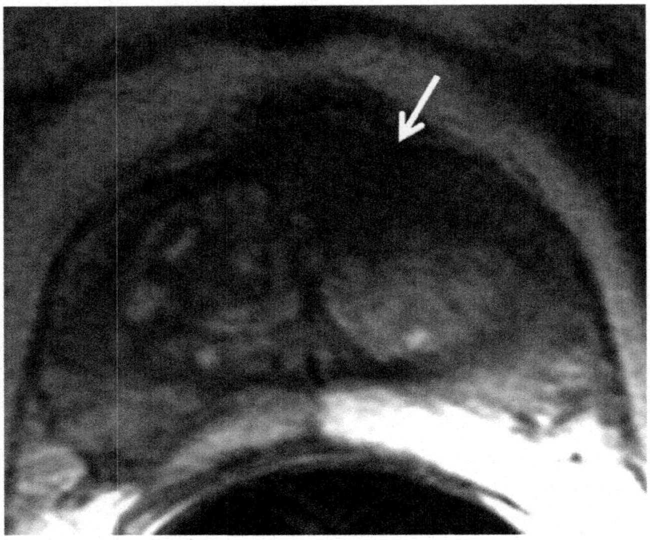

Fig. 4.19 PI-RADS 5. Transition zone. Axial T2WI showing a lenticular non-circumscribed homogeneous lesion (*arrow*) on the anterior left TZ >1.5 cm assigning a final PI-RADS score of 5. Histologic diagnosis was adenocarcinoma Gleason 4 + 3

4.12 Reporting mpMRI

Interpretation of mpMRI and assignment of the PI-RADS overall assessment category is based only on MRI findings [5]. In order to increase the influence and benefit of mpMRI for patient's management, especially to indicate or not biopsy, the results of mpMRI with PI-RADS assessment should always be combined with clinical data like PSA kinetics, family history, DRE findings, and previous biopsy results [6]. Targeted MR biopsy should be considered for PI-RADS assessment category 4 or 5 lesions but not for PI-RADS 1 or 2 [7]. If it is felt that the assessment underestimates the presence of a significant prostate cancer, interpretation quality of the examination should be carefully evaluated. Clinical factors became very important for PI-RADS 3 assessment. If there is low clinical suspicion of significant PCa, then repeat mpMRI in 9–12 months can be considered (Fig. 4.20). On the other hand, if there is high clinical suspicion of significant PCa, a biopsy should be considered (Fig. 4.20).

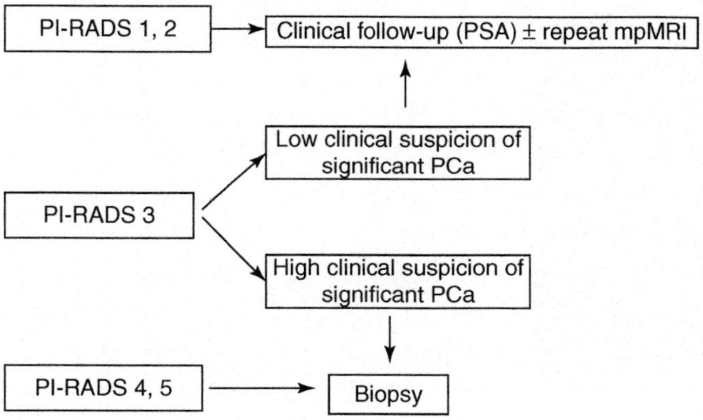

Fig. 4.20 Reasonable management of the outcome for mpMRI assessment category PI-RADS 3, intermediate (the presence of clinically significant cancer is equivocal); should assess the clinical risk of significant cancer to decide whether to perform biopsy or clinical follow-up by PSA and/or mpMRI

The report should include PI-RADS lesion description location-based scoring, indicated on the 39-sector map (Fig. 4.4), lesion measurement, measurement of prostate gland volume (it can be combined with PSA to calculate PSA density), T1WI analysis, extraglandular extension, lymph nodes and bone evaluation, final PI-RADS assessment score (1 to 5) for the likelihood (probability) of clinically significant prostate cancer, and the final conclusion and recommendations (Table 4.3).

Computer-aided evaluation (CAE) technology improves workflow post-process [8] mpMRI analysis (display, analysis, interpretation, reporting, and communication), provides quantification data, and enhances lesion detection and discrimination performance for radiologists (Fig. 4.21). Assignment of the PI-RADS overall assessment category is based on mpMRI findings only (Fig. 4.22). Nevertheless, patient's management should always combine the results of mpMRI with PI-RADS assessment and the clinical factors like serum kinetics, family history, DRE findings, and previous biopsy results (Fig. 4.20) [9, 10].

Table 4.3 PI-RADS v2 structured report

Checklist information to be included on a structured MRI report
– Clinical data: PSA, PSA history, previous biopsy/surgery with its results
– Technical details: sequences, planes, contrast, b value for DWI
– Measurement of the prostate gland and volume: multiplication 3 diameters × 0.52
– Analysis of T1 WI: rule out hemorrhage post-biopsy
– Lesion/s description/s: PI-RADS assessment criteria for T2 and DWI
Mapping: zonal and sector map
Tumor size: specify the plane measured
T2 and DWI score
Extraglandular extension
– Lymph nodes
– Pelvic bones
– PI-RADS assessment: score 1–5 likelihood for presence or absence of clinically significant prostate cancer
– Conclusion and recommendations

a

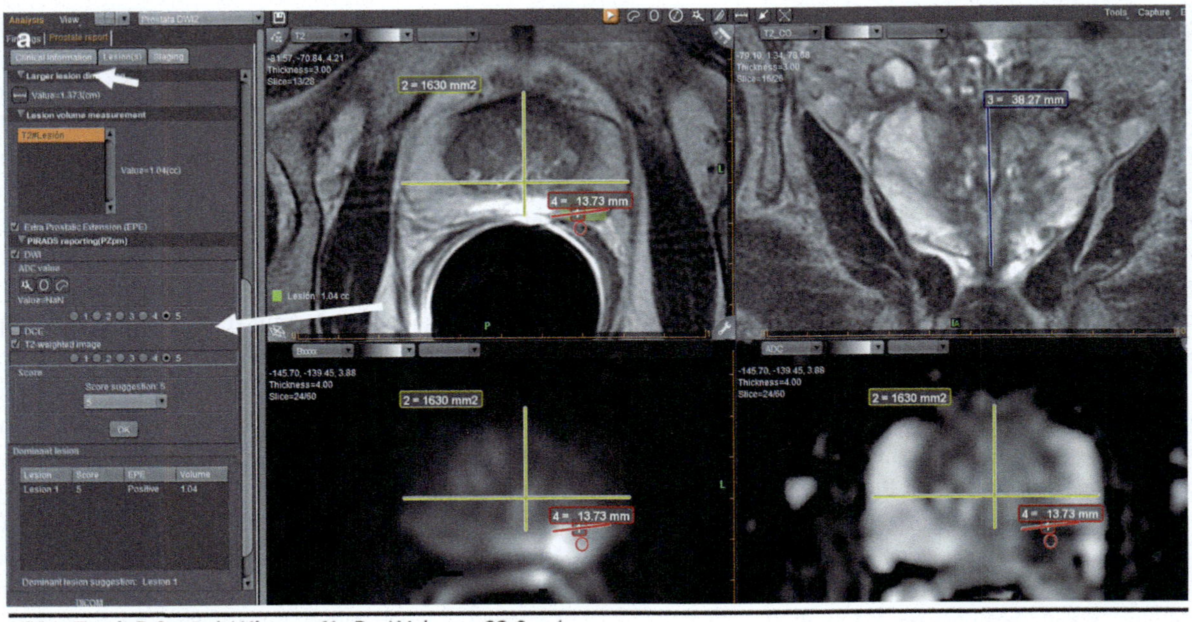

b

PSA: Total: 5.6ng/ml / History: No Bx / Volume: 33.0cc / Density: 0.17ng/mL/cc

Max axial tranverse and height: 16.295cm2
Max sagittal length: 3.827cm
Volume: 32.428cc

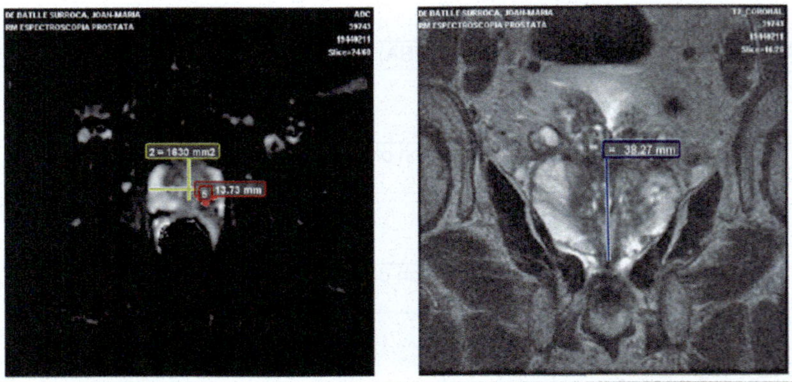

PIRADS

Dominant lesion: Lesion 1

Lesion	Score	EPE	Volume
Lesion 1	5	Positive	1.04

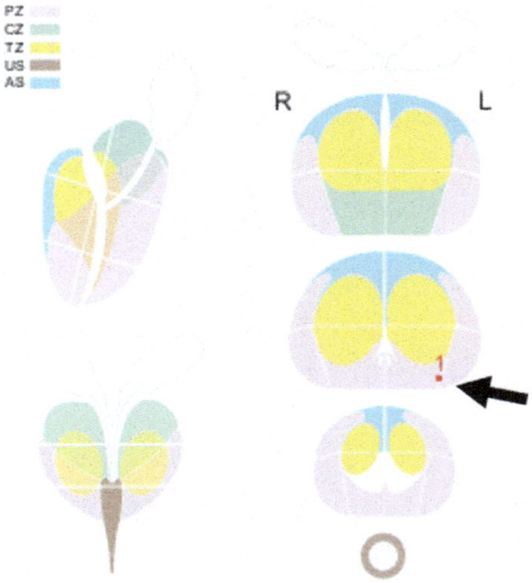

Fig. 4.21 Computer-aided evaluation technology helps to read and analyze mpMRI and perform a standardized report. (**a**) An automatic post-process software can display the significant sequences (T2 and DWI/ADC) on different planes with combined clinical data (*short arrow*) and the mpMRI PI-RADS category assessment according to the DWI and T2 scores (*long arrow*) within the same window. (**b**) All the data and the figures selected can generate automatically a PDF structured report to provide the final PI-RADS category assessment (*long arrow*) within the location according to the sector map (*short arrow*) previously selected

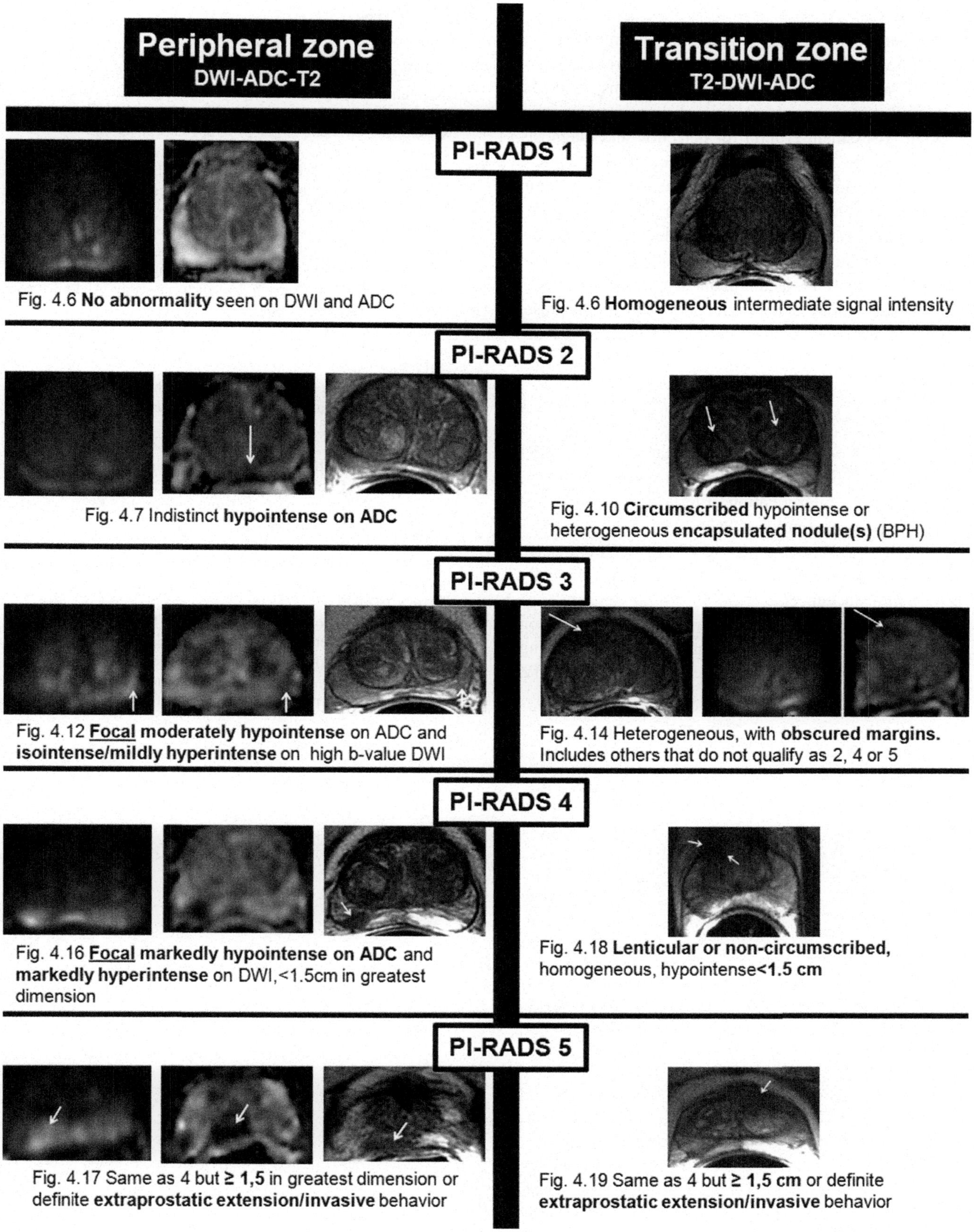

Fig. 4.22 PI-RADS v2 assessment categories for the peripheral and transition zone with the corresponding typical examples for Figs. 4.6, 4.7, 4.10, 4.12, 4.14, 4.16, 4.17, 4.18 and 4.19. The corresponding figure captions of these figures are described in the corresponding same figures shown within the chapter

Conclusion

The current PI-RADS v2 guidelines for mpMRI should be followed considering the information provided on clinical considerations, technical specifications for mpMRI, normal anatomy, and benign findings to perform appropriate assessment criteria for detection and diagnosis of significant PCa. The PI-RADS v2 guidelines are intended for diagnostic evaluation and risk assessment of patients with suspected PCa prior to or after TRUS. PI-RADS v2 assessment uses a final 5-point scale based on the likelihood (probability) that a combination of mpMRI findings on T2W and DWI, as dominant sequences depending on the zonal location of a lesion, correlates with the presence of a clinically significant cancer for each lesion in the prostate gland.

Key Points

- PI-RADS v2 guidelines for prostate cancer mpMRI should be followed to perform an appropriate acquisition and interpretation criteria for detection and diagnosis of significant PCa.
- PI-RADS v2 assessment uses a final 5-point scale based on the likelihood (probability) of a clinically significant cancer.
- PI-RADS combines information in mpMRI on T2W and DWI, as dominant sequences depending on the zonal location of a lesion; T2W for the TZ and DWI for the PZ.

References

1. Prostate MRI: www.esur.org [Internet]. [cited 8 April 2017]. Available at: http://www.esur.org/esur-guidelines/prostate-mri.
2. Weinreb JC, Barentsz JO, Choyke PL, Cornud F, Haider MA, Macura KJ, et al. PI-RADS prostate imaging - reporting and data system: 2015, version 2. Eur Urol. 2016;69(1):16–40.
3. Professionals S-O. Uroweb - European Association of Urology (EAU) [Internet]. Uroweb. 2017 [cited 8 April 2017]. http://uroweb.org/.
4. Barentsz JO, Weinreb JC, Verma S, Thoeny HC, Tempany CM, Shtern F, et al. Synopsis of the PI-RADS v2 guidelines for multiparametric prostate magnetic resonance imaging and recommendations for use. Eur Urol. 2016;69(1):41–9.
5. Horn GL, Hahn PF, Tabatabaei S, Harisinghani M. A practical primer on PI-RADS version 2: a pictorial essay. Abdom Radiol (NY). 2016;41(5):899–906.
6. Vilanova JC, Catalá V. Magnetic resonance imaging in the new paradigm for the diagnosis of prostate cancer. Radiologia. 2017;59(2):94–9.
7. Panebianco V, Barchetti F, Sciarra A, Ciardi A, Indino EL, Papalia R, et al. Multiparametric magnetic resonance imaging vs. standard care in men being evaluated for prostate cancer: a randomized study. Urol Oncol. 2015;33(1):17.e1–7.
8. Lemaître G, Martí R, Freixenet J, Vilanova JC, Walker PM, Meriaudeau F. Computer-Aided Detection and diagnosis for prostate cancer based on mono and multi-parametric MRI: a review. Comput Biol Med. 2015;60:8–31.
9. De Visschere PJL, Briganti A, Fütterer JJ, Ghadjar P, Isbarn H, Massard C, et al. Role of multiparametric magnetic resonance imaging in early detection of prostate cancer. Insights Imaging. 2016;7(2):205–14.
10. Alberts AR, Roobol MJ, Drost F-JH, van Leenders GJ, Bokhorst LP, Bangma CH, et al. Risk-stratification based on magnetic resonance imaging and prostate-specific antigen density may reduce unnecessary follow-up biopsy procedures in men on active surveillance for low-risk prostate cancer. BJU Int. 2017, on line first, in press.

Multiparametric MRI and Prostate Cancer: Pitfalls and Tricks

5

Violeta Catalá, Jonathan Hernández, Ferran Algaba, Oscar Laucirica, and Joan C. Vilanova

Contents

V. Catalá, M.D., Ph.D. (✉) • J. Hernandez, M.D.
Radiology Department, Fundació Puigvert,
Cartagena, 340-350, 08025 Barcelona, Spain
e-mail: vcatala@fundacio-puigvert.es; violetacatala@yahoo.com.ar; jhernandez.md@gmail.com

F. Algaba, M.D., Ph.D.
Pathology Department, Fundació Puigvert,
Carrer Cartagena, 340-350, 08025 Barcelona, Spain
e-mail: falgaba@fundacio-puigvert.es

O. Laucirica, M.D
Urology Department, Sant Joan Despí Moises Broggi Hospital,
Jacinto Verdaguer 90, 08970 Sant Joan Despí, Barcelona, Spain
e-mail: olauciricag@hotmail.com

J.C. Vilanova, M.D., Ph.D.
Radiology Department, Clínica Girona, Institute Catalan of Health-IDI, University of Girona,
Lorenzana 36, 17002 Girona, Spain
e-mail: kvilanova@comg.cat

5.1 Introduction

Prostate cancer (PCa) is the most common cancer in men [1]. Until a few years ago, digital rectal examination, serum prostate-specific antigen (PSA) measurement, and prostate biopsy were the main tools in the diagnosis of PCa. Now, the role of multiparametric MR (mpMR) in the detection of PCa is widely accepted, but it is also recognized that prostate mpMR probably represents one of the most demanding challenges in radiology. The technique has relatively high variability in intra- and interobserver agreement [2], and its learning curve is not easy [3]. At the same time, a wide spectrum of technical MR parameters influence the mpMR evaluation. A major effort has been made to standardize the technical mpMR parameters and the mpMR reading model, as reflected in Prostate Imaging—Reporting and Data System version 2 (PI-RADS v2) [4]. PI-RADS v2 was developed by an international expert committee created by the American College of Radiology (ACR), the European Society of Urogenital Radiology (ESUR), and the AdMeTech Foundation with the aim of updating and improving upon PI-RADS v1. Certainly, the extended use of PI-RADS v2 has facilitated the reading of mpMR and improved the diagnosis of PCa [5]. However, anatomic variants and benign pathologies frequently make radiological evaluation difficult in daily practice [6].

To perform differential diagnosis between PCa and the normal/benign conditions that mimic it, the radiologist needs to have a sound knowledge of prostate anatomy and the most common behavior and imaging appearances of different benign pathologies. Even then, it is sometimes not possible to differentiate malignant from normal/benign conditions using only mpMR. Knowledge of clinical aspects and an interdisciplinary approach can be the key in many cases. In other cases only pathologic analysis can resolve the diagnostic question.

The aim of this chapter is to provide the reader with a succinct overview of potential pitfalls in the diagnosis of PCa and to identify tricks that may be regularly employed to aid differential diagnosis.

J.C. Vilanova et al. (eds.), *Atlas of Multiparametric Prostate MRI*, DOI 10.1007/978-3-319-61786-2_5

5.2 Pitfalls and Tricks

The reader must be alert to potential pitfalls on mpMR in order to avoid mistakes. Table 5.1 shows a classification of such pitfalls in relation to the affected areas.

Table 5.1 Classification of mpMR pitfalls in relation to the affected areas

	Type	Area
Anatomic structures	Anterior fibromuscular stroma	Anterior zone
	Central zone	Prostatic base Posterior middle peripheral zone
	Surgical capsule	Area between transition and peripheral zone
	Periprostatic veins	Peripheral zone, frequently at the apex
Benign pathology	Stromal nodule of benign prostatic hyperplasia (SBPH nodule)	Transition zone and occasionally the peripheral zone
	Acute and chronic nonspecific prostatitis	Peripheral zone is more frequently affected, but adjacent transition zone may be involved
	Granulomatous prostatitis	
	Atrophy	Peripheral zone
Other	Hemorrhage	Peripheral or transition zone

5.2.1 Anatomic Structures

5.2.1.1 Anterior Fibromuscular Stroma

Anterior fibromuscular stroma (AFMS) is a dense fibrotic band without glandular elements located anterior to the transition zone that extends from the base to the apex of the prostate. It is anterior and anterolateral to the surface of the glandular prostate. Skeletal muscle fibers of the urogenital diaphragm are intertwined at the apex of the AFMS, whereas the smooth muscle fibers of the detrusor are fused at the base of that zone. This anatomic area must be recognized and must be distinguished from PCa (Table 5.2; Figs. 5.1 and 5.2).

Table 5.2 Multiparametric MR appearance of AFMS and key points to differentiate it from prostate cancer

mpMR sequences	Appearance	Tips and tricks
T2WI	Marked and homogeneous low signal (Fig. 5.1a) [7]	AFMS is usually symmetric with a regular margin (Fig. 5.1a) and more prominent in relatively young patients without significant benign prostatic hypertrophy
ADC	Hypointense signal may be present (Fig. 5.1b) [7]	
DWI	Isointense signal	PCa usually shows high signal (Fig. 5.2)
DCE	AFMS usually shows type 1 enhancement pattern (progressive enhancement) (Fig. 5.1d) [8]	PCa usually shows type 3 enhancement pattern (early enhancement and washout)

AFMS anterior fibromuscular stroma, *T2WI* T2-weighted image, *ADC* apparent diffusion coefficient, *DWI* diffusion-weighted imaging, *DCE* dynamic contrast enhancement, *PCa* prostate cancer

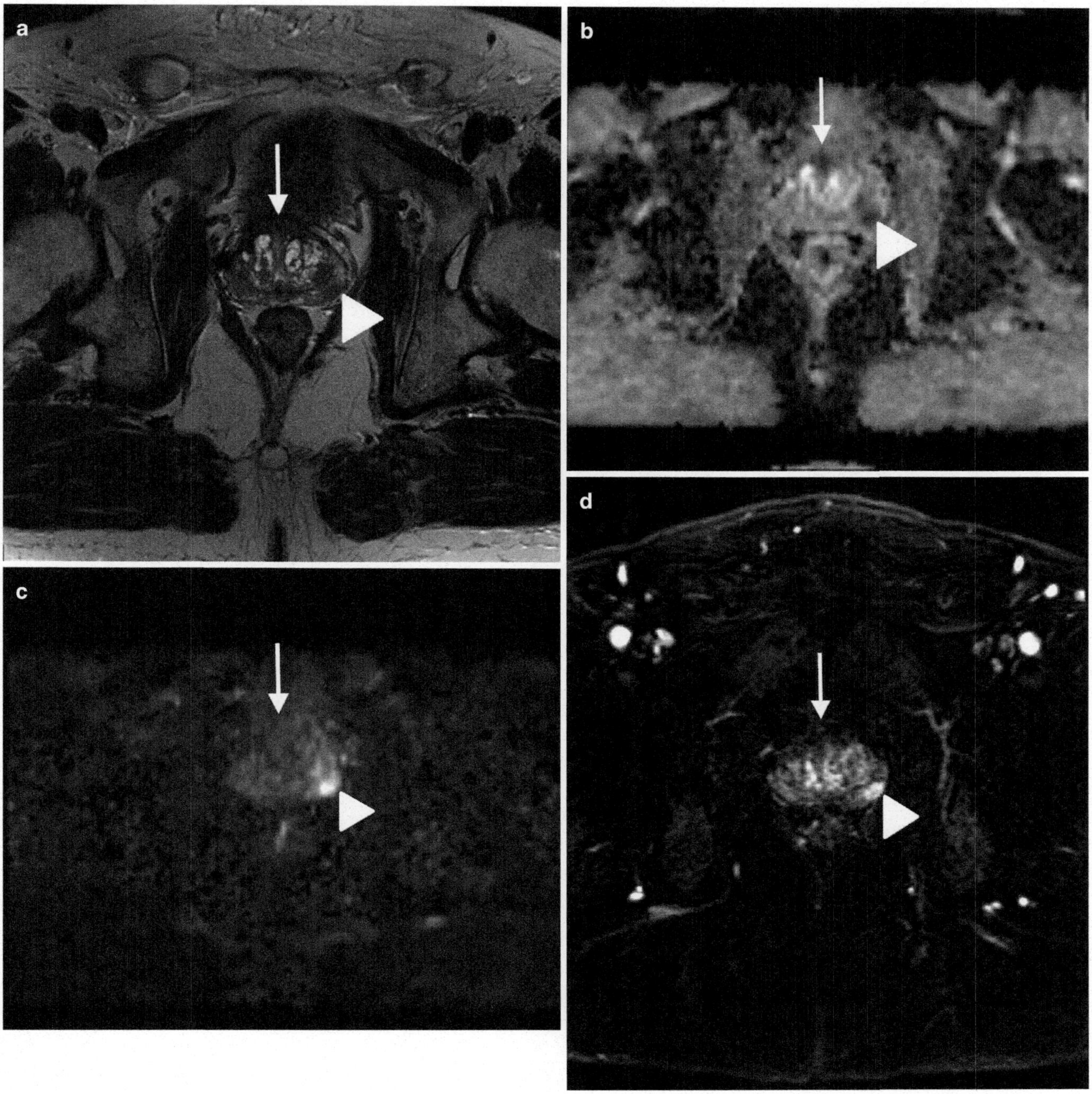

Fig. 5.1 Example of anterior fibromuscular stroma. (**a**) Axial T2-weighted image of the prostate at the midgland shows a hypointense area in the anterior parenchyma (*white arrow*). ADC map at the same level shows hypointensity (**b**) without hyperintensity in DW images (**c**) and no early enhancement after the administration of gadolinium (**d**). *White arrowhead* on (**a**–**d**) shows a left peripheral zone PI-RADS 4 lesion. (**e**) Surgical specimen correlating with axial MR images, showing area of anterior fibromuscular stroma (*black arrow*). *Dotted line* shows PCa correlating with mpMR findings

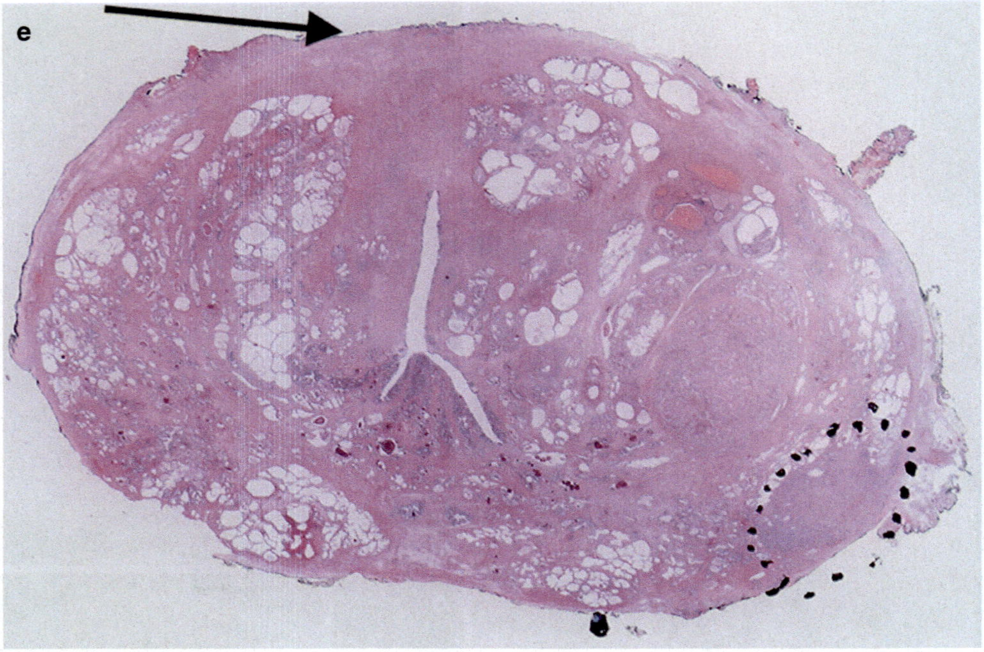

Fig. 5.1 (continued)

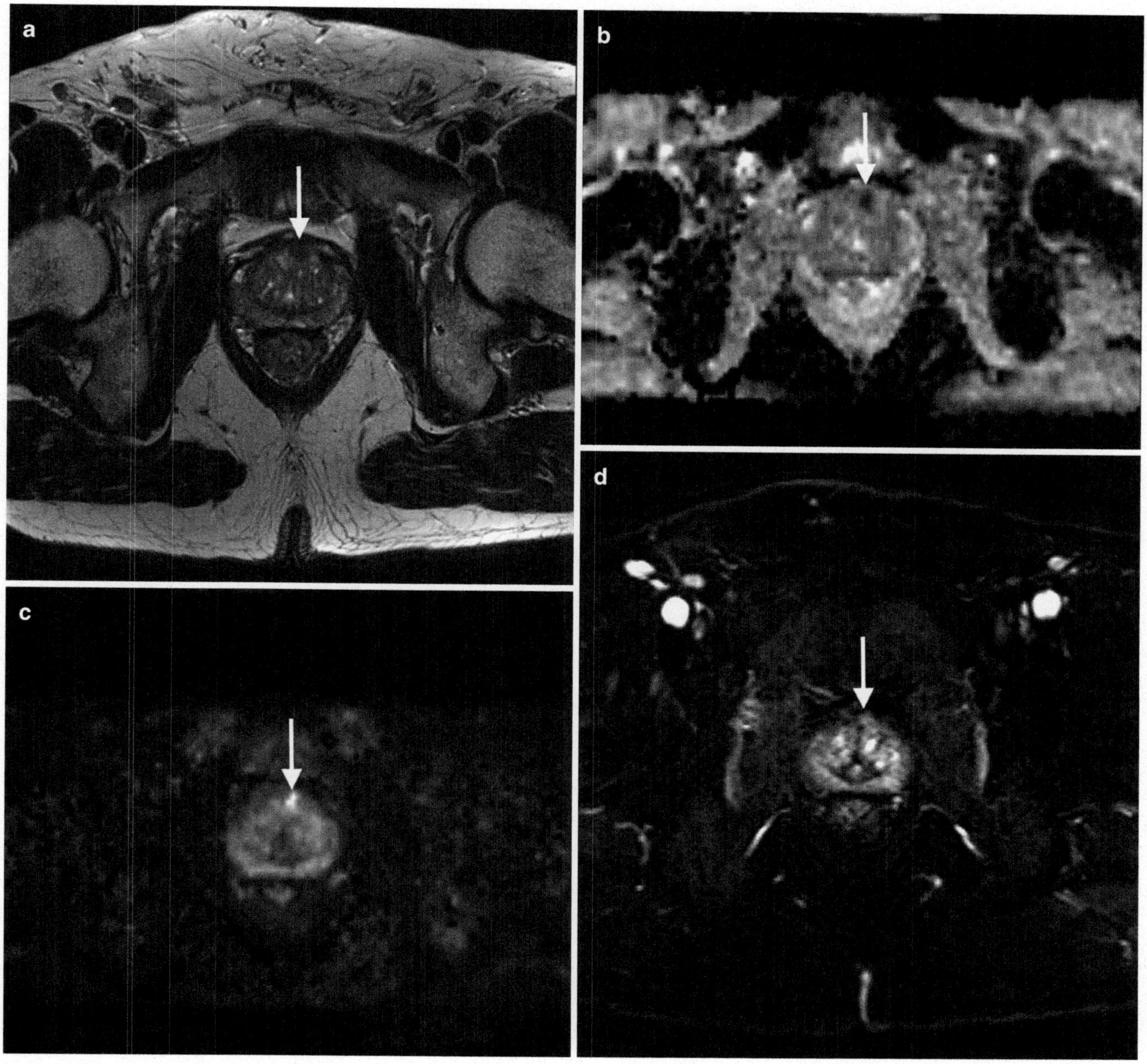

Fig. 5.2 PCa as an anterior fibromuscular stroma potential pitfall. (**a**) Axial T2-weighted image of the prostate at the midgland shows a subcentimetric, asymmetric, and hypointense nodular image in the most anterior part of the left prostatic lobe (*white arrow*). It has a marked diffusion restriction in ADC map (**b**) and DWI (**c**) and and shows slight early enhancement in DCE images (**d**). (**e**) Surgical specimen showed PCa in the anterior left prostatic lobe with extension to anterior fibromuscular stroma (Gleason 4 + 3, pT2c) (*black arrow*)

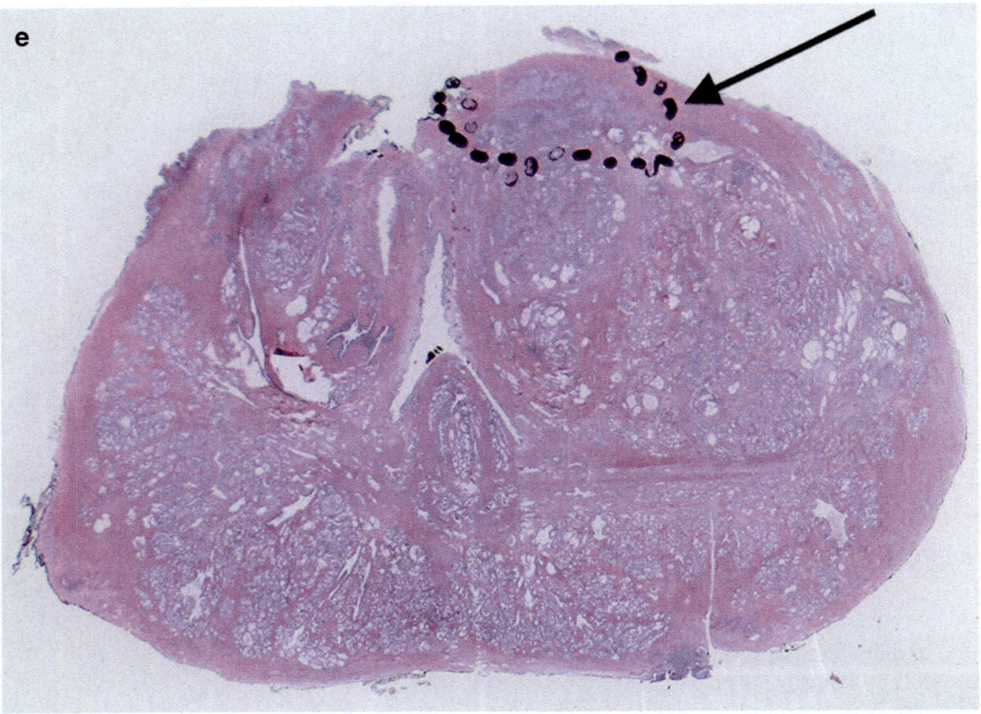

Fig. 5.2 (continued)

5.2.1.2 Central Zone

The central zone is defined anatomically as the region of the prostate surrounding the ejaculatory ducts from the prostatic base to the verumontanum (Fig. 5.3) [9]. Histological features suggest that the central zone is a derivative of the Wolffian duct, whereas the rest of the gland derives from the urogenital sinus [10]. Probably its particular histological characteristics, such as Roman bridge architecture, larger glands than those of the peripheral zone, intraglandular lacunae, and dense stroma, can explain its appearances on mpMR evaluation. Sound knowledge of central zone anatomy is the key to avoidance of diagnostic errors (Table 5.3, Fig. 5.3). PCa can involve the central zone (7% of cases) [11]. It is important to recognize such cases particularly because they are usually aggressive (higher Gleason score, extracapsular extension, and seminal vesicle invasion are more frequent) [11] (Fig. 5.6).

Table 5.3 Multiparametric MR appearance of central zone and key points to differentiate it from prostate cancer

mpMR sequences	Appearance	Tips and tricks
T2WI	The central zone can be seen as a hypointense area in the median posterior zone in the middle third of the gland (Fig. 5.3i, j) The central zone can be seen as a homogeneously hypointense area at the base of the prostate (mustache sign) (Fig. 5.4a)	The central zone has a conical shape with an usually well-defined margin (larger diameter at the base; smaller diameter at the verumontanum, like inverted tear). The coronal plane is useful to demonstrate this morphology (Figs. 5.3b and 5.5c)
		Frequently, the central zone is only seen at the base of the gland: it is visible throughout its length in 34–54% of cases [11] (Fig. 5.4b)
		The central zone is usually symmetric (80% of the cases) (Fig. 5.4), but asymmetry can be found (Fig. 5.5)
ADC	Hypointense signal in the areas mentioned above (Figs. 5.4c and 5.5b)	
DWI	Hyperintense signal in high b values in the areas mentioned above	
DCE	Associated with type 1 (progressive) and type 2 curve (early enhancement and plateau) rather than type 3 [12] (early enhancement and washout), which occasionally can be seen	PCa is more frequently associated with type 3 curve

T2WI T2-weighted image, *ADC* apparent diffusion coefficient, *DWI* diffusion-weighted imaging, *DCE* dynamic contrast enhancement

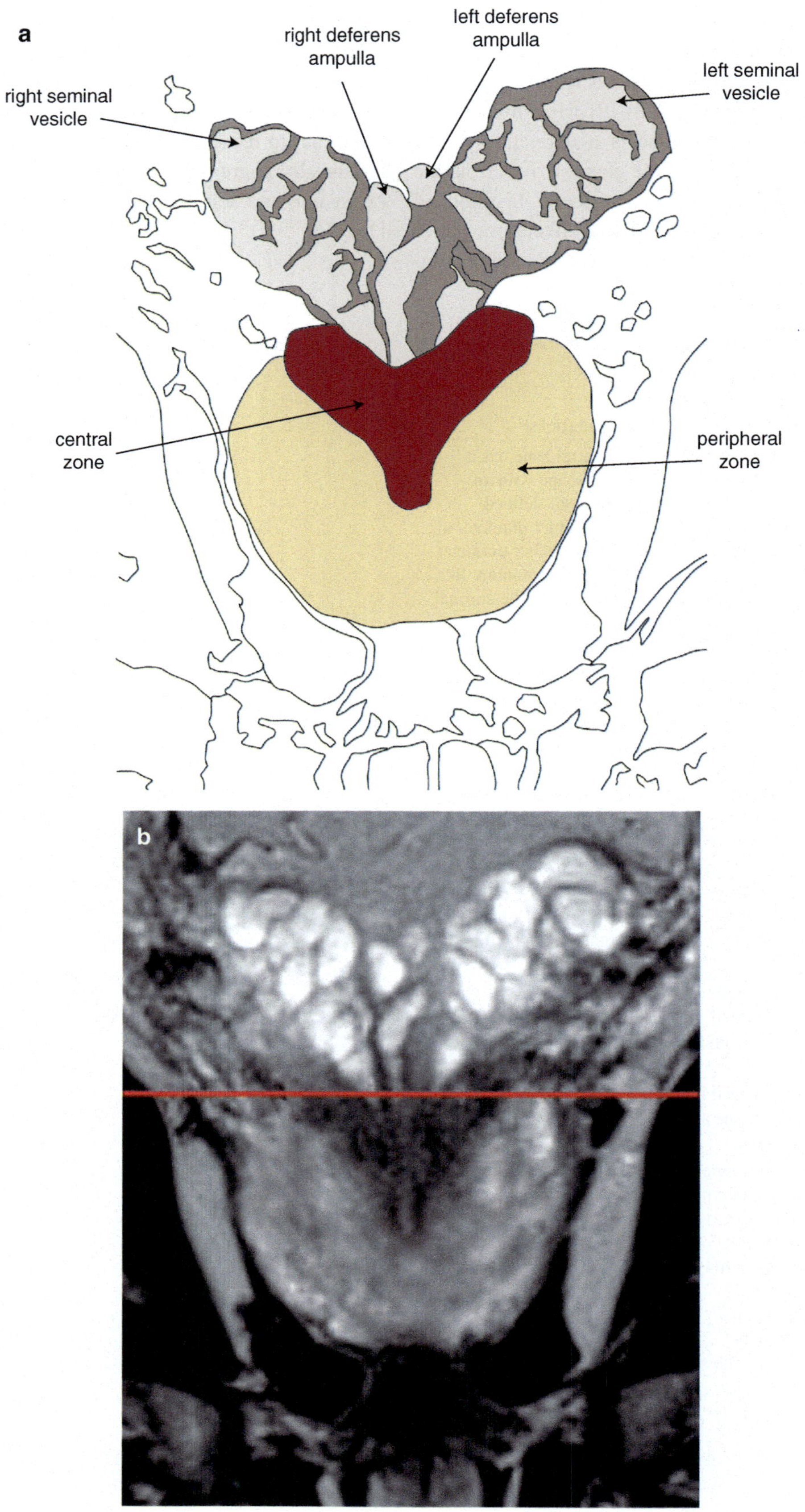

Fig. 5.3 Graphic representation of the central zone at different levels. (**a**) Coronal prostate graphic representation correlating with (**b**) coronal T2-weighted image. (**c**, **f**, and **i**) are axial T2-weighted images of the prostate and the central zone with its corresponding graphic representations in (**d**, **g**, and **j**) at the different levels depicted in (**b**, **e**, and **h**), respectively

c

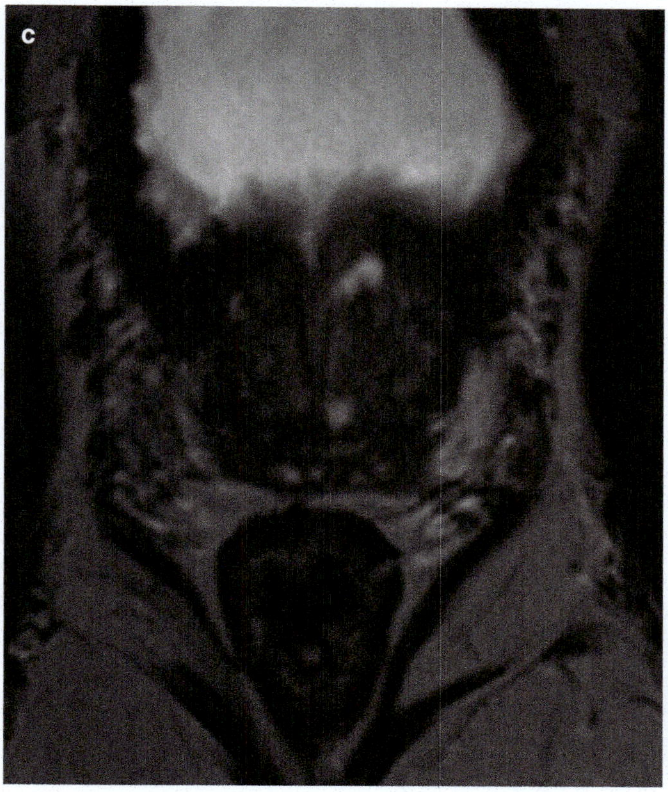

d

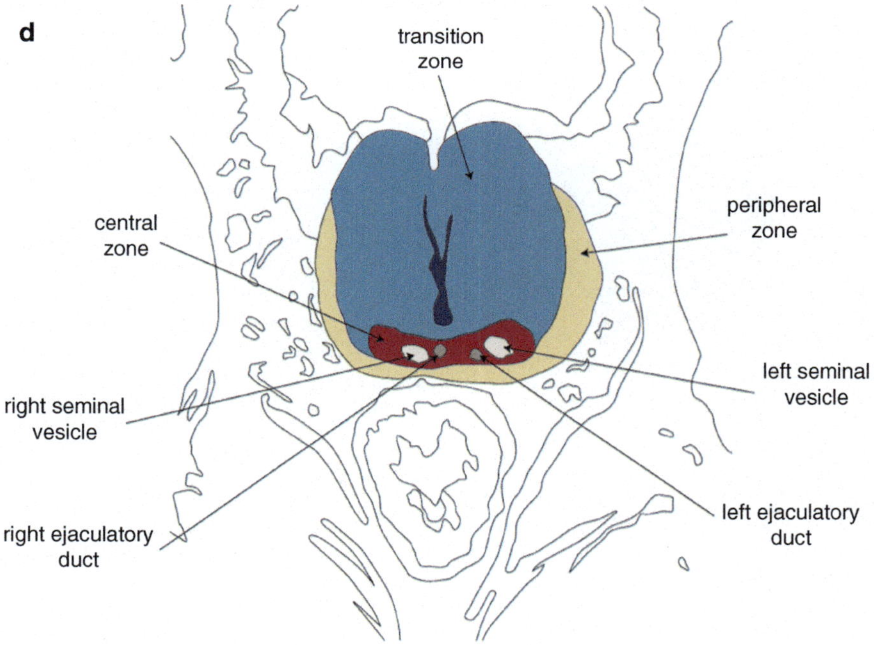

Fig. 5.3 (continued)

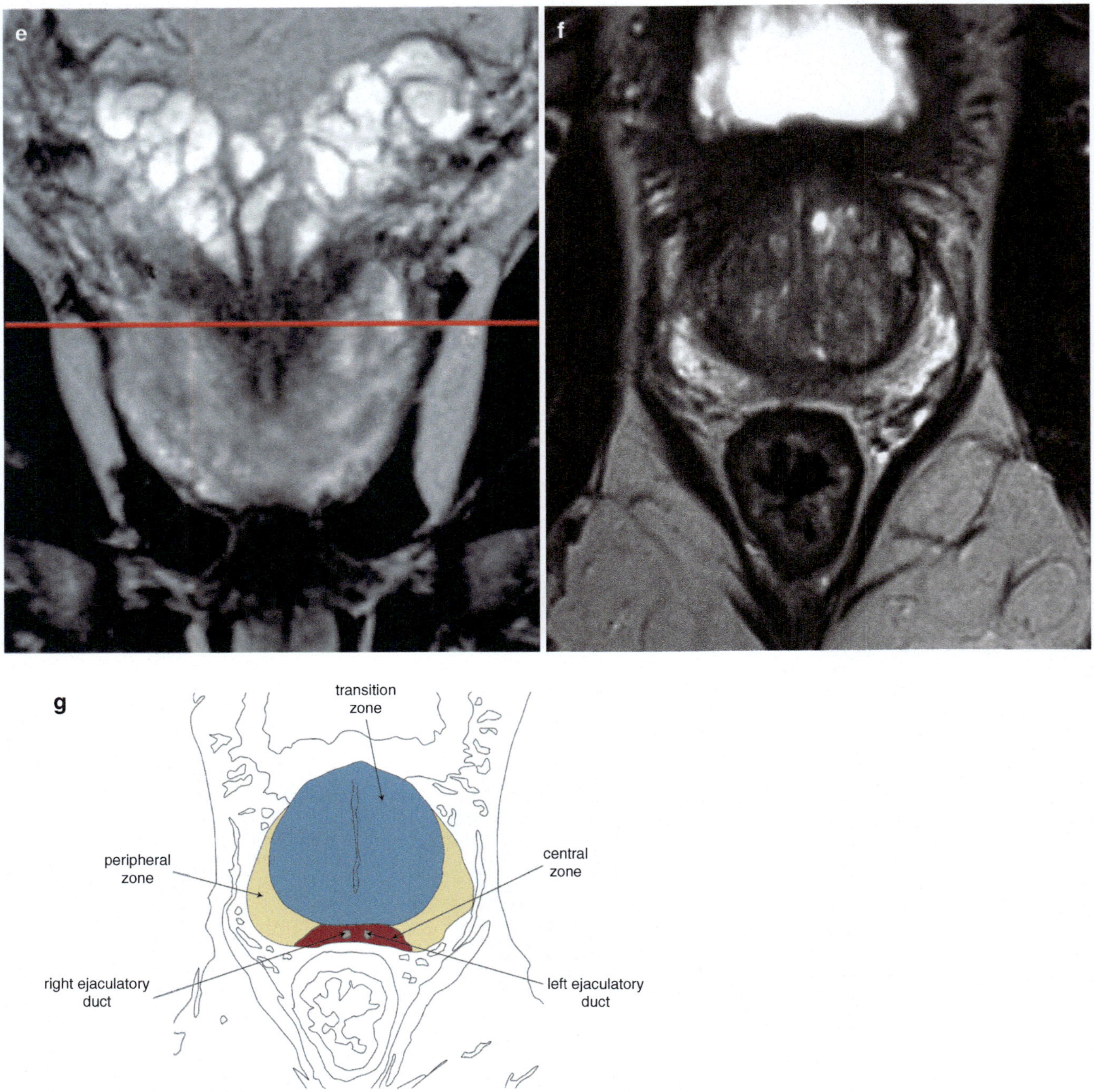

Fig. 5.3 (continued)

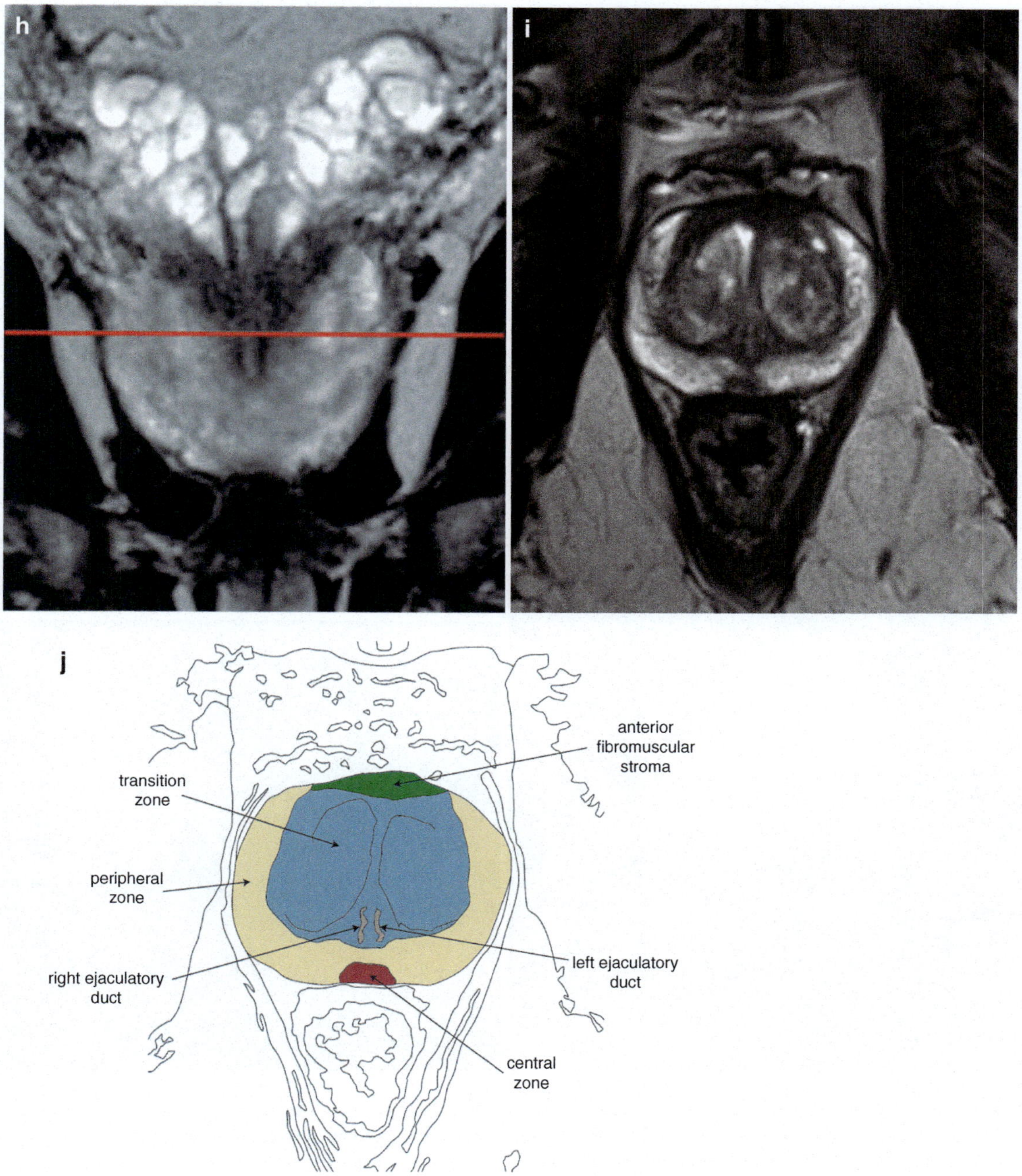

Fig. 5.3 (continued)

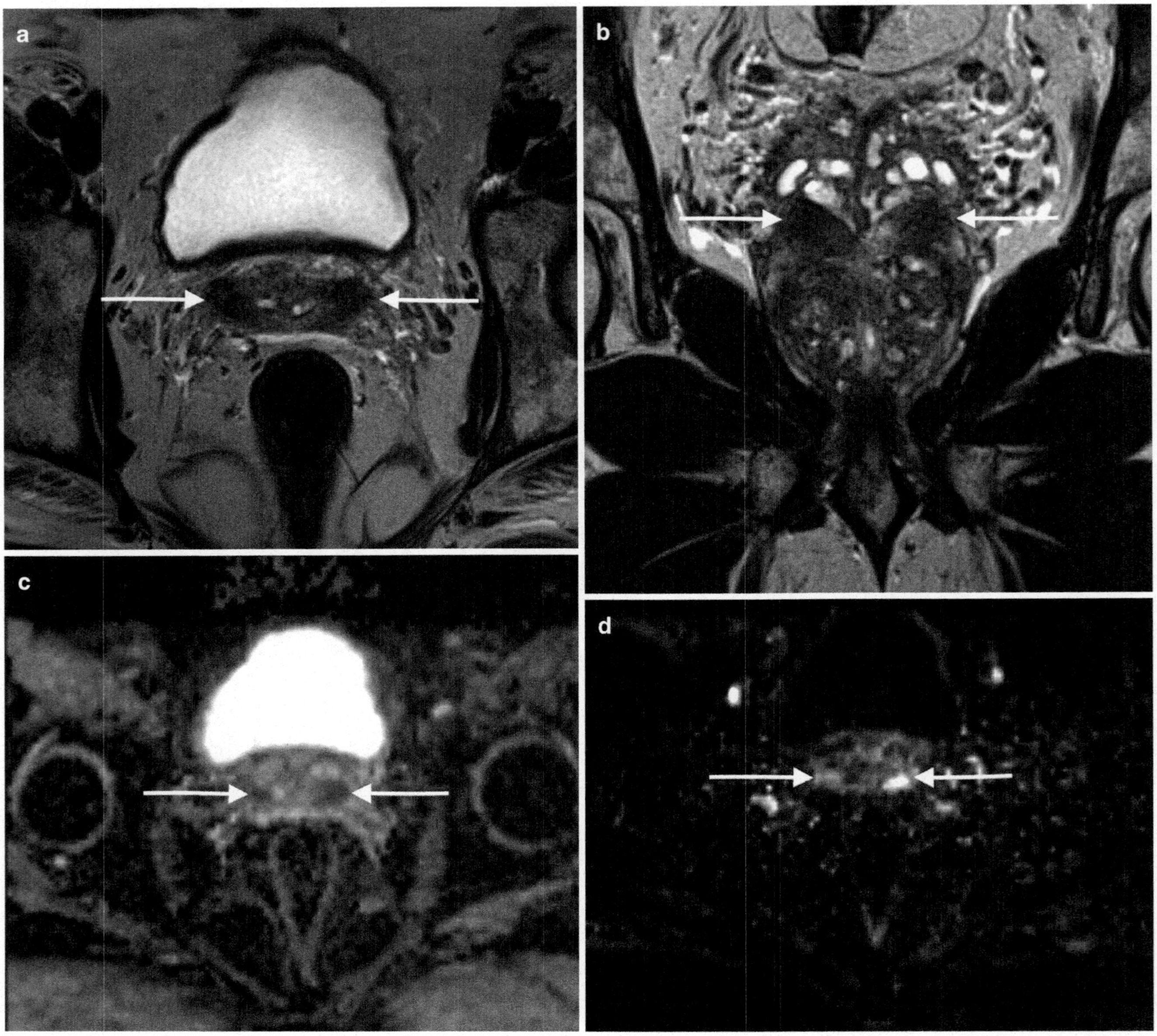

Fig. 5.4 Central zone of the prostate. (**a**) Axial T2-weighted image of the prostate at the base shows a bilateral and symmetric hypointense area lateral to both ejaculatory ducts, a finding also seen on the coronal T2-weighted images (**b**) (*white arrows*). (**c**) ADC map and (**d**) DCE axial images show discrete hypointensity and early enhancement, respectively (*white arrows*)

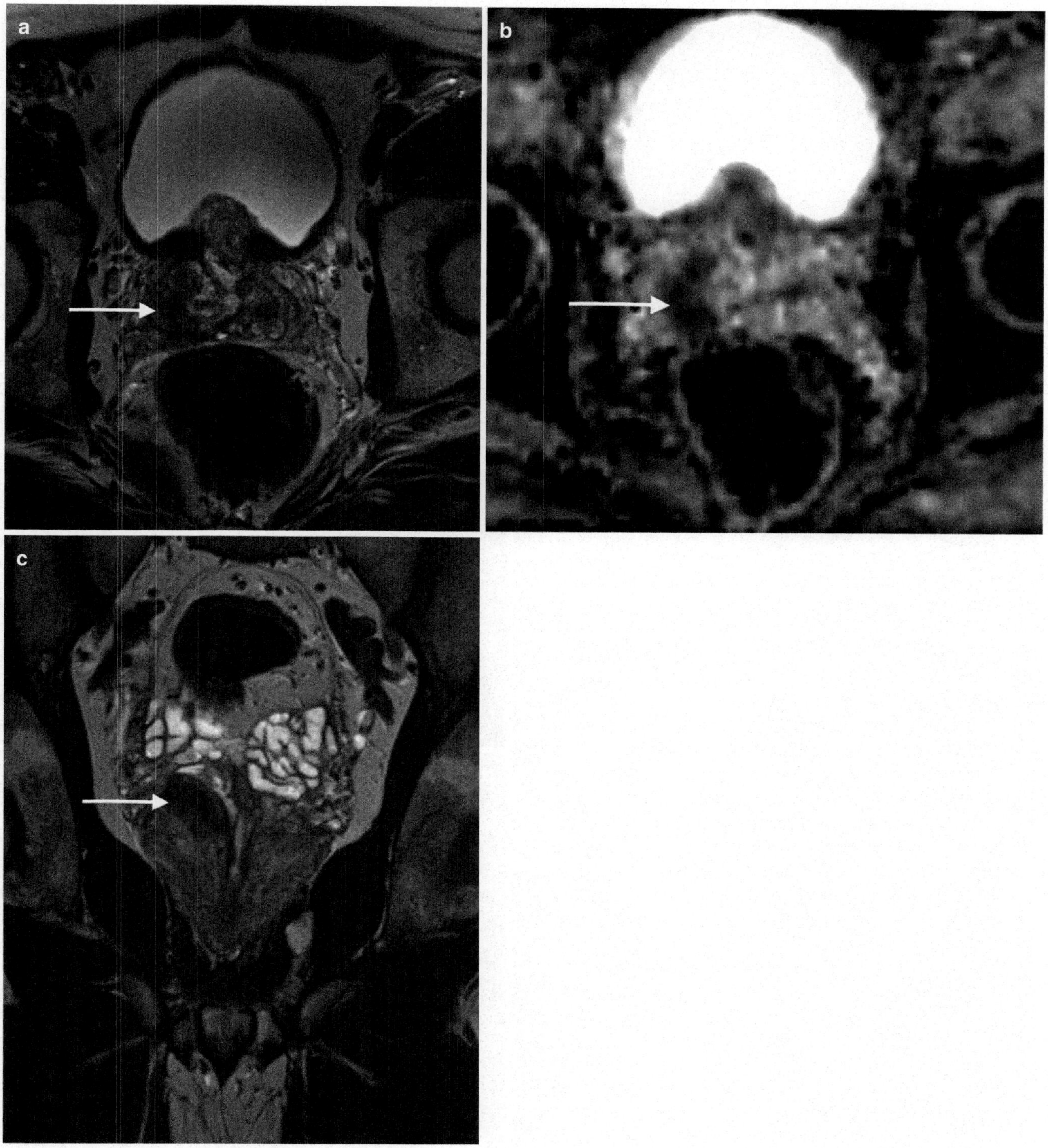

Fig. 5.5 Asymmetric central zone. (**a**) Axial T2-weighted image of the prostate at the base shows a hypointense area only in the right lobe (*white arrow*), with hypointensity on ADC map (**b**). (**c**) Coronal T2-weighted image of the prostate depicts the referred zone in the right lobe, with no similar image on the left lobe. This lesion was reported as PI-RADS 5. Surgical specimen of prostatectomy after demonstration of PCa in systematic biopsy (left lobe) showed this area to be an asymmetric central zone

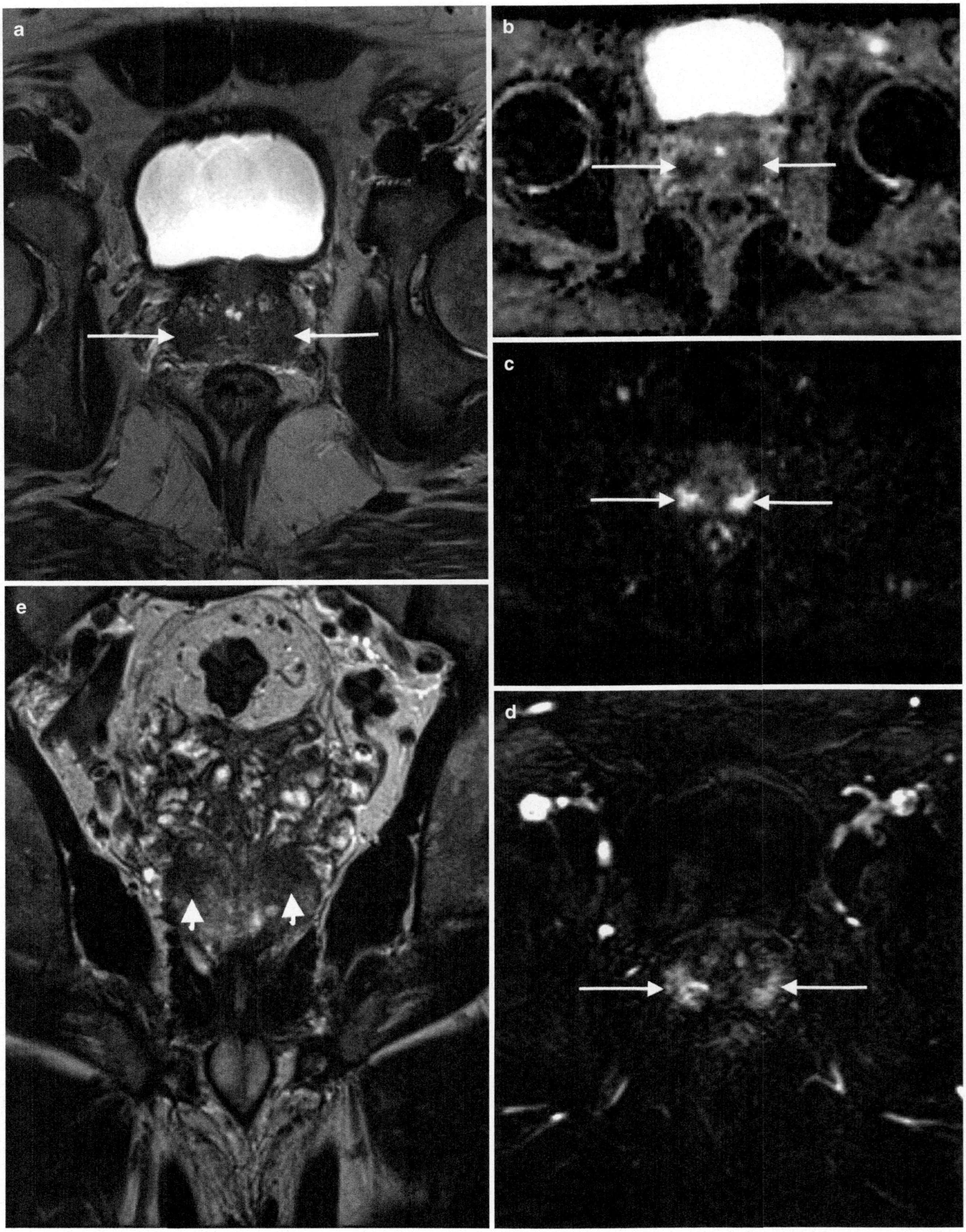

Fig. 5.6 PCa as a potential central zone pitfall. (**a**) Axial T2-weighted image at the base of the prostate shows a bilateral and symmetric oval area located lateral to both ejaculatory ducts (*arrows*). It has a significant restriction of the diffusion in ADC map (**b**) and DWI (**c**), with early enhancement after the administration of gadolinium (**d**), with a mustache-like disposition. However, in a coronal T2 reconstruction (**e**) it is seen slightly asymmetric, with a more lateral location of the right central zone, a finding that should alert the radiologist for the possibility of PCa (*white arrowheads*). (**f**) Surgical specimen confirmed a PCa Gleason 4 + 3 (*black arrows*)

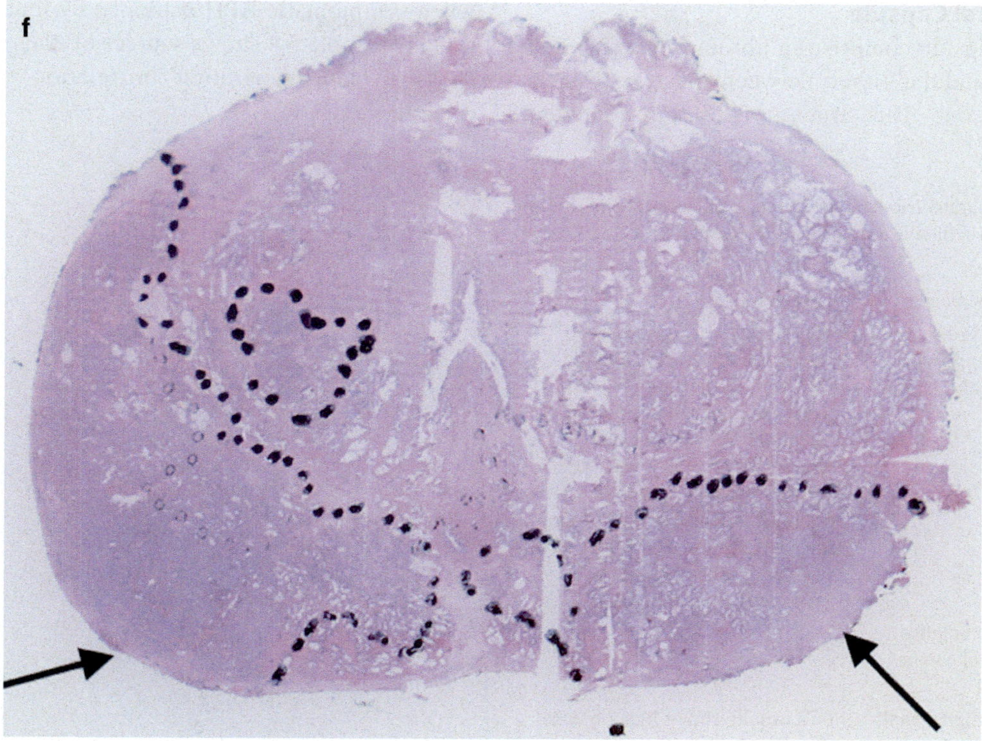

Fig. 5.6 (continued)

5.2.1.3 Surgical Capsule

The surgical capsule comprises a fibromuscular band and compressed glandular tissue between the transition and the peripheral zone. This structure is used as a landmark when symptomatic BPH is treated by transurethral resection [13]. Table 5.4 shows sources of diagnostic errors and tricks to aid recognition in relation to the surgical capsule.

Table 5.4 Multiparametric MR appearance of surgical capsule and key points to differentiate it from prostate cancer

mpMR sequences	Appearance	Tips and tricks
T2WI	Markedly hypointense signal	The surgical capsule is placed between the transition and the peripheral zone, and it has a band-like rather than a nodular morphology. Correlation of appearances on the axial and coronal planes is useful to establish the morphology of the surgical capsule (Fig. 5.7) The surgical capsule can be asymmetric in some cases
ADC	Hypointense signal can be seen	
DWI	No high signal	PCa usually shows hyperintense signal
DCE	Negative	PCa usually shows contrast enhancement

T2WI T2-weighted image, *ADC* apparent diffusion coefficient, *DWI* diffusion-weighted imaging, *DCE* dynamic contrast enhancement, *PCa* prostate cancer

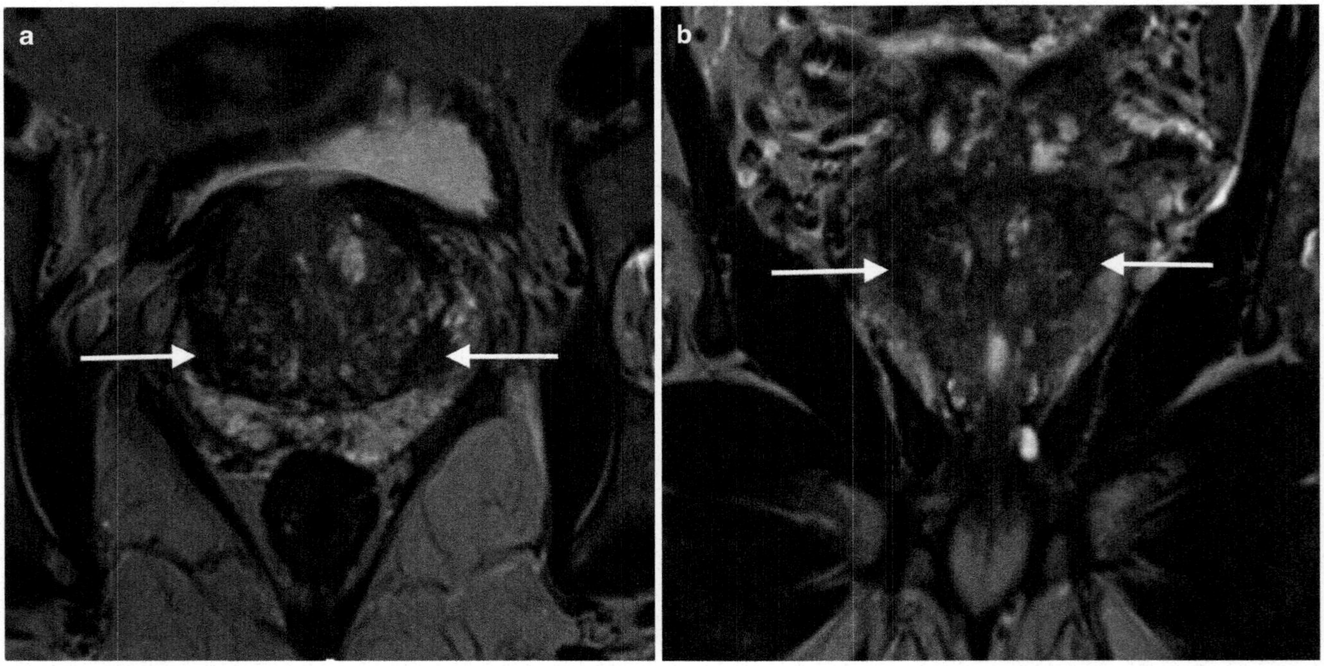

Fig. 5.7 Surgical capsule. (**a**) Axial and (**b**) coronal T2-weighted images of the prostate show the surgical capsule as a hypointense continuous band that separates the heterogeneous transition zone and the hyperintense peripheral zone (*white arrows*)

5.2.1.4 Periprostatic Veins

The prostate is surrounded by a periprostatic venous plexus, predominantly around the anterior and lateral faces [7]. Usually, the veins have a hyperintense signal on T2 sequences but, depending on the flow velocity, a hypointense signal may be seen. Because there is not a clear anatomic pseudocapsule at the apex, it is possible to confuse a rounded vein (axial diameter) that displays a hypointense appearance on T2-weighted images for a peripheral lesion of PCa (Fig. 5.8). Table 5.5 shows sources of diagnostic errors and tricks to aid recognition in relation to the periprostatic veins.

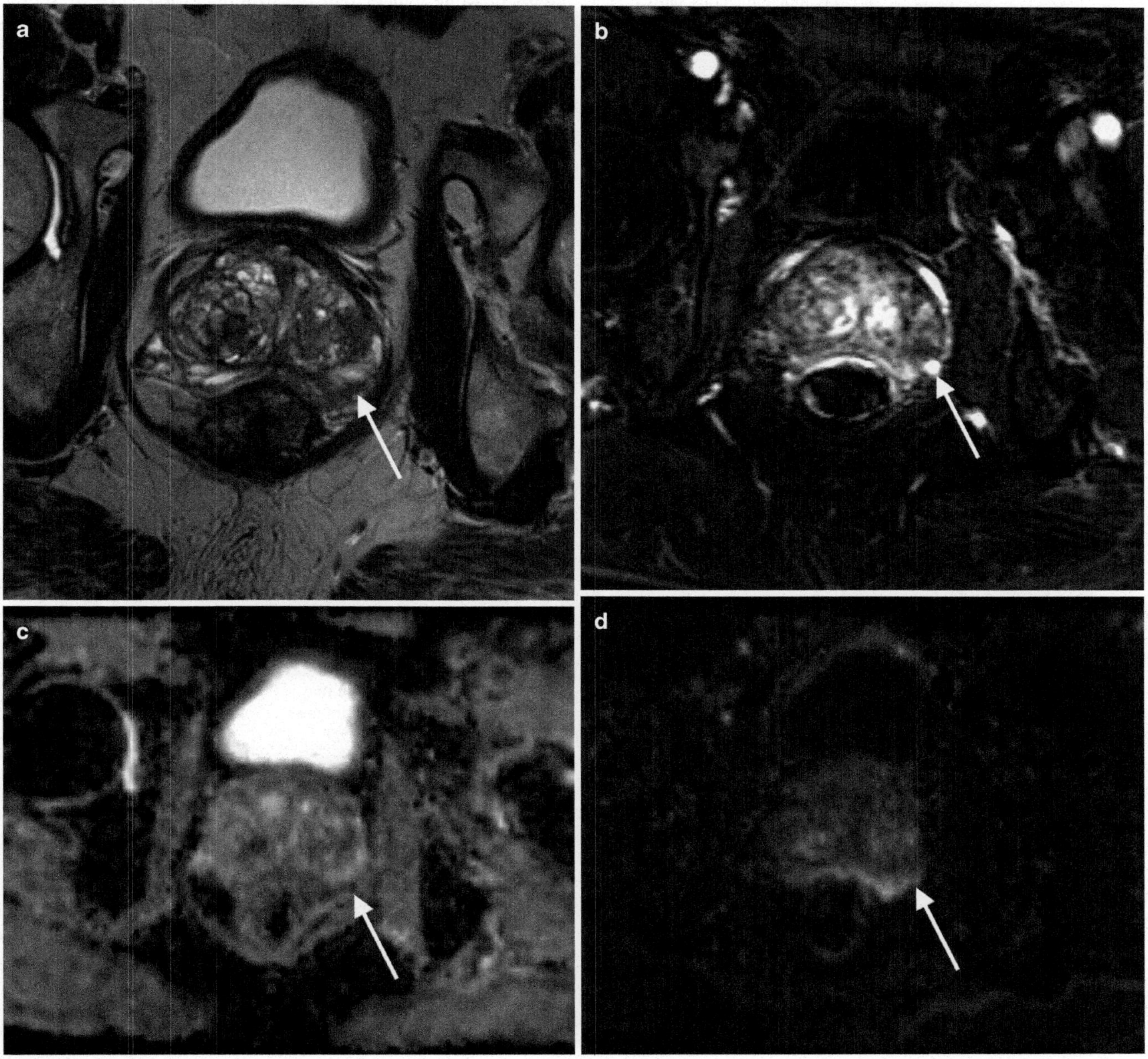

Fig. 5.8 Periprostatic veins. (**a**) Axial T2-weighed image of the prostate at the midgland shows a hypointense pseudonodular area in the left peripheral zone (*white arrow*). (**b**) DCE image at the same level depicts a hypervascular behavior of such lesion. (**c**) ADC map image shows moderated hypointense signal, and (**d**) DW image shows no significant restriction of diffusion. Surgical specimen showed this finding to correlate with a periprostatic vein

Table 5.5 Multiparametric MR appearance of periprostatic veins and key point to differentiate from PCa

mpMR sequences	Appearance	Tips and tricks
T2WI	A hypointense signal may be seen (Fig. 5.8a)	The periprostatic plexus is more prominent in younger men without marked BPH [14] Evaluate the consecutive planes and check the tubular morphology of the structure
ADC	A hypointense signal may be seen	
DWI	Isointense signal	PCa usually shows hyperintense signal
DCE	Positive enhancement	Check the vascular origin of the structure tubular structure with avid enhancement (Fig. 5.8b)

T2WI T2-weighted image, *ADC* apparent diffusion coefficient, *DWI* diffusion-weighted imaging, *DCE* dynamic contrast enhancement, *PCa* prostate cancer

5.2.2 Benign Abnormalities

5.2.2.1 Nodule of Benign Prostatic Hyperplasia

A BPH nodule is the result of the enlargement of the transition zone with variable proliferation of glandular and fibromuscular stromal components. When the proliferation of stromal components is dominant, the differential diagnosis with prostate cancer can be difficult (Table 5.6; Figs. 5.9, 5.10, and 5.11) [15].

Table 5.6 Multiparametric MR appearance of stromal BPH (SBPH) nodule and key points to differentiate them from PCa

mpMR sequences	Appearance	Tips and tricks
T2WI	SBPH nodule may appear as a hypointense nodule (Fig. 5.9a)	A SBPH nodule is usually located in the transition zone and shows a round shape with a well-defined margin and an encapsulated appearance (Fig. 5.9) In some cases, a BPH herniated nodule may be seen at the peripheral zone. The sagittal plane helps to define it (Fig. 5.10) Rarely, a BPH nodule can be ectopic, located in the peripheral zone without contact to the transition zone. In such cases, the characteristics of the nodule are similar to those of a typical BPH nodule located in the transition zone, as described above (Fig. 5.11)
ADC	SBPH nodule may show a hypointense signal (Fig. 5.9b)	
DWI	SBPH nodule may show a hyperintense signal in high b values (Fig. 5.9c)	
DCE	Early enhancement can be seen (Fig. 5.9d)	

T2WI T2-weighted image, *ADC* apparent diffusion coefficient, *DWI* diffusion-weighted imaging, *DCE* dynamic contrast enhancement, *SBPH* stromal benign prostatic hyperplasia

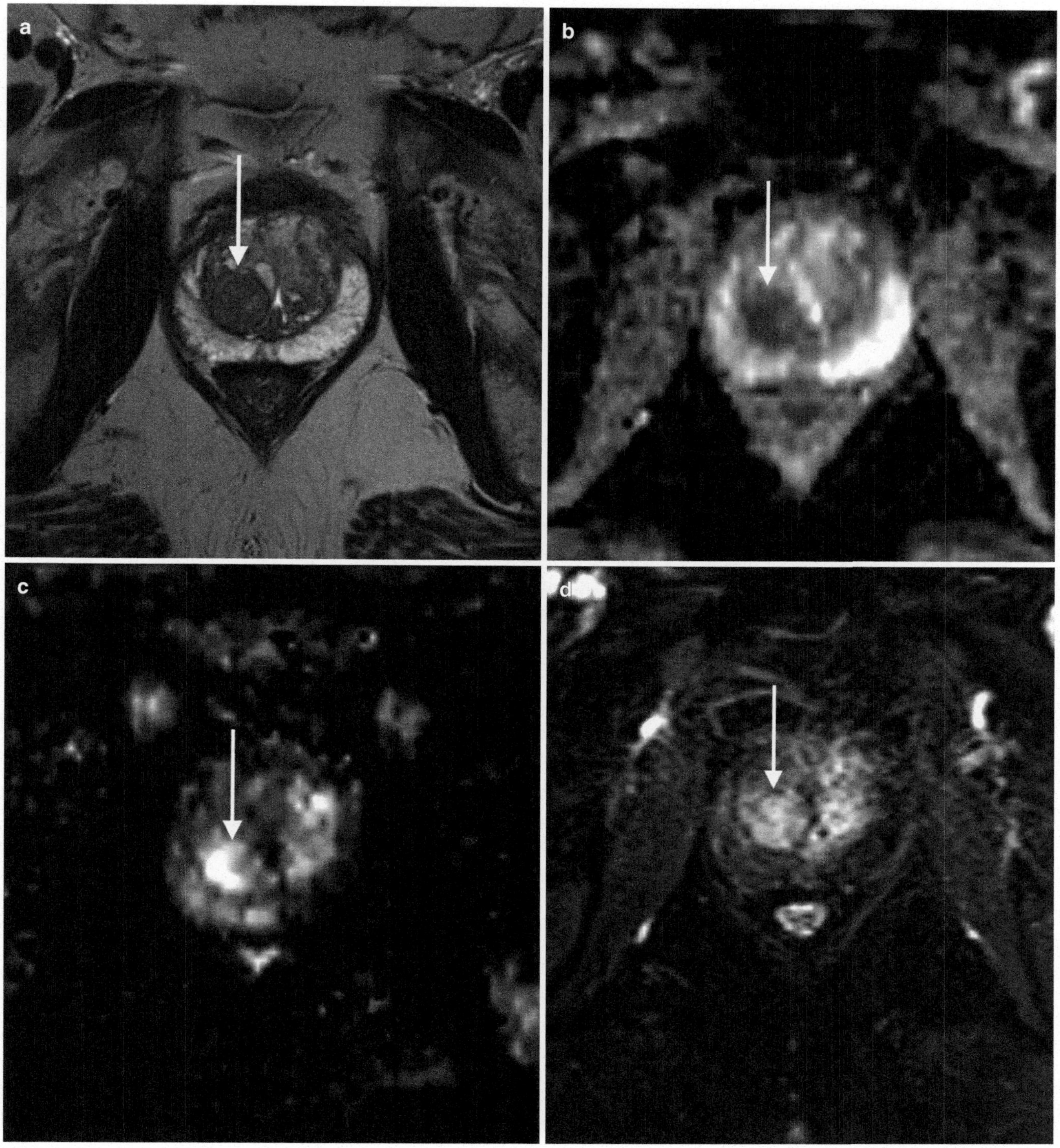

Fig. 5.9 Stromal benign prostatic hyperplasia (SBPH) nodule. (**a**) Axial T2-weighted image at the midgland shows a well-defined, round, encapsulated, hypointense nodule in the right transition zone (*white arrow*), with restriction of the diffusion in ADC map (**b**) and DWI (**c**). DCE image (**d**) demonstrates a moderate early enhancement. Despite the diffusion restriction and the enhancement after the administration of gadolinium, the morphologic characteristics in the T2 images strongly suggest a SBPH nodule. (**e**) Surgical specimen confirmed a benign prostatic hyperplasia nodule (*black arrow*)

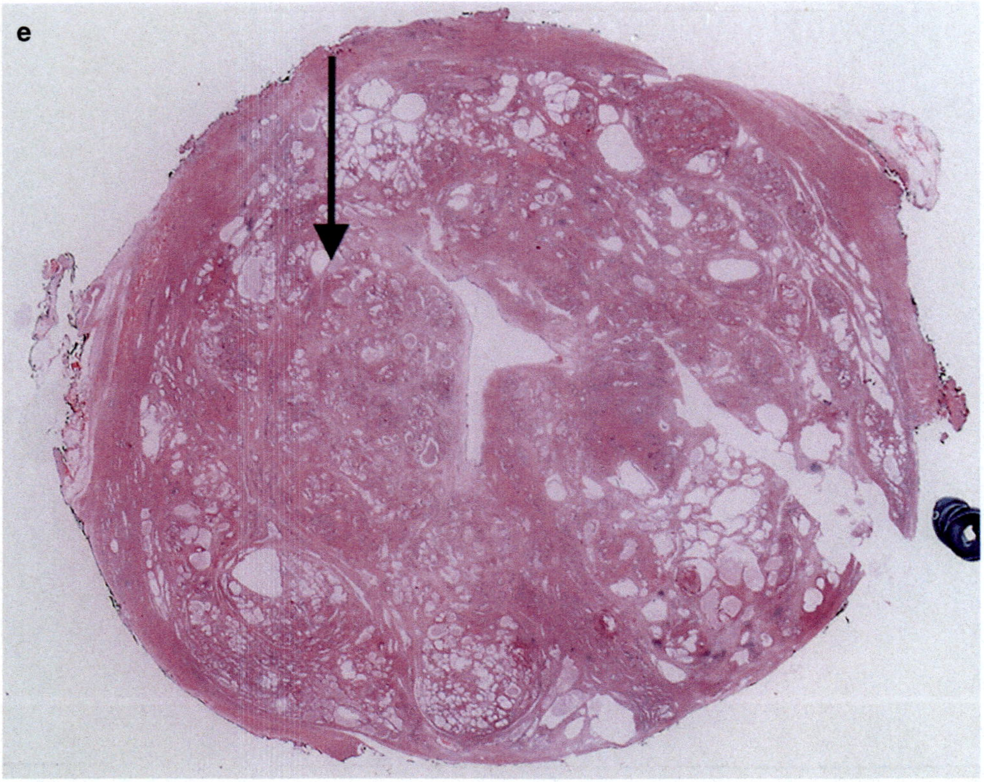

Fig. 5.9 (continued)

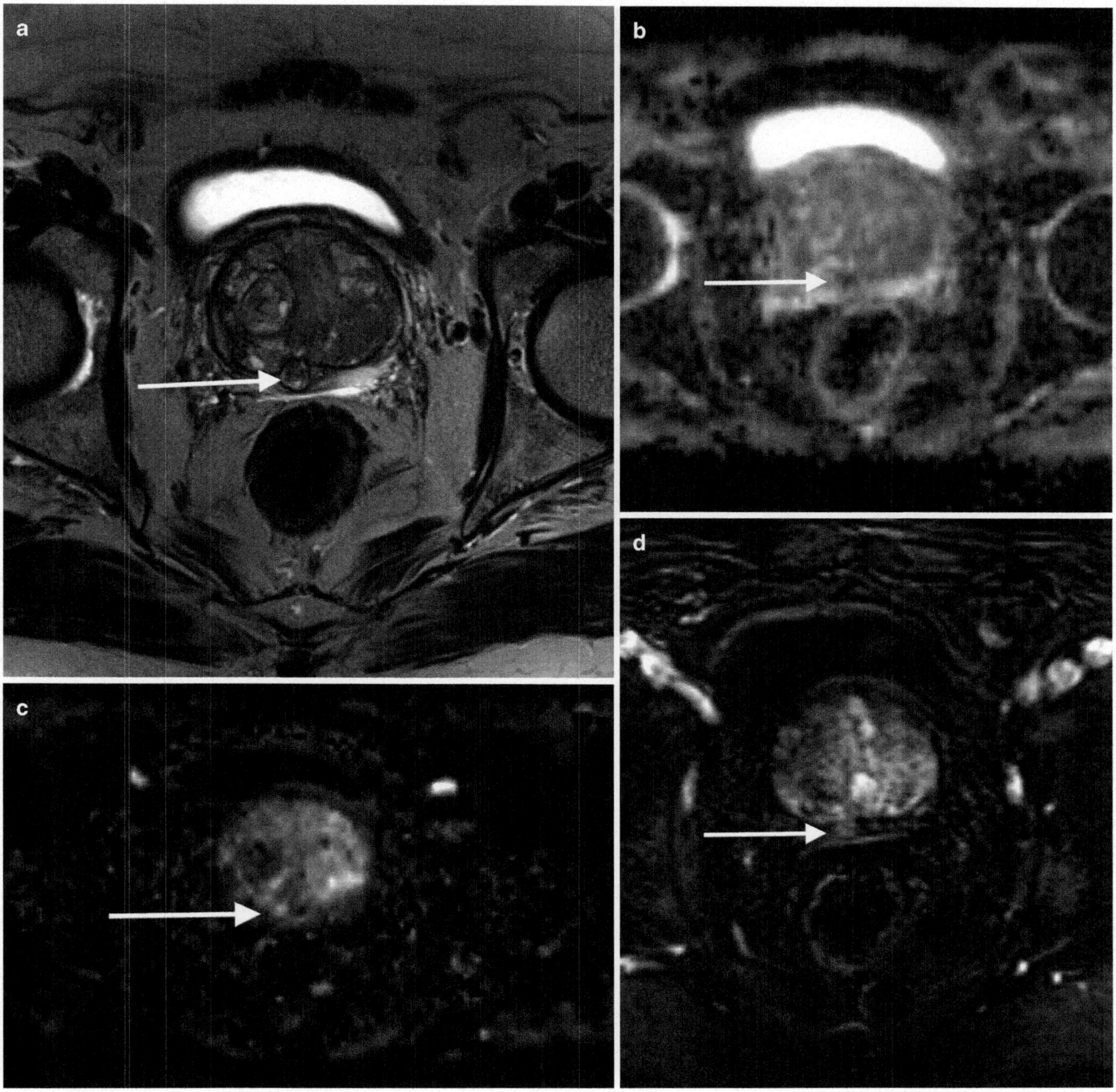

Fig. 5.10 Herniated benign prostatic hyperplasia nodule. (**a**) Axial T2-weighted image, (**b**) ADC map, (**c**) DWI, and (**d**) DCE images of the prostate at the midgland show a T2-hypointense encapsulated nodule in the right peripheral zone (*white arrow*), with restriction of diffusion in the central of the lesion. (**e**) Sagittal T2-weighted image depicts better the nodule (*white arrow*) as a herniated transition zone nodule and not a possible peripheral zone lesion

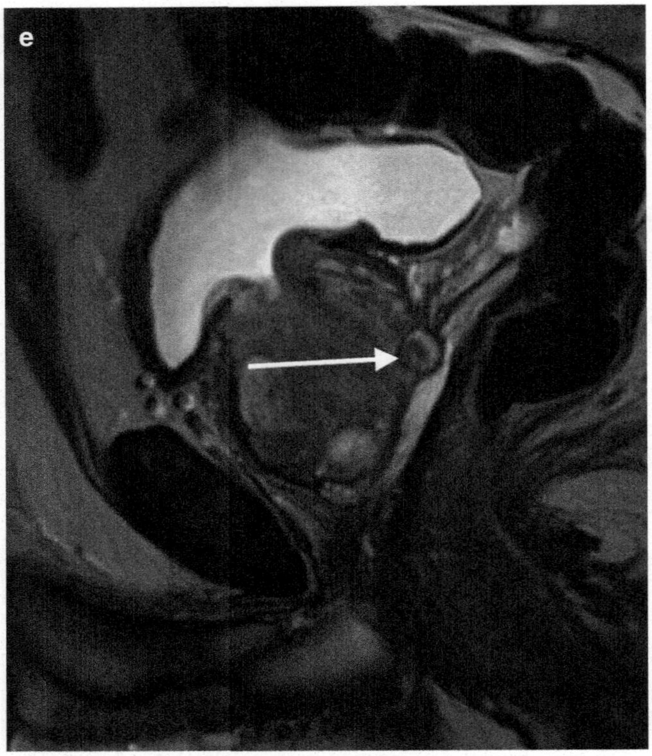

Fig. 5.10 (continued)

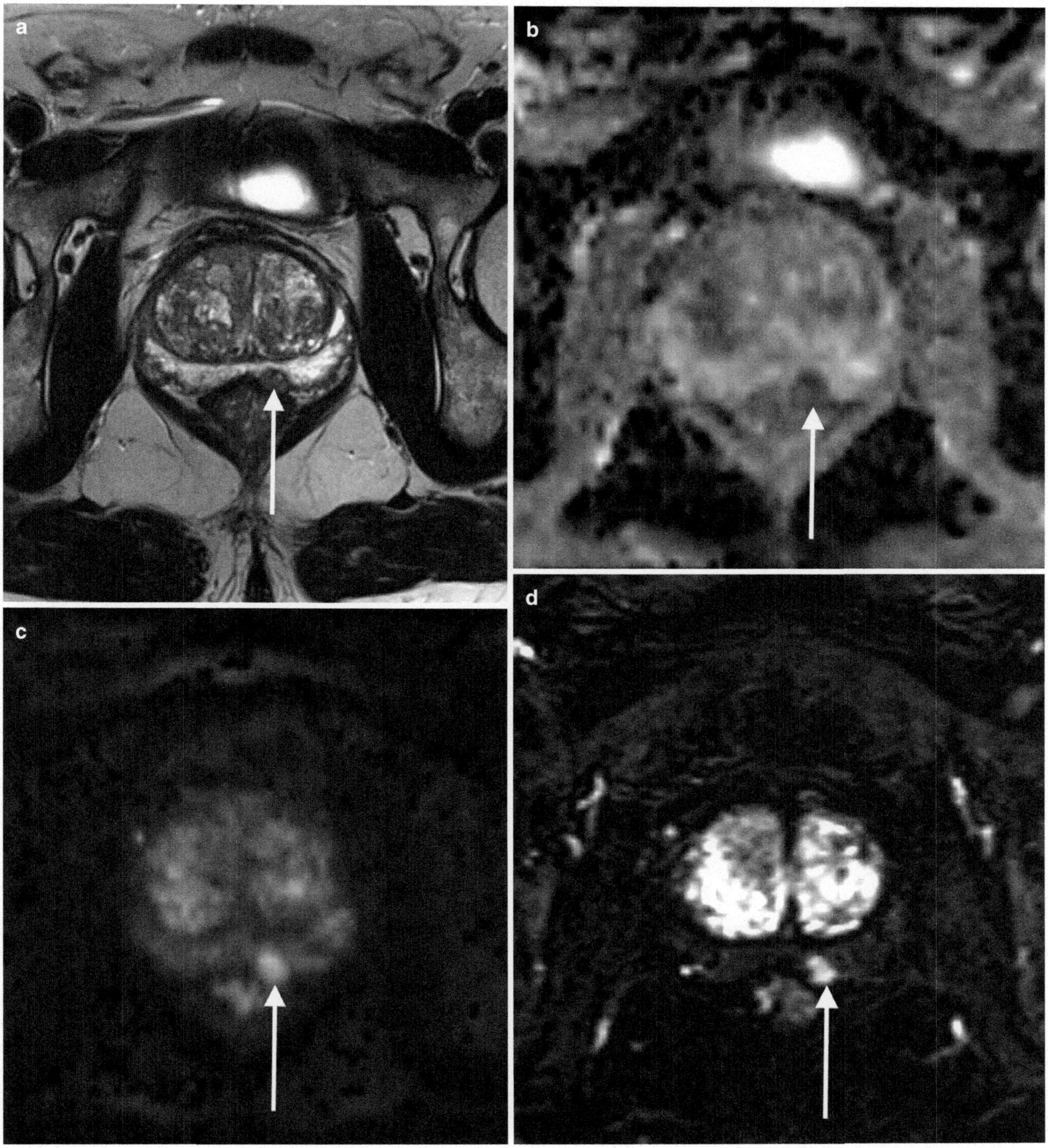

Fig. 5.11 Ectopic benign prostatic hyperplasia nodule. (**a**) Axial T2-weighted image at the midgland shows a well-defined, encapsulated, small, hypointense nodule in the medial left peripheral zone (*white arrow*). ADC map (**b**) and DWI (**c**) demonstrate a restriction of the diffusion, as well as early enhancement after gadolinium administration (**d**). (**e**) Surgical specimen confirmed an ectopic benign prostatic hyperplasia nodule (*black arrow*)

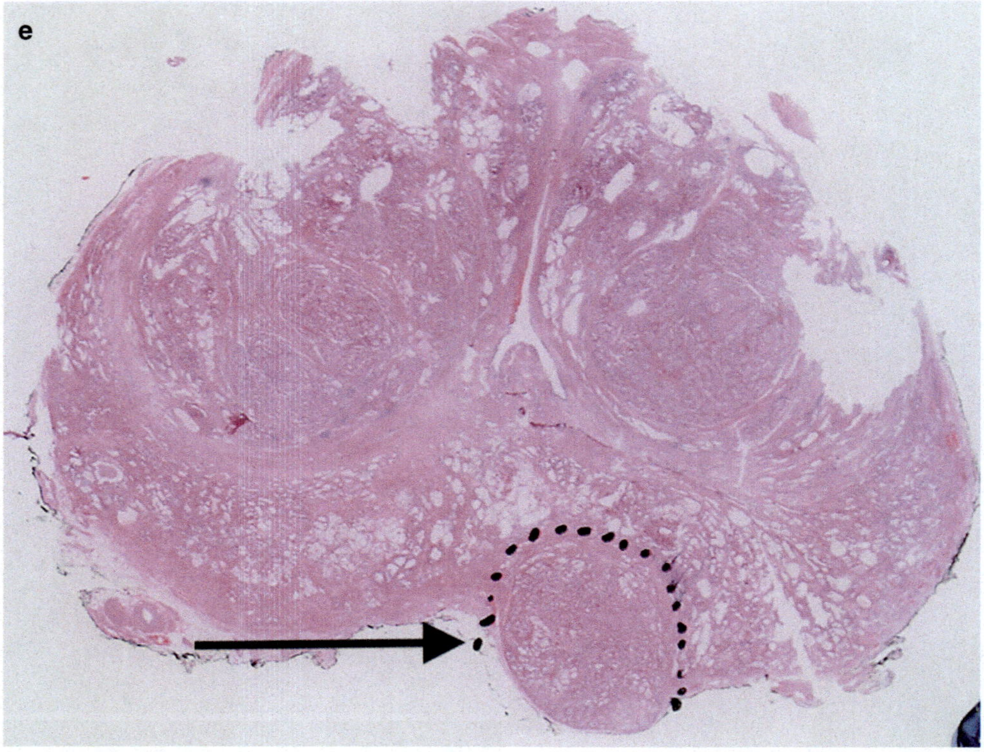

Fig. 5.11 (continued)

5.2.2.2 Acute and Chronic Nonspecific Prostatitis

Prostatitis includes a wide spectrum of acute and chronic conditions (Table 5.7).

Bacterial Acute and Chronic Prostatitis

Bacterial acute and chronic prostatitis is a cause of elevated PSA. The clinical presentation is variable. In some cases, no symptoms are present. When they are present, acute prostatitis tends to be more symptomatic (local and systemic symptoms) than chronic prostatitis (lower urinary tract symptoms and no systemic symptoms) [16]. Clinical behavior can aid diagnosis: a fluctuating PSA level and PSA response to antibiotics guide one to a diagnosis of prostatitis.

Usually, when prostatitis is symptomatic, imaging techniques are not necessary for diagnosis. However, in cases of indolent and asymptomatic prostatitis with elevated PSA, when imaging is deemed necessary, the mpMR diagnosis can be challenging for the radiologist (Table 5.8, Figs. 5.12, 5.13, and 5.14) [15, 17].

Prostatitis can show inflammatory changes in the periprostatic fat and simulate clinical and MR T3a staging. Likewise, enlarged reactive lymph nodes may also be seen in the context of prostatitis.

Table 5.7 Classification of different types and subtypes of prostatitis [16]

Type	Subtype	Clinical presentation
Bacterial	Acute	Local and systemic symptoms are usually present
	Chronic	Local symptoms can be present, but asymptomatic cases are also possible
Granulomatous	Idiopathic	Usually is asymptomatic, but local symptoms can be present
	Iatrogenic (transurethral resection of the prostate or bladder)	
	Infective (*Mycobacterium tuberculosis* or develop after intravesical bacillus Calmette-Guérin therapy for bladder cancer)	
	Malacoplakia	

Table 5.8 Multiparametric MR appearance of bacterial acute and chronic prostatitis and key points to differentiate them from PCa

mpMR sequences	Appearance	Tips and tricks
T2WI	Usually, bacterial acute and chronic prostatitis is seen as a hypointense area in the peripheral (more frequent) and/or transition zone (Fig. 5.12a)	Signal changes tend to be more diffuse and ill-defined than in PCa (Fig. 5.12)
	When necrosis is present, low-intensity signal on the T2 sequence can be seen	The low signal intensity is more pronounced than in PCa, in cases of necrosis (Fig. 5.13a)
ADC	Prostatitis may show a hypointense signal (Fig. 5.12b)	The hypointense signal tends to be less evident in prostatitis than in PCa (mild to moderate diffusion restriction) (Fig. 5.12b) [18]
	Marked low signal intensity can be seen, when necrosis is present (Fig. 5.13b)	Low signal intensity on ADC is more pronounced than in PCa in cases of necrosis. ADC usually >0.9mm2/s
DWI	Prostatitis may show a hyperintense signal in high b values (Fig. 5.12c)	The hyperintense signal tends to be less evident in prostatitis than in PCa (mild to moderate diffusion restriction) (Fig. 5.12c) [18]
DCE	Usually, prostatitis areas show contrast enhancement	An area without contrast enhancement can be seen when necrosis is present (Fig. 5.13d)

T2WI T2-weighted image, *ADC* apparent diffusion coefficient, *DWI* diffusion-weighted imaging, *DSC* dynamic contrast enhancement, *PCa* prostate cancer

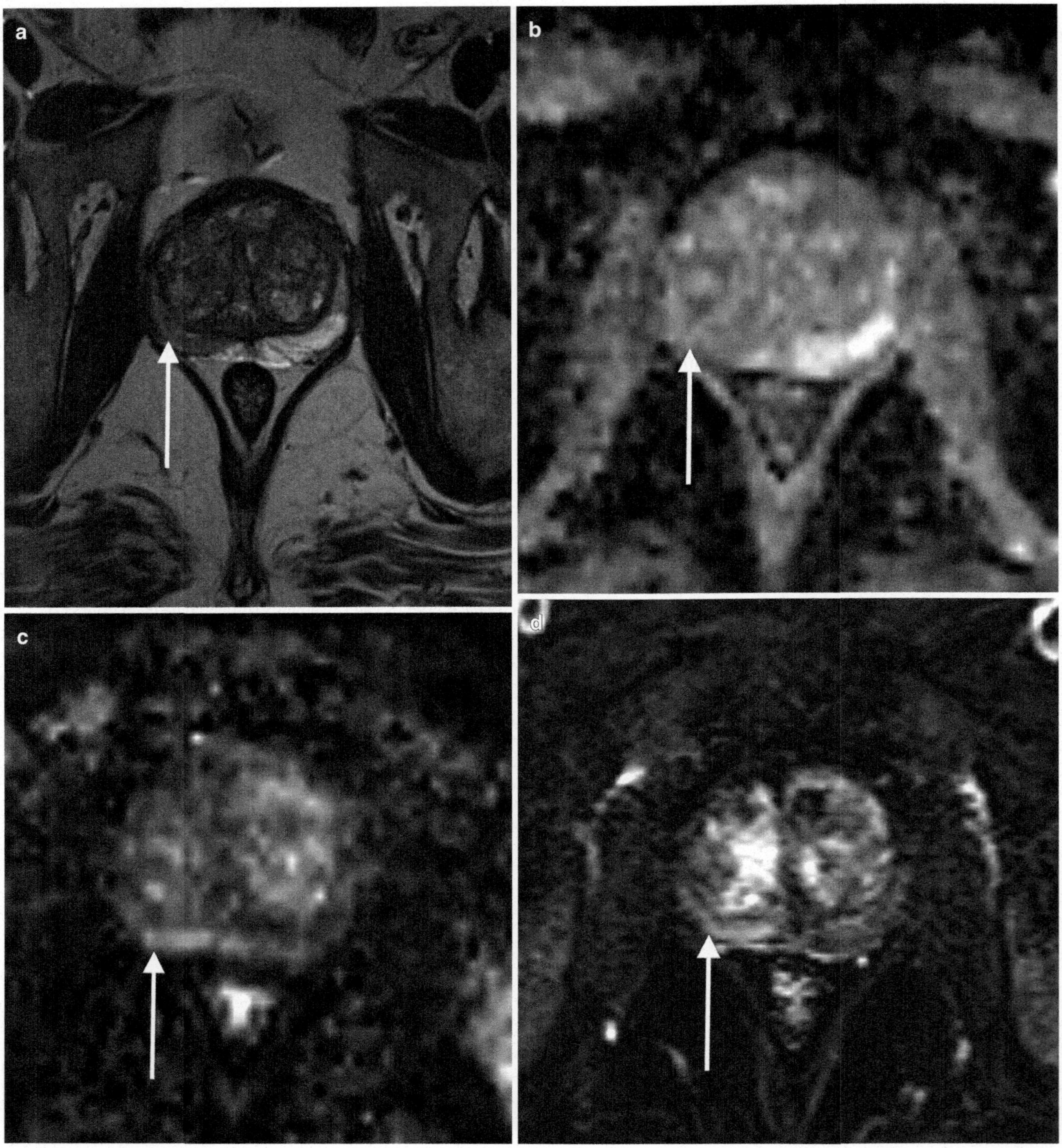

Fig. 5.12 Prostatitis of the right lobe. (**a**) Axial T2-weighted image at the midgland shows a homogeneous hypointensity of the right peripheral zone (*white arrow*), with a small medial area preserving the typical peripheral zone hyperintensity. ADC map (**b**) and DWI (**c**) present a discrete restriction of the diffusion in the right peripheral zone, as well as slight enhancement in DCE images (**d**)

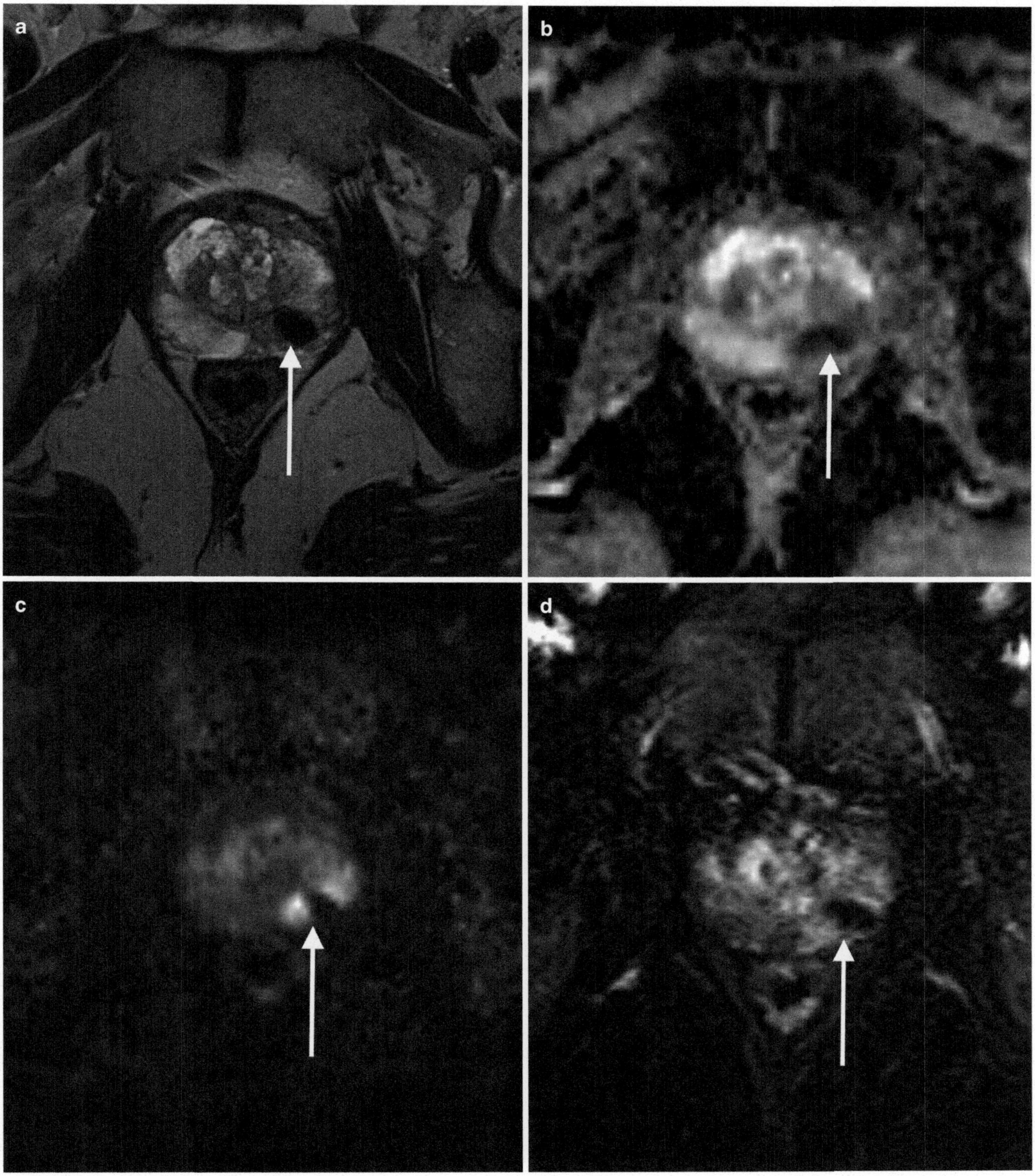

Fig. 5.13 Purulent acute prostatitis. (**a**) Axial T2-weighted image at the midgland shows a diffuse hypointensity of the left peripheral zone (white arrow), with an oval area of severe hypointensity in the middle. ADC map (**b**) and DWI (**c**) show a significant restriction of the diffusion and an early enhancement after gadolinium administration (**d**). Note that in all sequences, there is a persistence of the severe hypointensity/absence of signal in the middle of the left peripheral zone, a finding that could represent the presence of necrosis/air bubbles in a severe infection. (**e**) Surgical specimen showed acute prostatitis with extensive glandular substitution for neutrophils compatible with purulent prostatitis (*black arrow*)

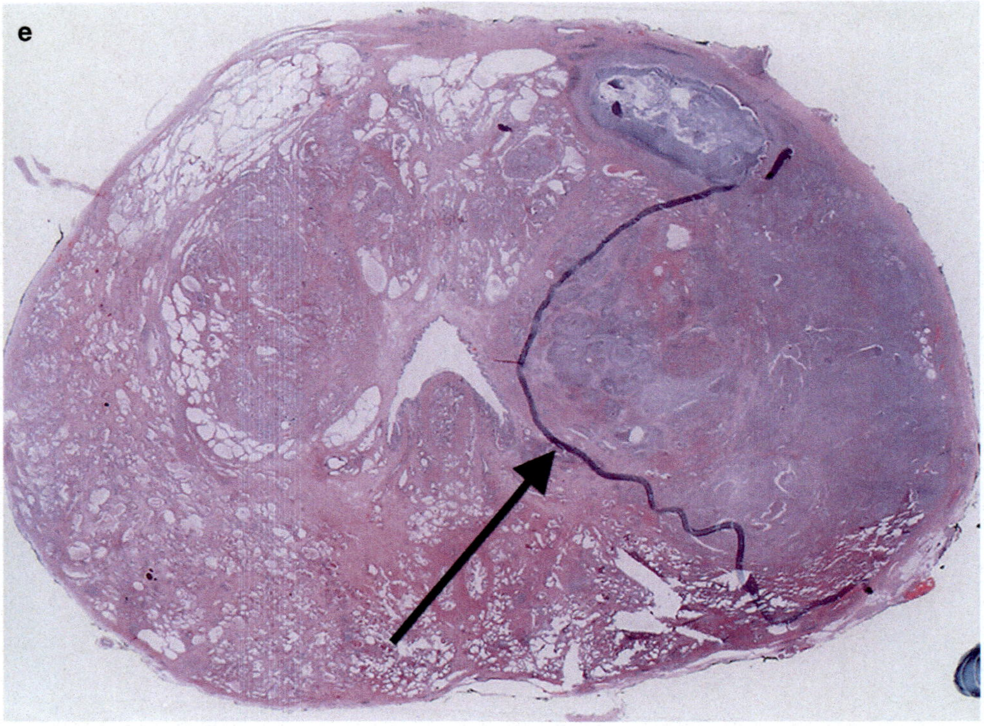

Fig. 5.13 (continued)

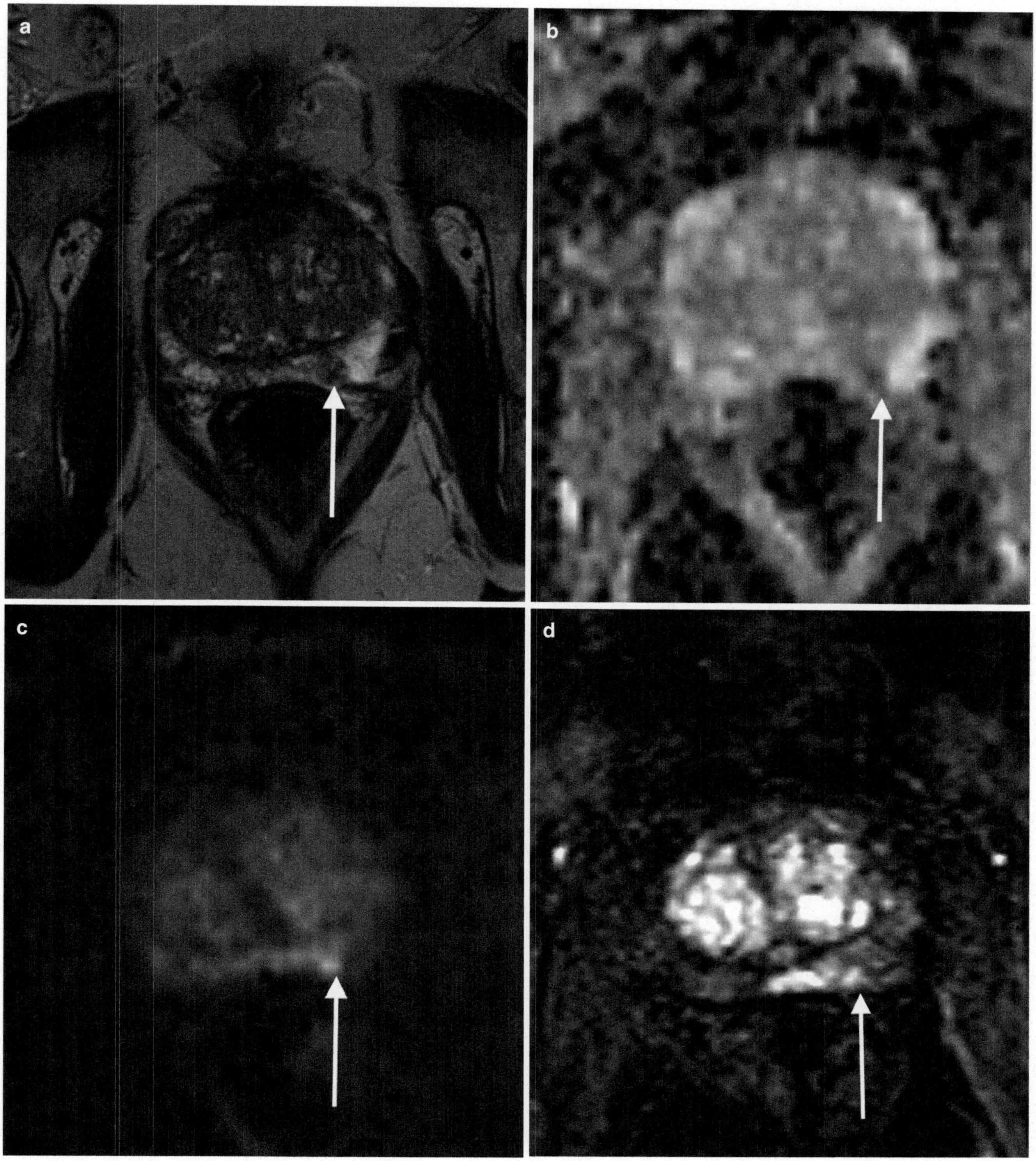

Fig. 5.14 Focal acute prostatitis. (**a**) Axial T2-weighted image at the midgland shows a round, ill-defined hypointense area in the medial left peripheral zone (*white arrow*). ADC map (**b**) and DWI (**c**) show a moderate restriction of the diffusion that correlates with the area seen in the T2 images and discrete enhancement after the administration of gadolinium (**d**). MRI-guided TRUS biopsy showed a focal nonspecific prostatitis

Granulomatous Prostatitis

Granulomatous prostatitis is an uncommon pathology, but it is important to take it into account because it is a great simulator of PCa (Table 5.9) [19]. This entity can occur secondary to bladder cancer therapy with bacillus Calmette-Guérin (BCG) (intravesical instillation), tuberculous prostatitis, or prostate interventions (e.g., transurethral resection of the prostate); in most cases, however, no cause can be found [20].

Table 5.9 Multiparametric MR appearance of granulomatous prostatitis and key points to differentiate it from PCa

mpMR sequences	Appearance	Tips and tricks
T2WI	Usually granulomatous prostatitis is seen as a hypointense area (Figs. 5.15a and 5.16a)	
ADC	Granulomatous prostatitis shows a hypointense signal (this appearance is more common than other causes of prostatitis) (Figs. 5.15b and 5.16b)	
DWI	Granulomatous prostatitis shows a hyperintense signal in high b values (this appearance is more common than other causes of prostatitis) (Figs. 5.15c and 5.16c)	
DCE	Usually contrast enhancement is shown (Figs. 5.15d and 5.16d)	Necrotic areas without contrast enhancement may be seen (caseous abscess) (Fig. 5.16d)

T2WI T2-weighted image, *ADC* apparent diffusion coefficient, *DWI* diffusion-weighted imaging, *DCE* dynamic contrast enhancement, *PCa* prostate cancer

Clinical features can contribute to diagnostic confusion between granulomatous prostatitis and PCa: an elevated PSA and a firm nodule on digital rectal examination can be found in both pathologies [19]. The inflammatory component of periprostatic fat can simulate extracapsular extension in clinical and MR evaluation (T3a stage) (Figs. 5.15 and 5.16). An option when mycobacterial granulomatous prostatitis is suspected is to perform a short-term follow-up after the specific treatment in order to evaluate the therapeutic response.

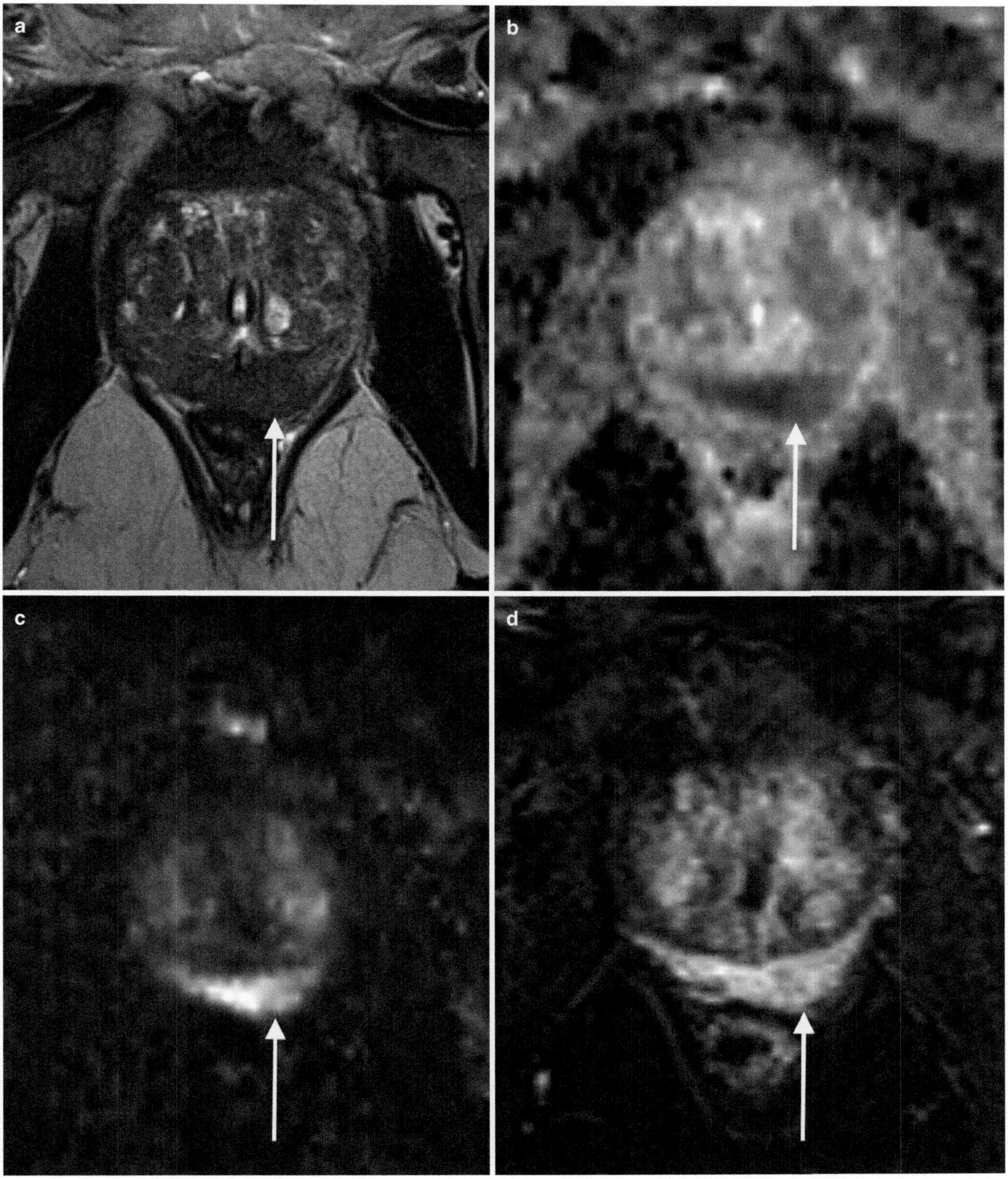

Fig. 5.15 Granulomatous prostatitis. (**a**) Axial T2-weighted image at the midgland/apex shows an area of hypointensity affecting the medial border of both peripheral zones (*white arrow*). ADC map (**b**) and DWI (**c**) demonstrate a significant restriction of diffusion in the same area, along with some degree of enhancement in DCE images (**d**). This area bulges the capsule, a finding suggestive of extracapsular extension (ESUR Score 4, see Chap. 6). (**e**) Surgical specimen showed severe chronic granulomatous prostatitis at this level (*black arrow*)

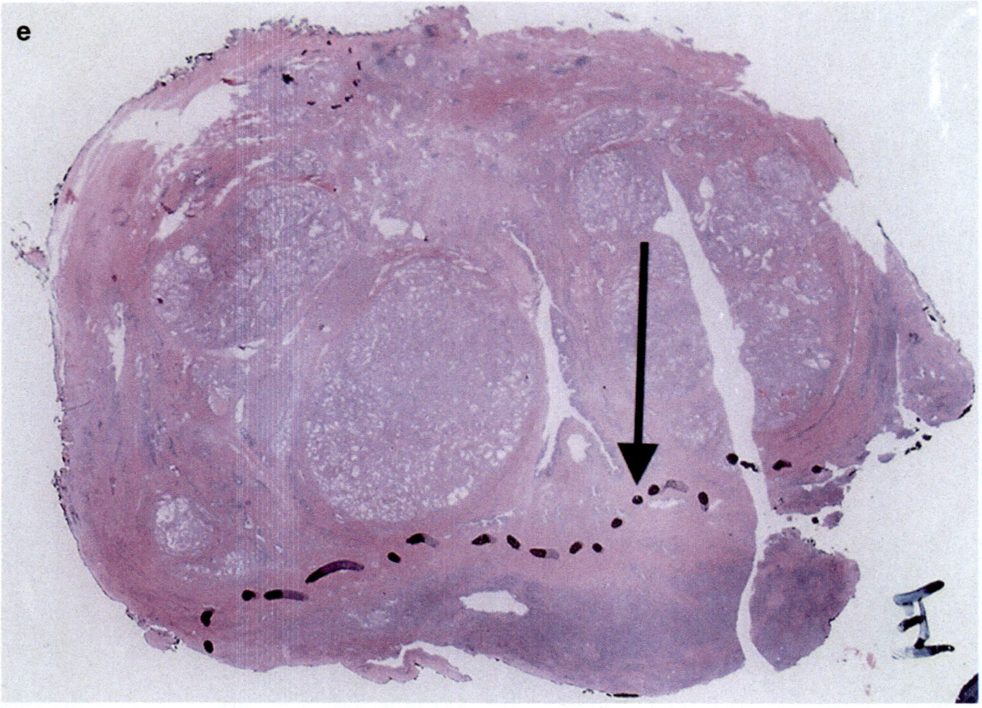

Fig. 5.15 (continued)

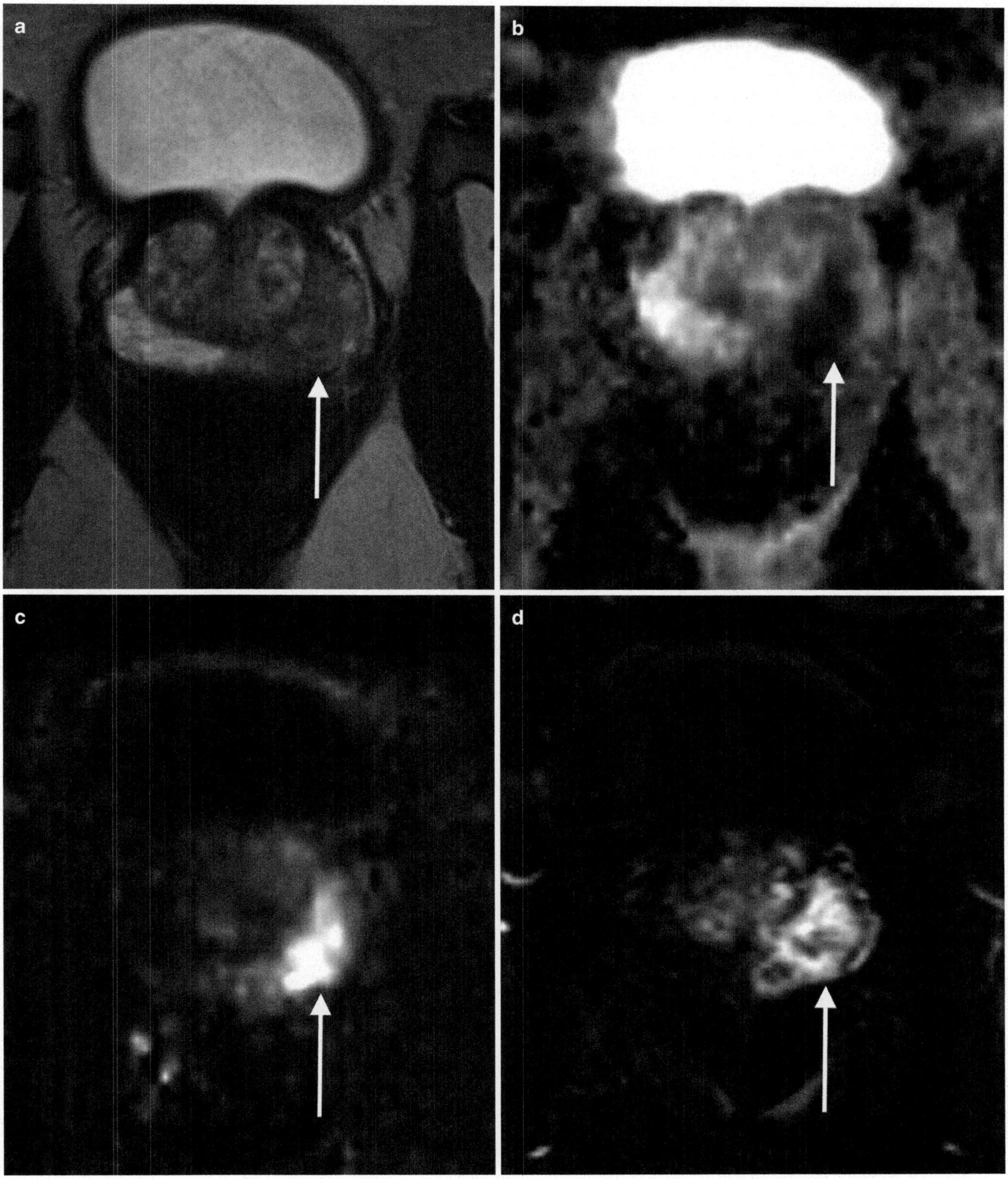

Fig. 5.16 Necrotizing chronic granulomatous prostatitis. (**a**) Axial T2-weighted image at the prostate base shows a diffuse hypointensity of the whole left peripheral zone (*white arrow*), with a marked restriction of diffusion in ADC map (**b**) and DWI (**c**), and early enhancement after the administration of gadolinium with necrotic areas without contrast enhancement can be seen (**d**). Prostate biopsy showed a chronic necrotizing granulomatous prostatitis

5.2.2.3 Atrophy

Atrophy is characterized by distortion of the prostatic architecture, with crowded glandular tissue. The histological alterations associated with atrophy are the cause of its mpMR appearance. Focal atrophic areas may simulate PCa and give rise to a false-positive diagnosis (Table 5.10). Perhaps because prostatic atrophy is a common alteration without clinical consequences, the pathological report frequently does not report this entity specifically. However, the radiologist must know that atrophy is a cause of elevated PSA [21]. If no suspicious lesion is found, prostatic atrophy may explain the abnormal PSA.

5.2.2.4 Hemorrhage

Hemorrhage is commonly seen in the prostate after prostate biopsy, and its appearance can simulate PCa (Table 5.11).

Citrate has anticoagulant properties. A particularity of non-tumoral prostate tissue is the high level of citrate, while prostate tumors have a lower level. These characteristics can explain the "MRI exclusion sign": where there is hemorrhage, there is probably not a tumor and vice versa (Fig. 5.18). Even though the majority of institutions recommend that an interval of 6–8 weeks is allowed between biopsy and mpMR to avoid potential mistakes, in daily practice such a delay is not always possible. For this reason, it is very important that the radiologist knows the keys to differentiating between hemorrhage and PCa.

Table 5.10 Multiparametric MR appearance of atrophy and key points to differentiate it from PCa

mpMR sequences	Appearance	Tips and tricks
T2WI	May cause decreased signal intensity	Usually focal prostatic atrophy is seen in the peripheral zone, frequently as a zone with geometric limits and reduced parenchyma
ADC	A hypointense signal may be seen	Commonly less low signal than in PCa
DWI	A hyperintense signal may be seen	Commonly less high signal than in PCa
DCE	Contrast enhancement may be seen in high b values	

T2WI T2-weighted image, *ADC* apparent diffusion coefficient, *DWI* diffusion-weighted imaging, *DCE* dynamic contrast enhancement

Table 5.11 Multiparametric MR appearance of hemorrhage and key points to differentiate it from PCa

mpMR sequences	Appearance	Tips and tricks
T1WI	Hyperintense signal	It is always important to read the T1 sequence to avoid false-positive diagnosis of PCa secondary to the presence of hemorrhage (Fig. 5.17)
T2WI	Hypointense signal may be seen	
ADC	Hypointense signal may be seen	
DWI	Hyperintense signal may be seen in high b values	
DCE	Usually hemorrhage shows a hyperintense signal on DCE without subtraction	The post-contrast subtraction imaging is mandatory to depict the suspicious focus of PCa because the hyperintensity of the hematoma is eliminated and the enhancing PCa nodule persists (Fig. 5.18e)

T1WI T2-weighted image, *T2WI* T2-weighted image, *ADC* apparent diffusion coefficient, *DWI* diffusion-weighted imaging, *DCE* dynamic contrast enhancement

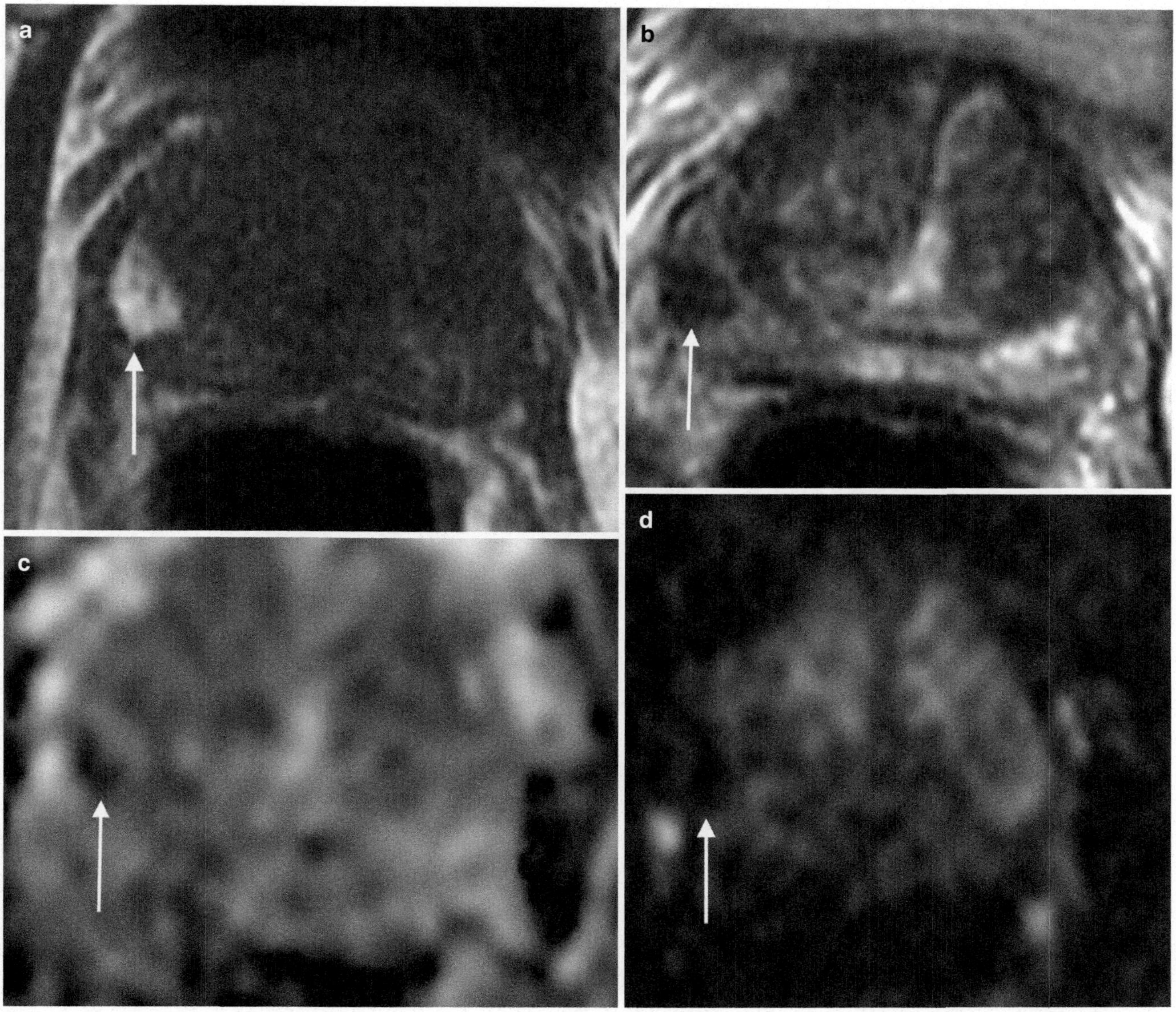

Fig. 5.17 Post-biopsy hemorrhage. (**a**) Axial T1-weighted image at the midgland of the prostate shows a hyperintense area in the right peripheral zone (*white arrow*). This finding correlates with an area of hypointensity at the same level in T2-weighted images (**b**) and a hypointense signal on ADC map (**c**) and DW image (**d**) (*arrows*). These findings are suggestive of intraprostatic hemorrhage

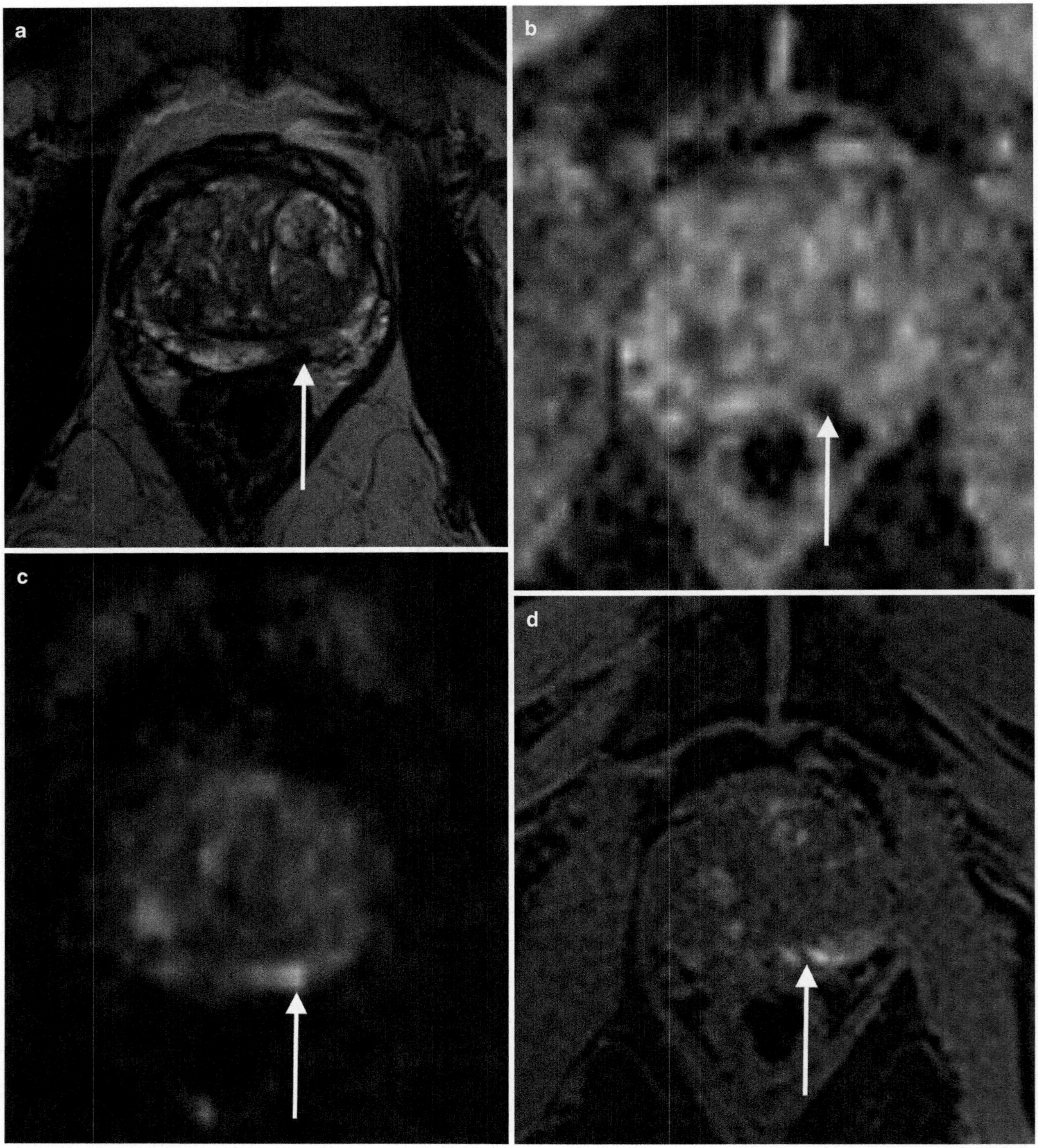

Fig. 5.18 Example of "exclusion sign." (**a**) Axial T2-weighted image at the midgland of the prostate shows a hypointense nodule (*white arrow*) in the left peripheral zone. (**b**) ADC map and (**c**) DW images show restriction of diffusion. These findings would suggest a PI-RADS 4 lesion. However, in the T1-weighted images (**d**) there is a hyperintensity in the left peripheral zone that suggests bleeding, but it is located surrounding a hypointense nodule corresponding to the lesion seen on the rest of the images ("exclusion sign"). There is also an early enhancement of the nodule in DCE images (**e**). MRI-guided biopsy of this area showed a Gleason 3 + 4 PCa

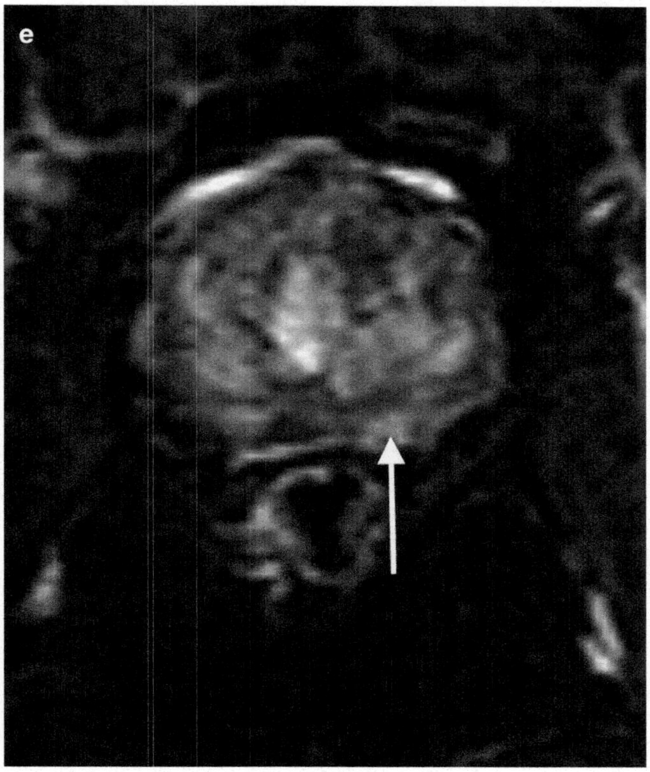

Fig. 5.18 (continued)

Key Points

- Radiologist must be aware of the different anatomical structures and benign conditions that may mimic PCa on mpMR.
- PCa may also arise from normal structures such as anterior fibromuscular stroma and the central zone, hence the need for an adequate knowledge of the normal MRI characteristics of these areas.
- Prostatitis is a common cause of false-positive diagnosis of PCa. The correlation with clinical history must be performed whenever possible (e.g., intravesical BCG instillation); however, sometimes only prostate biopsy can enable the correct diagnosis to be reached.
- Prostatitis can show inflammatory changes in the periprostatic fat and simulate T3a staging.
- Enlarged reactive lymph nodes may also be seen in the context of prostatitis.
- Post-biopsy hemorrhage can simulate PCa, but it may also help define PCa when present ("MRI exclusion sign").

References

1. Torre L, Bray F, Siegel R, et al. Global cancer statistics, 2012. CA Cancer J Clin. 2015;65(2):87–108.
2. Ghai S, Haider M. Multiparametric-MRI in diagnosis of prostate cancer. Indian J Urol. 2015;31(3):194.
3. Gaziev G, Wadhwa K, Barrett T, et al. Defining the learning curve for multiparametric magnetic resonance imaging (MRI) of the prostate using MRI-transrectal ultrasonography (TRUS) fusion-guided transperineal prostate biopsies as a validation tool. BJU Int. 2015;117(1):80–6.
4. Weinreb J, Barentsz J, Choyke P, et al. PI-RADS prostate imaging – Reporting and Data System: 2015, version 2. Eur Urol. 2016;69(1):16–40.
5. Kasel-Seibert M, Lehmann T, Aschenbach R, et al. Assessment of PI-RADS v2 for the detection of prostate cancer. Eur J Radiol. 2016;85(4):726–31.
6. Panebianco V, Barchetti F, Barentsz J, et al. Pitfalls in interpreting mp-MRI of the prostate: a pictorial review with pathologic correlation. Insights Imaging. 2015;6(6):611–30.
7. Hricak H, Dooms G, McNeal J, et al. MR imaging of the prostate gland: normal anatomy. AJR. 1987;148(1):51–8.
8. Bouyé S, Potiron E, Puech P, et al. Transition zone and anterior stromal prostate cancers: zone of origin and intraprostatic patterns of spread at histopathology. Prostate. 2009;69(1):105–13.
9. McNeal J. The zonal anatomy of the prostate. Prostate. 1981;2(1):35–49.
10. Quick C, Gokden N, Sangoi A, et al. The distribution of PAX-2 immunoreactivity in the prostate gland, seminal vesicle, and ejaculatory duct: comparison with prostatic adenocarcinoma and discussion of prostatic zonal embryogenesis. Hum Pathol. 2010;41(8):1145–9.
11. Vargas H, Akin O, Franiel T, et al. Normal central zone of the prostate and central zone involvement by prostate cancer: clinical and MR imaging implications. Radiology. 2012;262(3):894–902.
12. Hansford B, Karademir I, Peng Y, et al. Dynamic contrast-enhanced MR imaging features of the normal central zone of the prostate. Acad Radiol. 2014;21(5):569–77.
13. Semple J. Surgical capsule of the benign enlargement of the prostate. BMJ. 1963;1(5346):1640–3.
14. Allen K, Kressel H, Arger P, et al. Age-related changes of the prostate: evaluation by MR imaging. AJR. 1989;152(1):77–81.
15. Watanabe Y, Nagayama M, Araki T, et al. Targeted biopsy based on ADC map in the detection and localization of prostate cancer: a feasibility study. J Magn Reson Imaging. 2012;37(5):1168–77.
16. Ramakrishnan K, Salinas R. Prostatitis: acute and chronic. Prim Care. 2010;37(3):547–63.
17. Hambrock T, Fütterer J, Huisman H, et al. Thirty-two-channel coil 3T magnetic resonance-guided biopsies of prostate tumor suspicious regions identified on multimodality 3T magnetic resonance imaging: technique and feasibility. Investig Radiol. 2008;43(10):686–94.
18. Meier-Schroers M, Kukuk G, Wolter K, et al. Differentiation of prostatitis and prostate cancer using the prostate imaging—Reporting and Data System (PI-RADS). Eur J Radiol. 2016;85(7):1304–11.
19. Bour L, Schull A, Delongchamps N, et al. Multiparametric MRI features of granulomatous prostatitis and tubercular prostate abscess. Diagn Interv Imaging. 2013;94(1):84–90.
20. Mohan H, Bal A, Punia R, et al. Granulomatous prostatitis - an infrequent diagnosis. Int J Urol. 2005;12(5):474–8.
21. Prando A, Billis A. Focal prostatic atrophy: mimicry of prostatic cancer on TRUS and 3D-MRSI studies. Abdom Imaging. 2008;34(2):271–5.

Prostate Cancer and MRI: Local Staging

6

Violeta Catalá, Oscar Laucirica, Jhonatan Hernandez,
Ferrán Algaba, Joan C. Vilanova,
and Francesco Sanguedolce

Contents

V. Catalá, M.D., Ph.D. (✉) • J. Hernandez, M.D.
Radiology Department, Fundació Puigvert, Autonomous University of Barcelona,
Cartagena 340-350, 08025 Barcelona, Spain
e-mail: violetacatala@yahoo.com.ar; vcatala@fundacio-puigvert.es; falgaba@fundacio-puigvert.es

F. Algaba, M.D.
Pathology Department, Fundació Puigvert, Autonomous University of Barcelona, Carrer Cartagena 340-350, 08025 Barcelona, Spain
e-mail: falgaba@fundacio-puigvert.es

O. Laucirica, M.D.
Urology Department, Sant Joan Despí Moises Broggi Hospital, Jacinto Verdaguer 90, 08970 Sant Joan Despí, Barcelona, Spain
e-mail: lauciricag@hotmail.com

J.C. Vilanova, M.D., Ph.D.
Radiology Department, Clínica Girona, Institute Catalan of Health-IDI, University of Girona,
Lorenzana 36, 17002 Girona, Spain
e-mail: kvilanova@comg.cat

F. Sanguedolce, M.D., Ph.D.
Urology Department, Fundació Puigvert, Autonomous University of Barcelona, Cartagena 340-350, 08025 Barcelona, Spain
e-mail: fsangue@hotmail.com; fsanguedol@fundacio-puigvert.es

6.1 Introduction

Correct staging of prostate carcinoma (PCa) is important for therapeutic management as it allows selection of an appropriate therapeutic option and correct therapeutic planning. The detection of extracapsular extension (ECE) of a PCa is an essential part of tumor staging because the absence of ECE (organ-confined disease) positively affects long-term prognosis, while the converse is true for the presence of ECE (non-organ-confined/pathologic stage ≥T3 disease) [1, 2].

Clinical nomograms have been developed to assess the risk of ECE [3, 4]. Most of them have been based on prostate-specific antigen (PSA), biopsy information, and clinical stage. Magnetic resonance imaging (MRI) is, however, recognized to be the best imaging tool in local tumor staging of PCa and is clearly superior to digital rectal examination, ultrasound, and CT in determining T stage [5]. Recent studies have demonstrated that multiparametric (mp) MRI information can improve the accuracy of clinical nomograms and probably these nomograms will include such information in the near future [6]. Despite the advantages of prostate MRI, however, its reading entails a significant learning curve, and its diagnostic efficacy depends on dedicated training and experience [7–9].

The aim of this chapter is to provide a synthesis of the main aspects of PCa staging involving a combination of clinical and radiological approaches in order to enable the reader to understand the utility of mpMRI in this setting and to facilitate tumor staging by mpMRI.

J.C. Vilanova et al. (eds.), *Atlas of Multiparametric Prostate MRI*, DOI 10.1007/978-3-319-61786-2_6

6.2 Tumor Staging

The staging of PCa is performed using the tumor, node, and metastasis (TNM) classification (Table 6.1). Local tumor staging is illustrated in Fig. 6.1.

Various therapeutic options are available for PCa. As already mentioned, tumor extension is one of the most important aspects to consider when choosing and planning treatment. Table 6.2 indicates the importance of tumor staging and other clinical and mpMR factors in therapeutic decision-making.

In daily practice, the use of mpMR focuses mainly on the differentiation of T2 and T3 tumor stages. Its utility in the discrimination between the different subcategories of T2 stages is limited because while mpMR has a relatively high sensitivity for detection of the index lesion (the larger and usually more aggressive lesion), it has relatively low sensitivity for detection of multifocal, smaller, and/or nonaggressive tumors [10, 11].

In the past, T3 tumors were considered unsuitable for surgery, but this attitude has changed. In this scenario, the surgeon encounters three main problems when performing radical prostatectomy: oncologic safety, preservation of urinary continence, and preservation of erectile function. The radiologist plays an important role in this setting and must provide the surgeon with useful information to allow avoidance of positive margins and to assist decision-making regarding neurovascular sparing, bearing in mind the aim of preserving urinary continence and erectile function. However, it is important to recognize the scope and limitations of mpMR. There are certain mpMR signs which are associated with a greater or lesser probability of ECE, but these signs are only indicative and not definitive. The surgeon must be aware of this when making surgical decisions.

Table 6.1 Tumor, node, and metastasis (TNM) classification of PCa (Sobin LH, G.M., Wittekind C., TNM classification of malignant tumors. UICC International Union Against Cancer. 7th edn. 2009. http://www.uicc.org/resources/tnm)

T – Primary tumor	
TX T0 T1	Primary tumor cannot be assessed No evidence of primary tumor Clinically inapparent tumor not palpable or visible by imaging
	T1a Tumor incidental histological finding in 5% or less of tissue resected T1b Tumor incidental histological finding in more than 5% of tissue resected T1c Tumor identified by needle biopsy (e.g., because of elevated PSA level)
T2	Tumor confined within the prostate[a]
	T2a Tumor involves one half of one lobe or less T2b Tumor involves more than half of one lobe, but not both lobes T2c Tumor involves both lobes
T3	Tumor extends through the prostatic capsule[b]
	T3a Extracapsular extension (unilateral or bilateral) including microscopic bladder neck involvement T3b Tumor invades seminal vesicle(s)
T4	Tumor is fixed or invades adjacent structures other than seminal vesicles: external sphincter, rectum, levator muscles, and/or pelvic wall
N – Regional lymph nodes[c]	
NX N0 N1	Regional lymph nodes cannot be assessed No regional lymph node metastasis Regional lymph node metastasis[d]
M – Distant metastasis[e]	
MX M0 M1	Distant metastasis cannot be assessed No distant metastasis Distant metastasis
	M1a Non-regional lymph node(s) M1b Bone(s) M1c Other site(s)

[a]*Tumor found in one or both lobes by needle biopsy, but not palpable or visible by imaging, is classified as T1c*

[b]*Invasion into the prostatic apex, or into (but not beyond) the prostate capsule, is not classified as pT3, but as pT2*

[c]*The regional lymph nodes are the nodes of the true pelvis, which essentially are the pelvic nodes below the bifurcation of the common iliac arteries*

[d]*Laterality does not affect the N-classification*

[e]*When more than one site of metastasis is present, the most advanced category should be used*

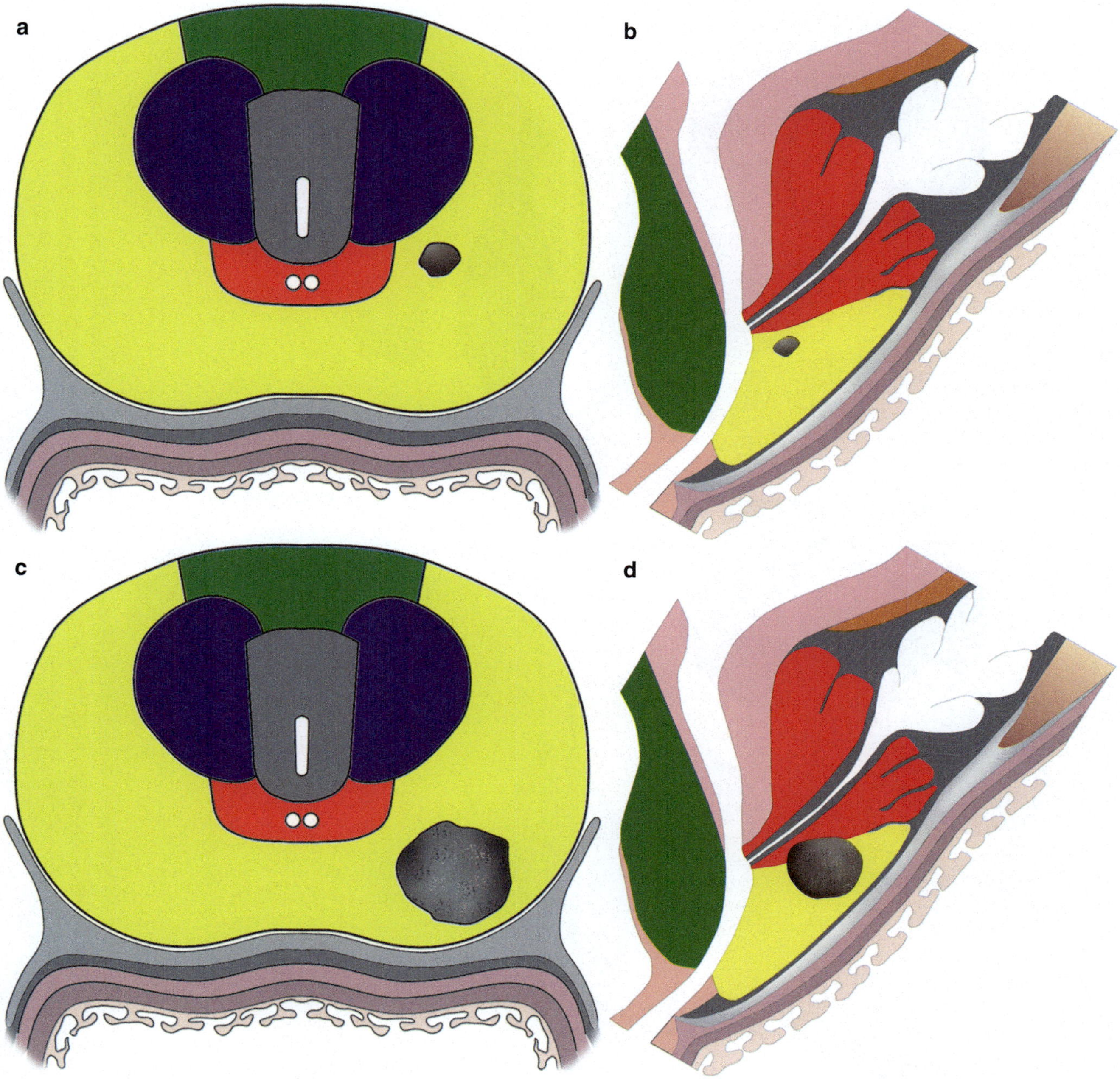

Fig 6.1 Graphic representation of the tumor score in TNM classification of PCa (as seen in Table 6.1). (**a**) Axial and (**b**) sagittal representation of T1PCa. (**c**) Axial and (**d**) sagittal representation of T2a PCa. (**e**) Axial and (**f**) sagittal representation of T2b PCa. (**g**) Axial representation of T2c PCa. (**h**) Axial and (**i**) sagittal representation of T3a PCa. (**j**) Sagittal representation of T3b PCa. (**k**) Axial and (**l**) sagittal representation of T4 PCa

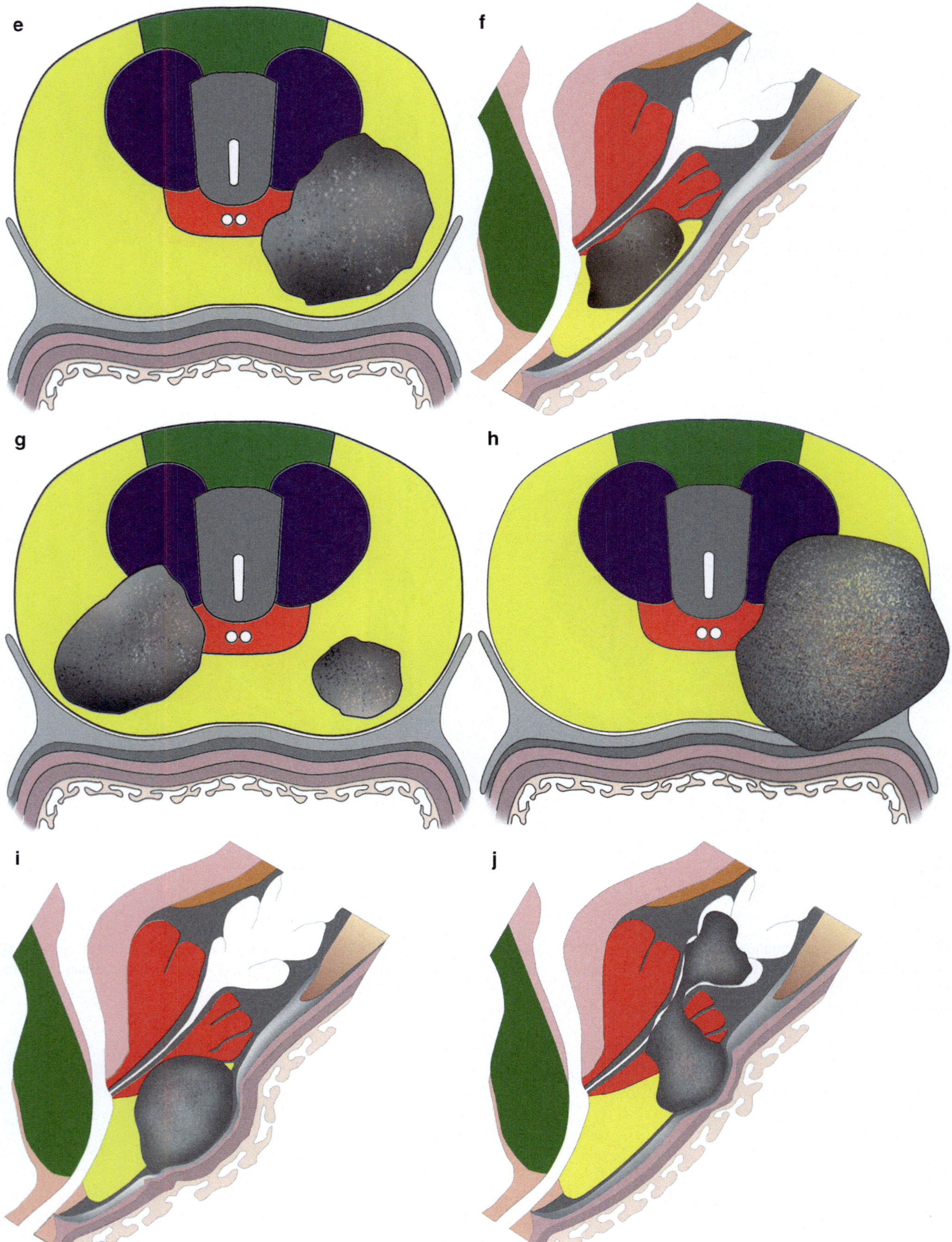

Fig 6.1 (continued)

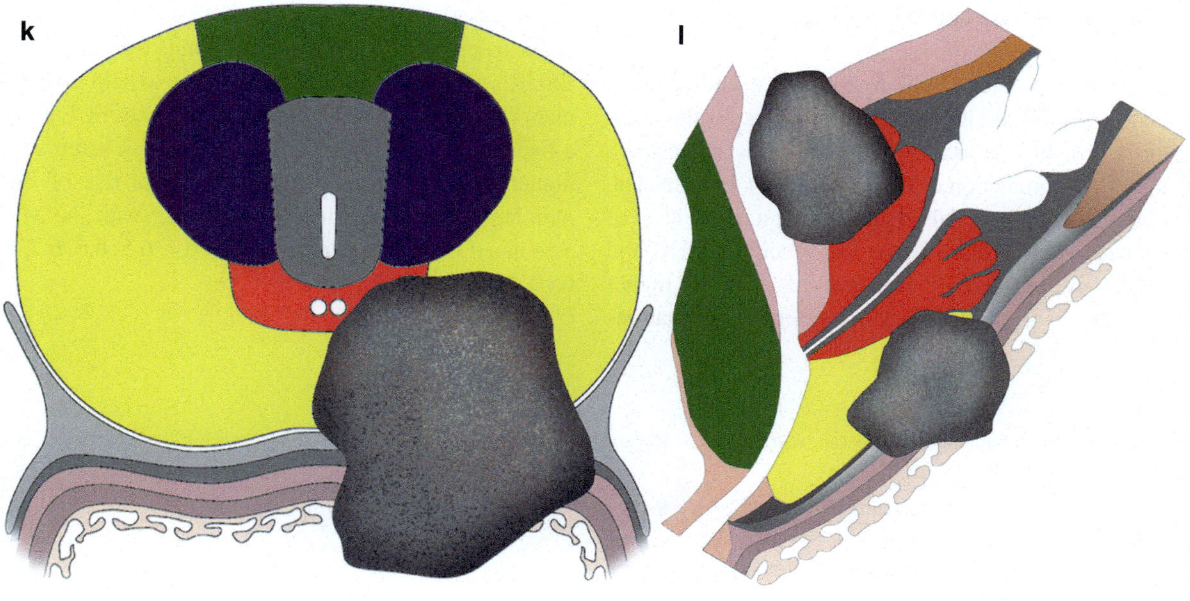

Fig 6.1 (continued)

Table 6.2 Implications of clinical and mpMRI factors for management of PCa, according to the EAU risk group classification

	Clinical factors	mpMRI factors	Clinical implications
Low risk – localized	PSA <10 ng/mL and GS <7 (ISUP grade 1) and cT1–2a	Characterization of lesion(s) size and PIRADS score Exclusion of cT3 disease	Suitability of patients for active surveillance protocols or focal therapy
Intermediate risk – localized	PSA 10–20 ng/mL or GS 7 (ISUP grade 2/3) or cT2b	Characterization of lesion(s) size, PIRADS score, and T stage (T2 vs. T3 disease) Exclusion of N+ disease	Suitability of patients for nerve-sparing approach during radical prostatectomy Assessment of lymphadenectomy extension during radical prostatectomy (if indicated) Planning of radiotherapy treatment and modality
High risk – localized	PSA >20 ng/mL or GS >7 (ISUP grade 4/5) or cT2c	Characterization of lesion(s) size, PIRADS score, and T stage (T2 vs. T3 disease) Identification of N+ Exclusion of M+ disease	Suitability of patients for curative treatment Assessment of lymphadenectomy extension during radical prostatectomy (if indicated) Assessment of EBRT treatment fields in prostatic fossa and pelvic areas
High risk – locally advanced	Any PSA Any GS cT3–4 or cN+ Any ISUP grade	Characterization of N+ number, volume, and sites Identification of M+ disease	Suitability of patients for multimodal treatment Assessment of lymphadenectomy extension during radical prostatectomy (if indicated) Assessment of EBRT treatment fields in prostatic fossa and pelvic areas
Metastatic	Any PSA Any T stage Any N+/M+ Any ISUP grade	Characterization and measurement of N+ and/or M+ disease	Indication for appropriate systemic treatment Assessment of response to systemic treatment

Abbreviation: Prostate-Specific Antigen (PSA), Gleason Score (GS), International Society of Urological Pathology (ISUP), External Beam Radiation Therapy (EBRT)

6.3 Signs associated with ECE

The evaluation of possible ECE is qualitative and requires expert readers [9]. While a complete consensus on the signs related to ECE of PCa is lacking, the ESUR has suggested a scoring system for prediction of ECE (Table 6.3). Boesen et al. [12] have evaluated this model and found that a cutoff level of ≥4 has the best relation of sensitivity and specificity (0.81 and 0.78, respectively) but that a cutoff level of ≥3 has a higher predictive negative value (0.95). More extensive evaluations are necessary in order to define the best way to predict ECE when using mpMRI. In the meantime, we consider that the ESUR's scoring system is a good option to help in the management of patients with PCa. The probability of ECE is scored on a five-point scale, providing an ordinal risk score scale, with higher scores corresponding to the higher risk of ECE. The radiologist must accordingly be familiar with the MRI signs associated with ECE (Figs. 6.2, 6.3, 6.4, 6.5, 6.6, 6.7, 6.8, 6.9, 6.10, 6.11, and 6.12).

Table 6.3 ESUR MRI prostate guidelines risk scoring of extracapsular extension [11]

Criteria	Tumor characteristics	Score
Extracapsular extension	Capsular abutment	1
	Capsular irregularity, retraction, or thickening	3
	Neurovascular bundle thickening	4
	Bulge or loss of capsule	4
	Measurable extracapsular disease	5

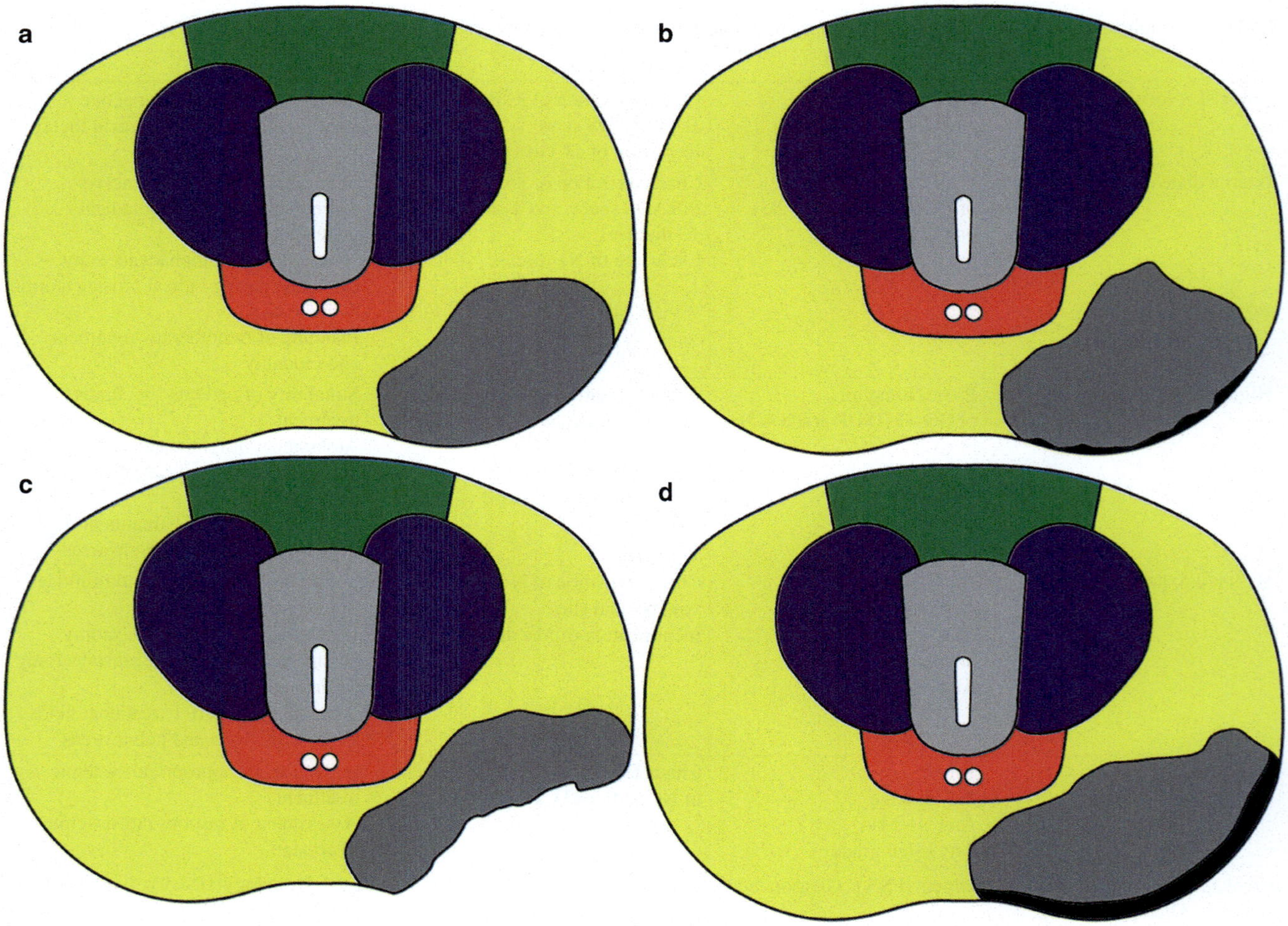

Fig 6.2 Graphic representation of the ESUR MR prostate guidelines risk scoring of ECE (as seen in Table 6.3). (**a**) Capsular abutment. (**b**) Capsular irregularity. (**c**) Capsular retraction. (**d**) Capsular thickening. (**e**) Neurovascular bundle thickening. (**f**) Bulge of capsule. (**g**) Loss of capsule. (**h**) Measurable extracapsular disease

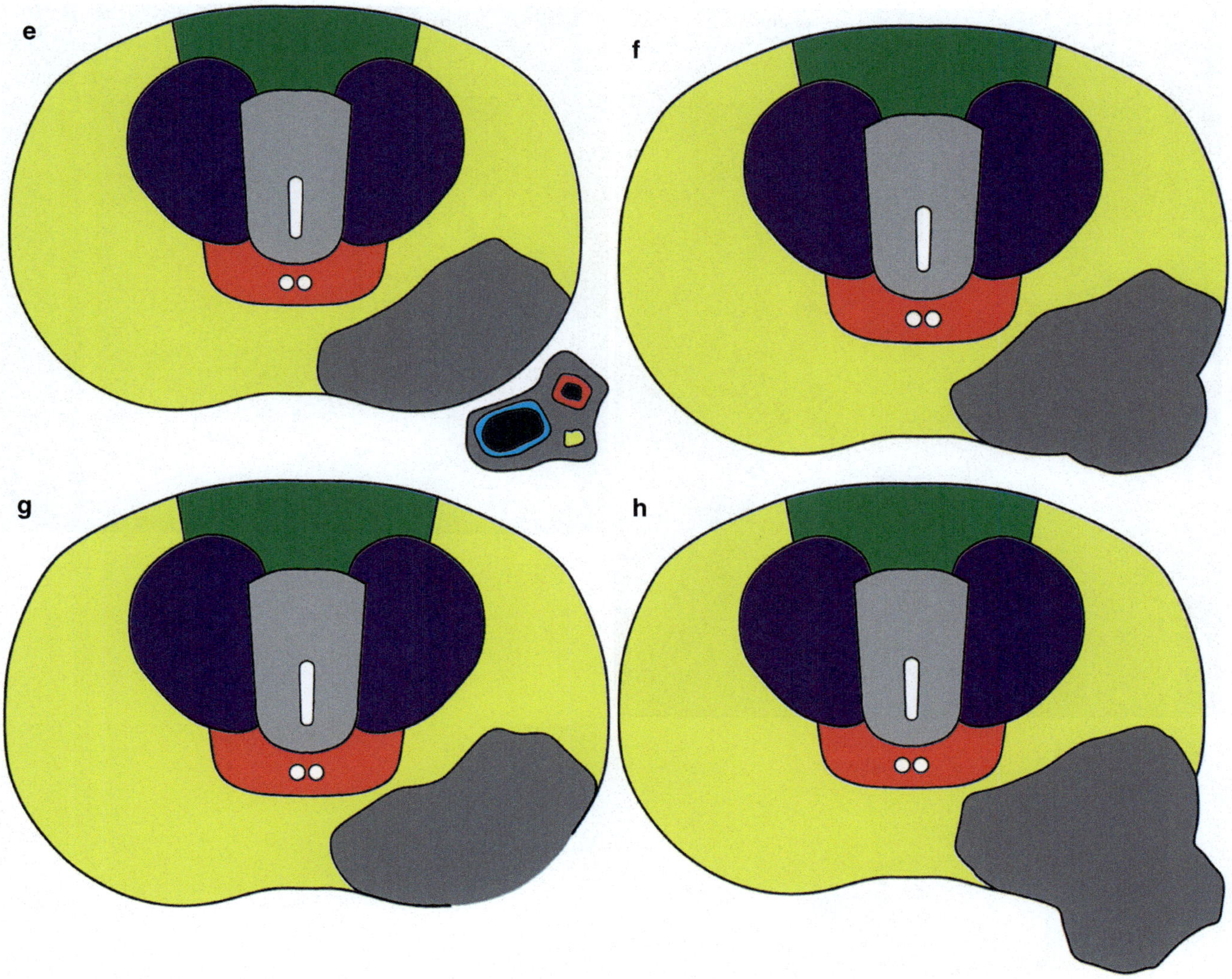

Fig 6.2 (continued)

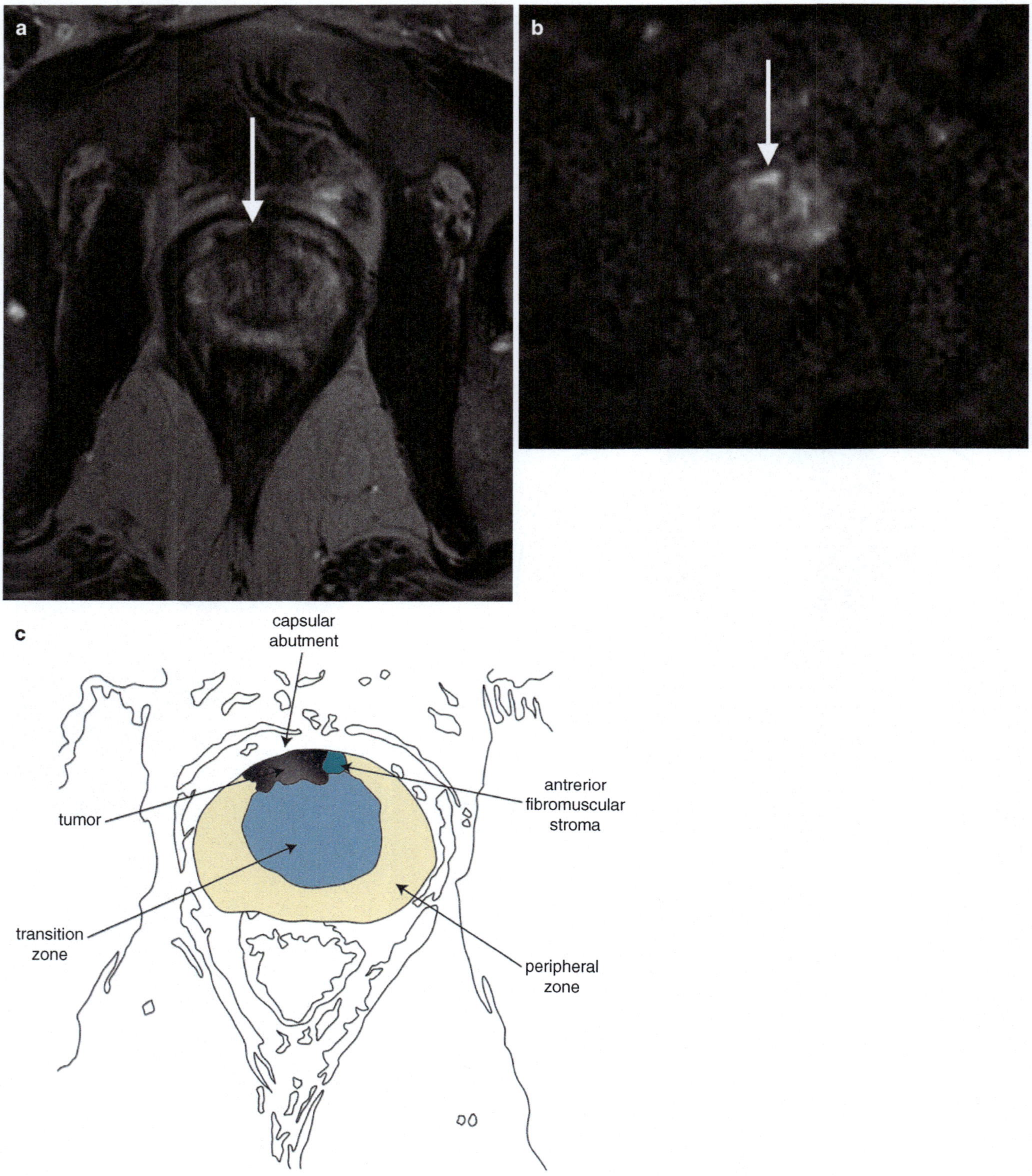

Fig 6.3 Example of possible extracapsular extension (ECE) in a 59-year-old patient with a PSA of 8 ng/ml. (**a**) Axial T2-weighted image of the prostate at the midgland shows an ill-defined and hypointense area in the anterior horn of the right peripheral zone, which also shows significant restriction of diffusion on DW images (**b**), compatible with a PIRADS 4 lesion (*white arrow*). Note that there is a contact between the suspicious lesion and the prostatic capsule in the anterior margin, a finding suggestive of ECE (capsular abutment – ESUR Score 1, low risk of ECE). (**c**) Graphic correlation. Surgical specimen (**d**) showed a pT2c Gleason 3 + 4 PCa with surgical limits free of tumor (*black arrow*)

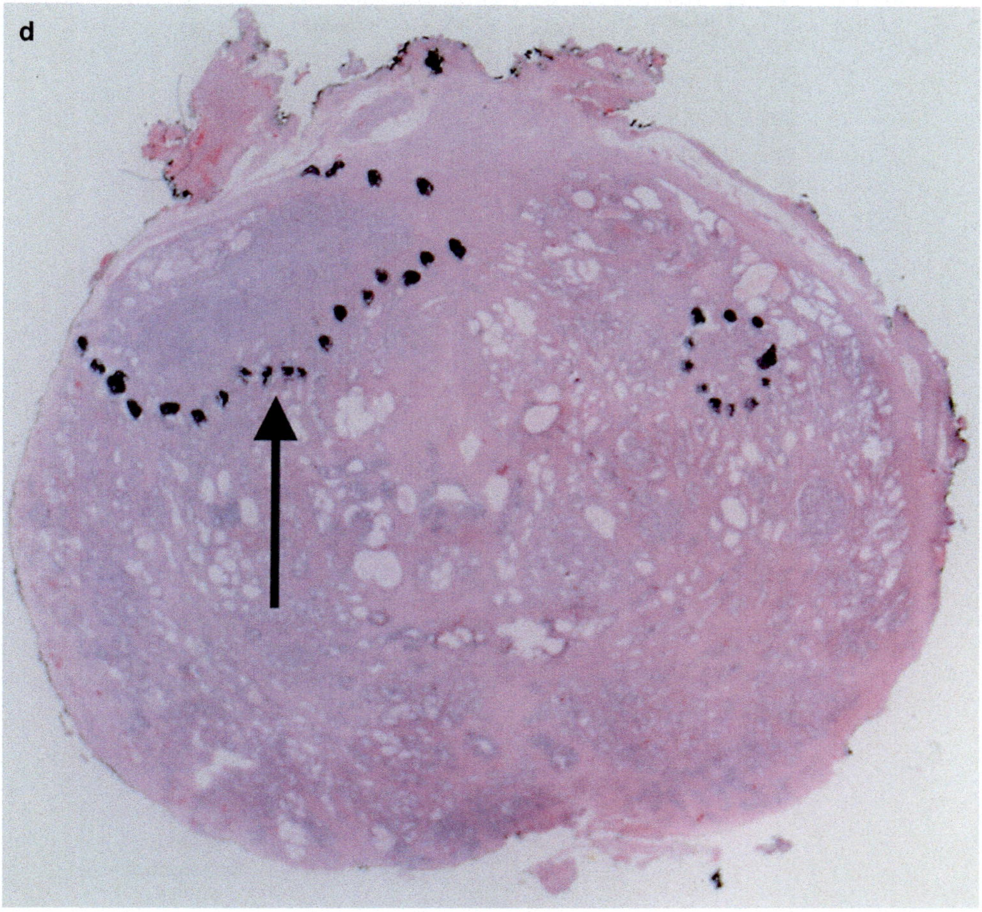

Fig 6.3 (continued)

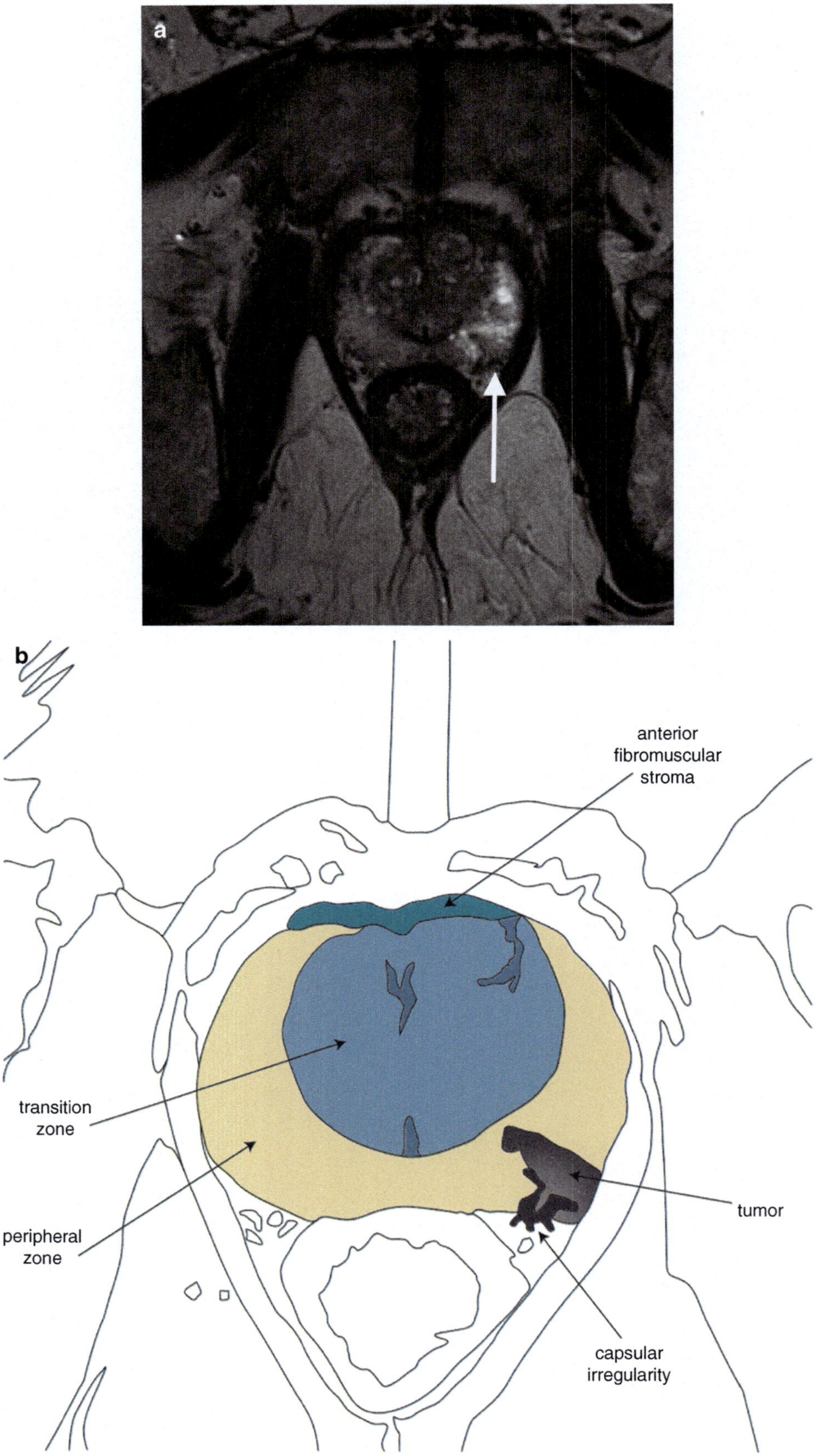

Fig 6.4 Example of capsular irregularity as a sign of ECE in a 63-year-old patient with a PSA of 6.39 ng/ml. (**a**) Axial T2-weighted image of the prostate at the midgland shows in the left peripheral zone a visible irregularity of the prostatic capsule (*white arrow*) that was reported as possible ECE (ESUR Score 3, moderate risk of ECE). (**b**) Graphic correlation. (**c**) Surgical specimen confirmed a pT3a Gleason 3 + 4 PCa, with minimal microscopic ECE (*black arrow*)

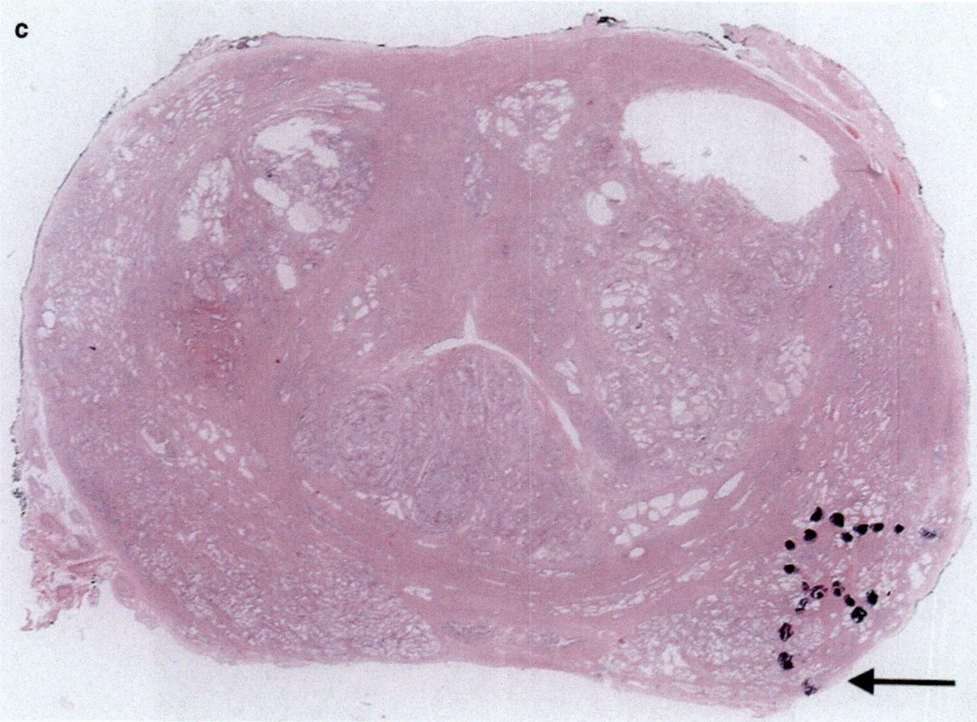

Fig 6.4 (continued)

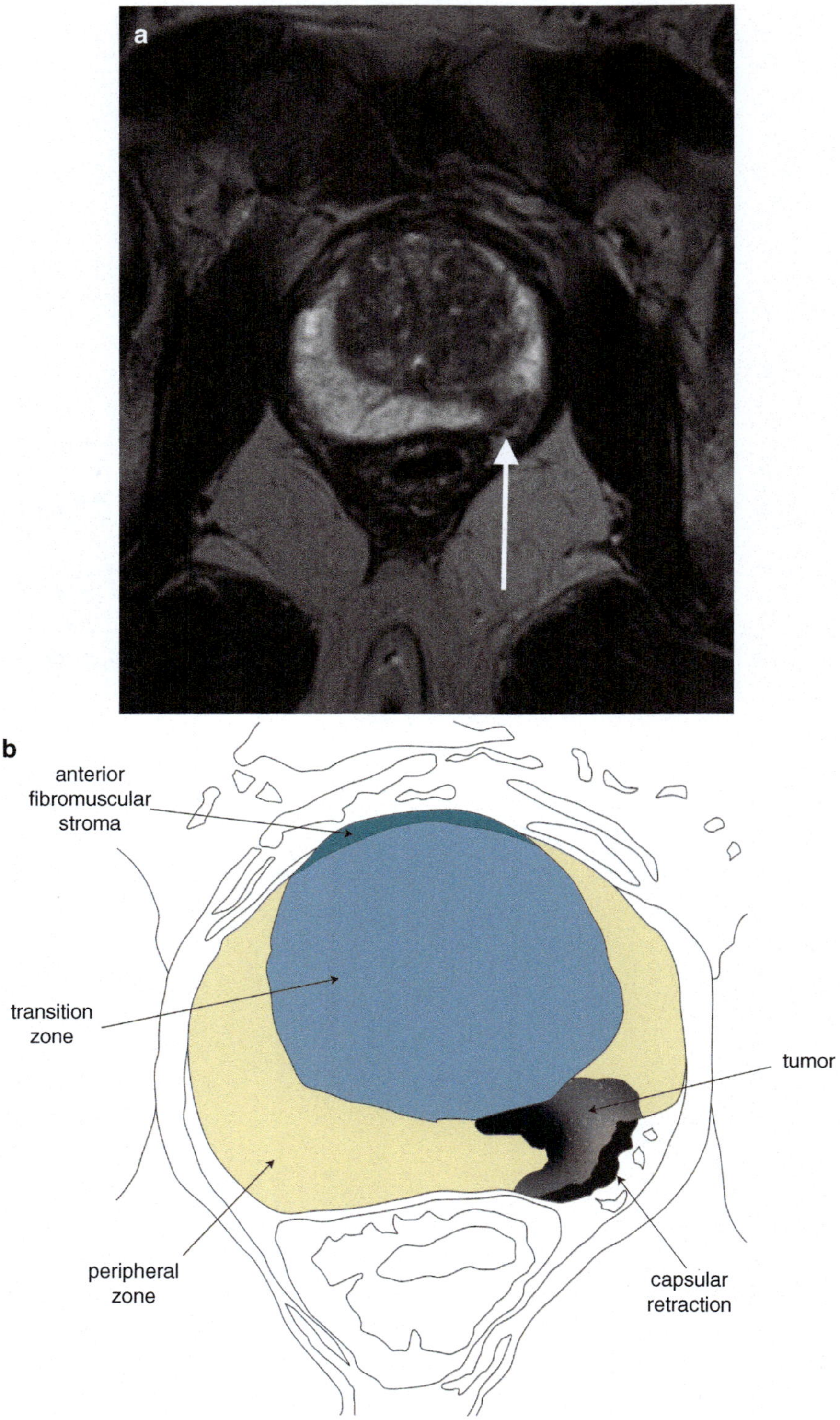

Fig 6.5 Capsular retraction as a sign of ECE in a 61-year-old patient with a PSA of 10 ng/ml. (**a**) Axial T2-weighted image of the prostate at the midgland-apex demonstrates a nodular hypointensity in the left peripheral zone with significant restriction of the diffusion (*not shown*), compatible with a PIRADS 4 lesion. There is a visible asymmetry in the margins of the peripheral zone of both lobes, with a notorious retraction of the left capsule (*white arrow*) that alters the contour of the left peripheral zone. This finding should be reported as a sign of ECE (ESUR Score 3, moderate risk of ECE). (**b**) Graphic correlation. (**c**) Surgical specimen confirmed a pT3b Gleason 4 + 3 PCa, with ECE in the periprostatic fat surrounding the area described in the MRI (*black arrow*)

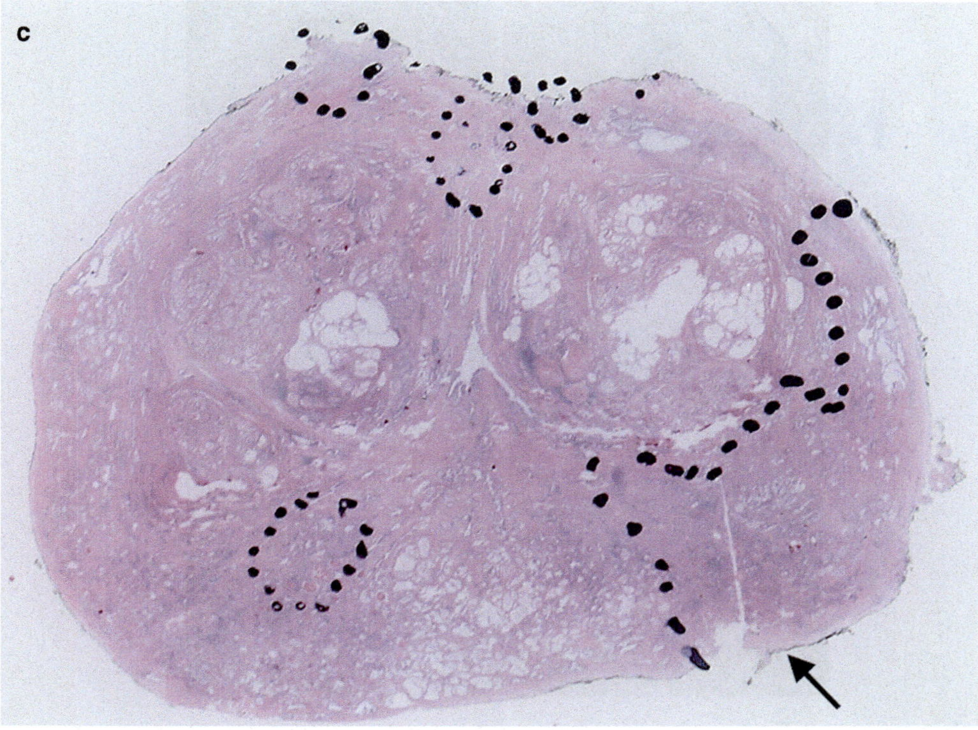

Fig 6.5 (continued)

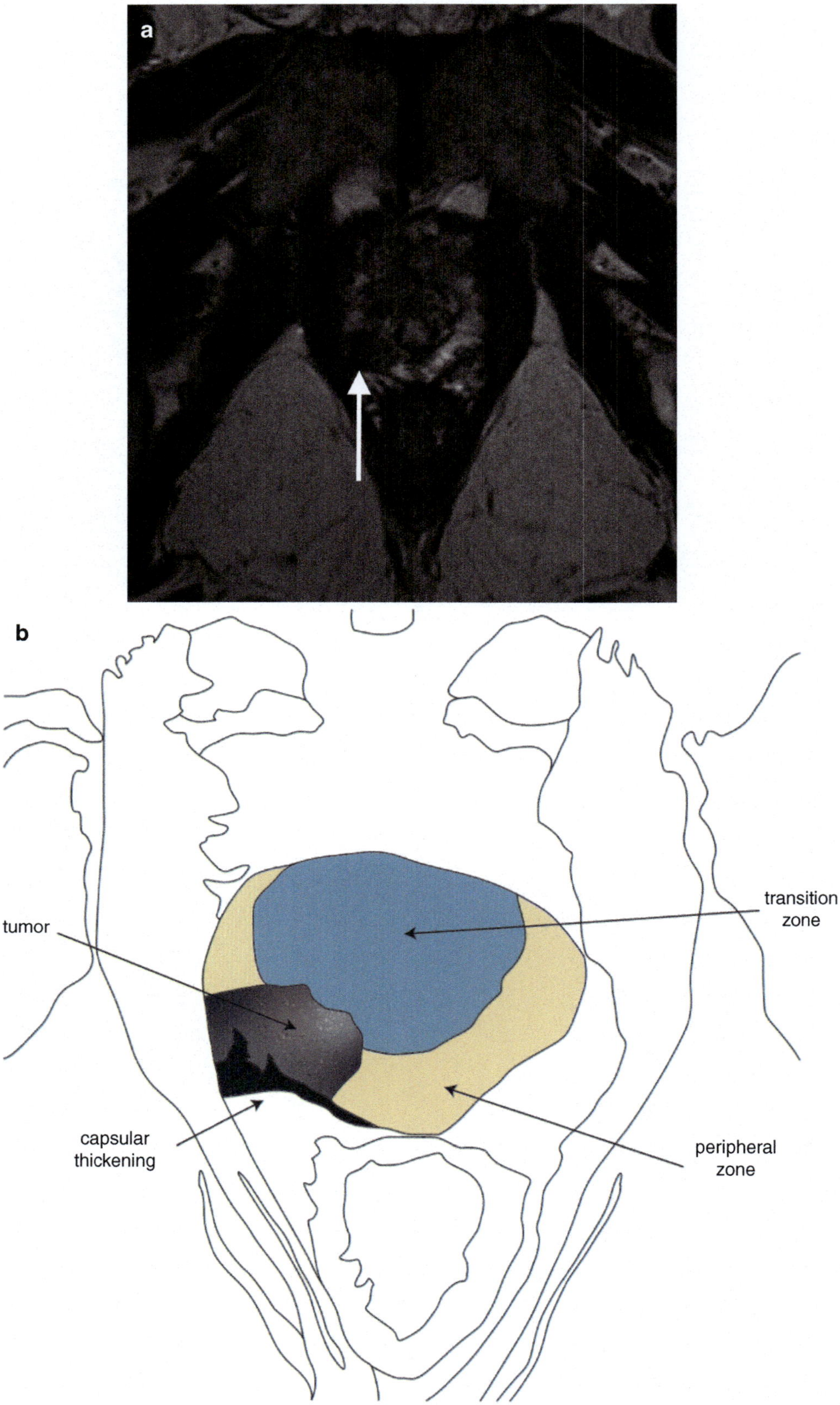

Fig 6.6 Thickening of the capsule in ECE in a 61-year-old patient with a PSA of 5.21 ng/ml. (**a**) Axial T2-weighted image of the prostate at the apex shows a hypointense nodule in the right peripheral zone, with characteristics on the rest of the MpMRI compatible with a PIRADS 4 lesion (*not shown*). White arrow points a focal thickening of the capsule in the right lobe that can be compared to the normal capsule surrounding the left peripheral zone (ESUR Score 3, moderate risk of ECE). (**b**) Graphic correlation. (**c**) Surgical specimen showed a pT2c Gleason 4 + 3 PCa with tumoral compromise of surgical limits in the referred zone (*black arrow*)

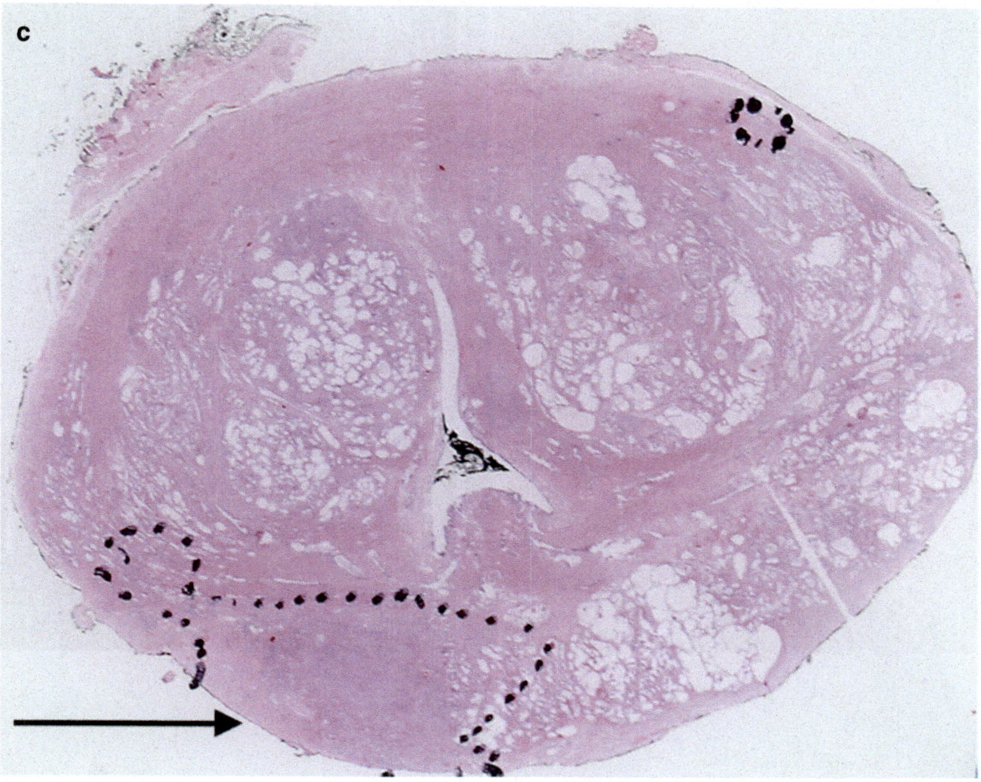

Fig 6.6 (continued)

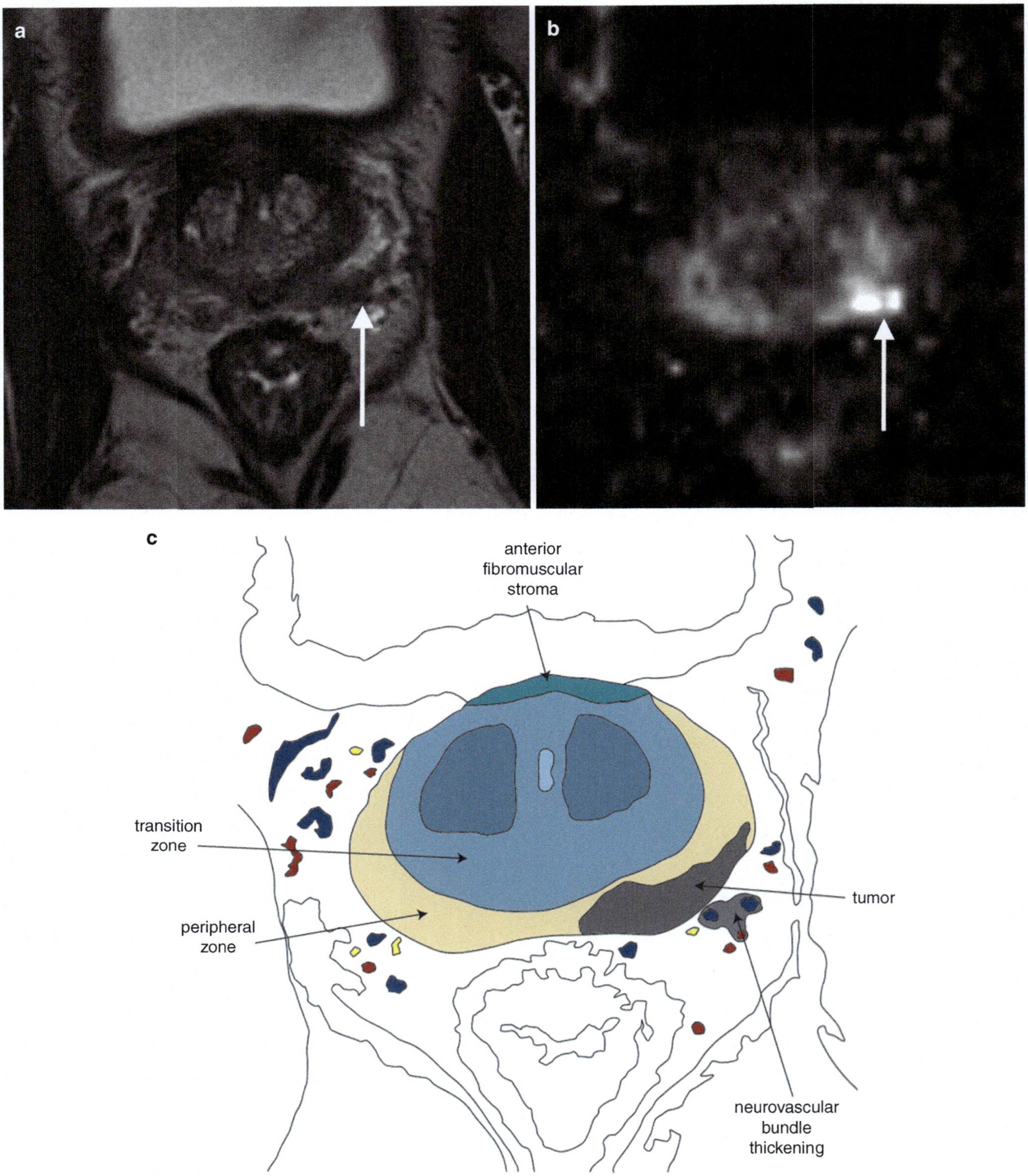

Fig 6.7 Neurovascular bundle thickening as a sign of ECE in a 68-year-old patient with a PSA of 4.76 ng/ml. (**a**) Axial T2-weighted image and (**b**) DW image of the prostate at the union of the base and the midgland show a T2-hypointense nodular lesion in the left peripheral zone, with significant restriction of diffusion in DWI, compatible with a PIRADS 4 lesion. There also is a thickening of the capsule that extends to the left neurovascular bundle (*white arrow*), which also seems enlarged compared to the contralateral bundle (ESUR Score 4, high risk of ECE). The normal right neurovascular bundle can be seen as hypointense dots in the fat located lateral to the right peripheral zone and the rectum. (**c**) Graphic correlation. (**d**) Surgical specimen confirmed a pT3a Gleason 4 + 3 PCa, with infiltration of the left neurovascular bundle (*black arrow*)

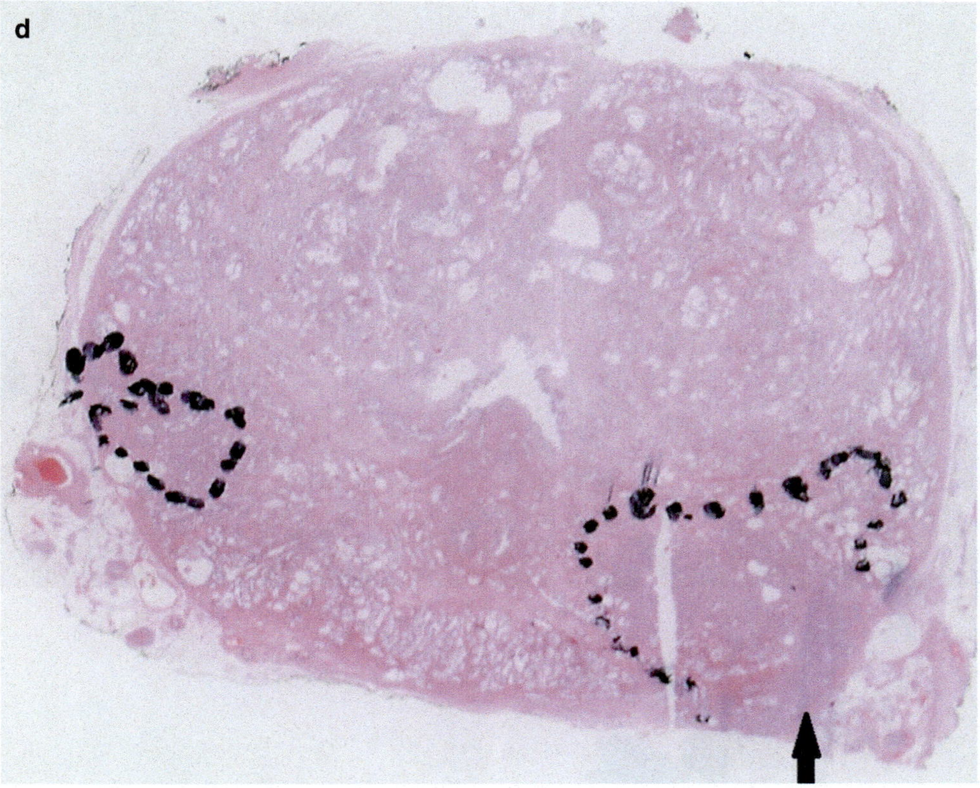

Fig 6.7 (continued)

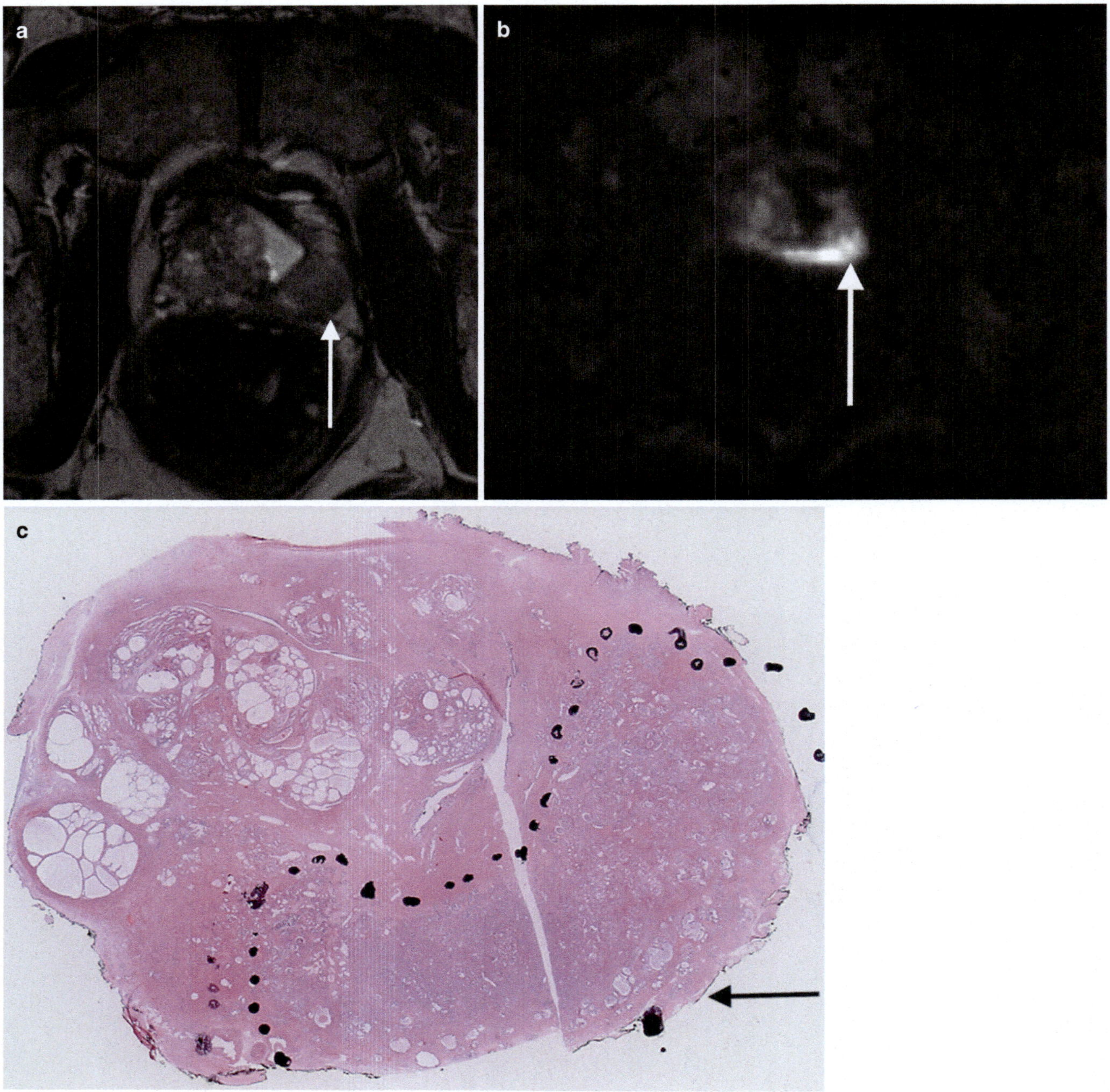

Fig 6.8 Capsular bulging in a 62-year-old patient with a PSA of 8.46 ng/ml. (**a**) Axial T2-weighted image and (**b**) DW image of the prostate at the midgland-apex level show a PIRADS 4 lesion in the left peripheral zone. There is also a notorious asymmetry between the two lobes, with an enlarged left lobe secondary to the referred lesion and an associated bulging of the capsule (*white arrow*), a finding that may suggest ECE (ESUR Score 4, high risk of ECE). (**c**) Surgical specimen confirmed a pT3a Gleason 3 + 4 PCa with extensive infiltration of the periprostatic fat (*black arrow*)

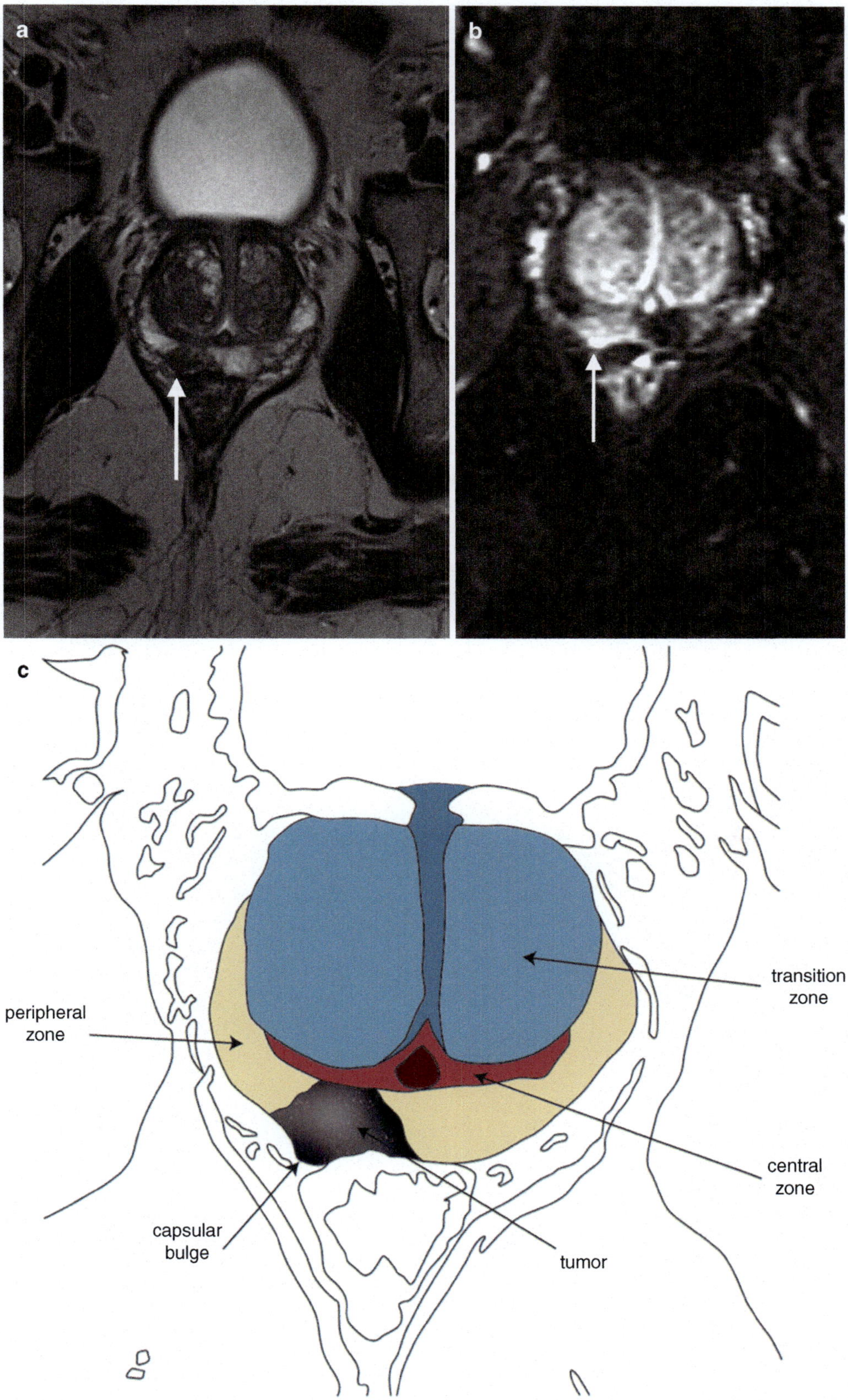

Fig 6.9 Example of capsular bulging as a predictor of ECE in a 68-year-old patient with a PSA of 9.26 ng/ml. (**a**) Axial T2-weighted image at the level of the midgland shows a nodular hypointense area in the right peripheral zone, with characteristics of a PIRADS 4 lesion in the MpMRI (*not shown*). Please note the focal capsular bulging (*white arrow*), a finding better seen on the DCE images (**b**) (ESUR Score 4, high risk of ECE). (**c**) Graphic representation. (**d**) Surgical specimen confirmed a pT3a Gleason 3 + 4 PCa with infiltration of the right periprostatic fat (*black arrow*)

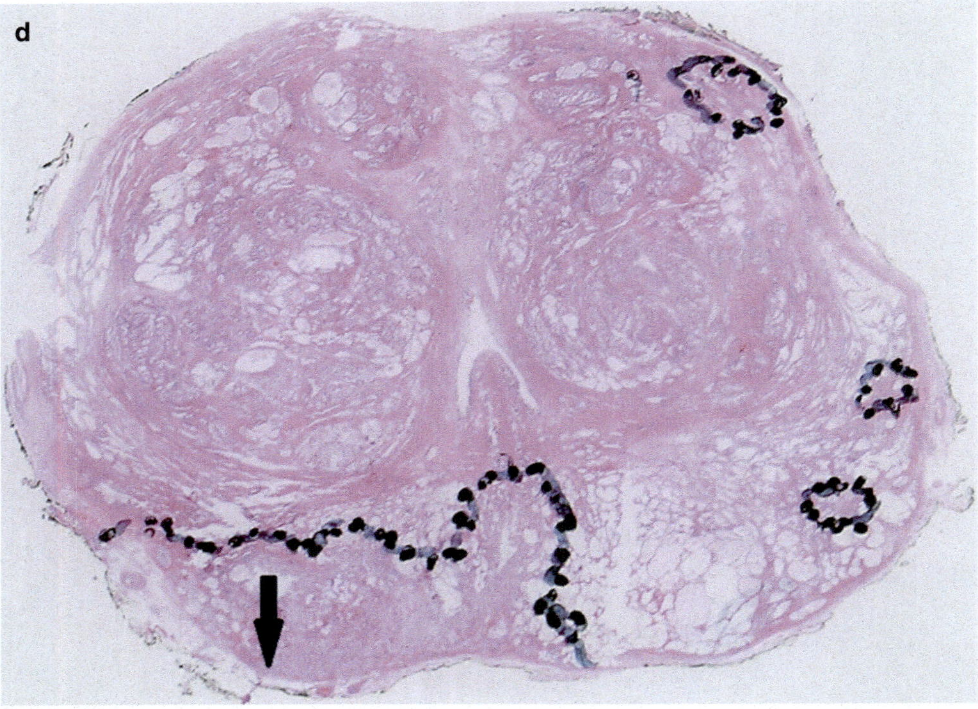

Fig 6.9 (continued)

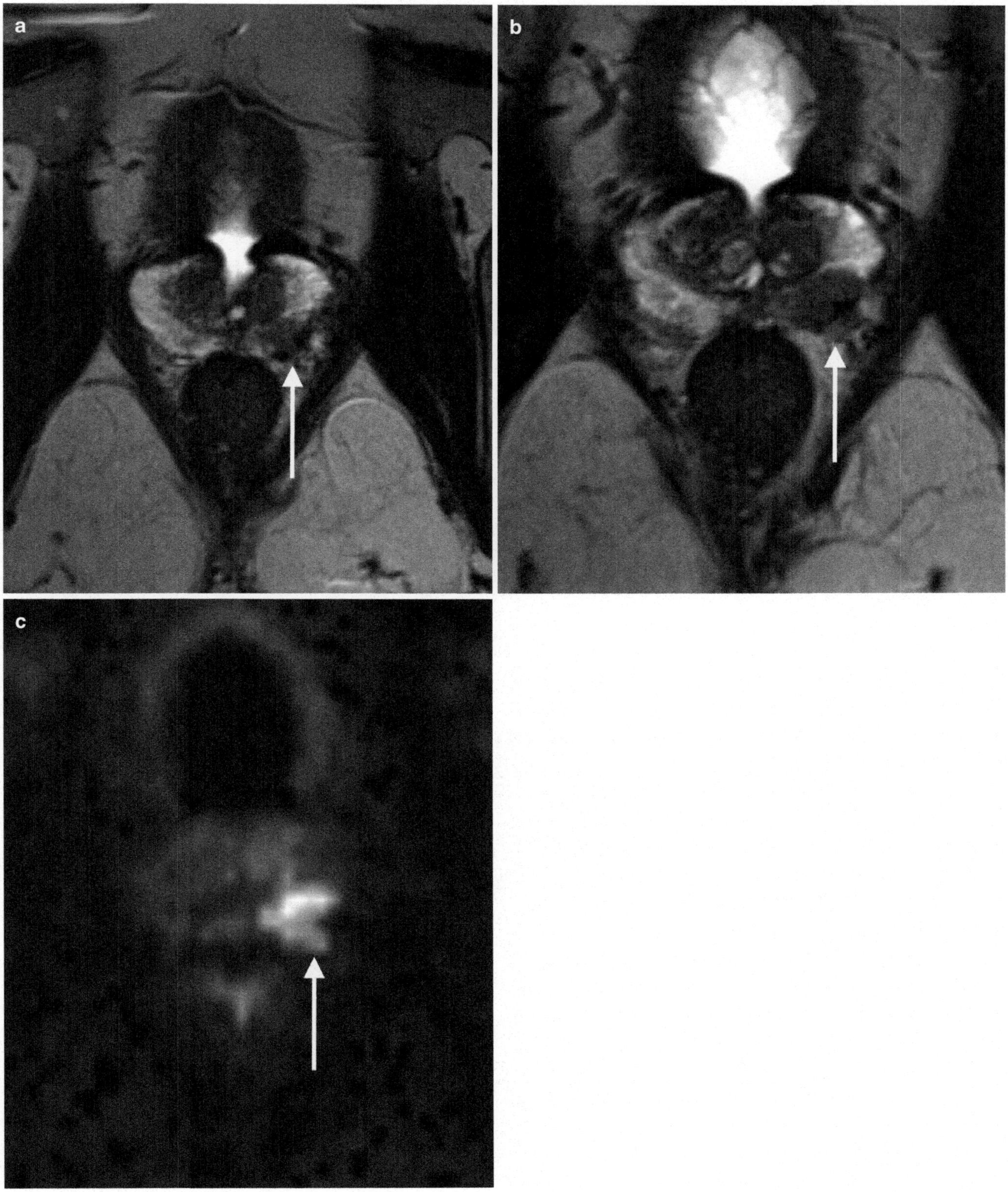

Fig 6.10 Measurable ECE in a 69-year-old patient with a PSA of 16 ng/ml. (**a**, **b**) Axial T2-weighted images and (**c**) DW images of the prostate at the midgland at different levels show a PIRADS 5 lesion in the left peripheral zone. However, in (**a**, **b**) the zone of hypointensity can be seen extending beyond the capsule toward the periprostatic fat with an interruption of the capsule (*white arrows*) (ESUR Score 4, high risk of ECE). In the DW images, the ECE can be measurable, a finding highly suggestive of ECE (ESUR Score 5, high risk of ECE). (**d**, **e**) Graphic representation at the level of (**a**, **b**), respectively. (**f**, **g**) Surgical specimen confirmed a pT3a Gleason 4 + 5 PCa with infiltration of the periprostatic fat of up to 4 mm (*black arrows*)

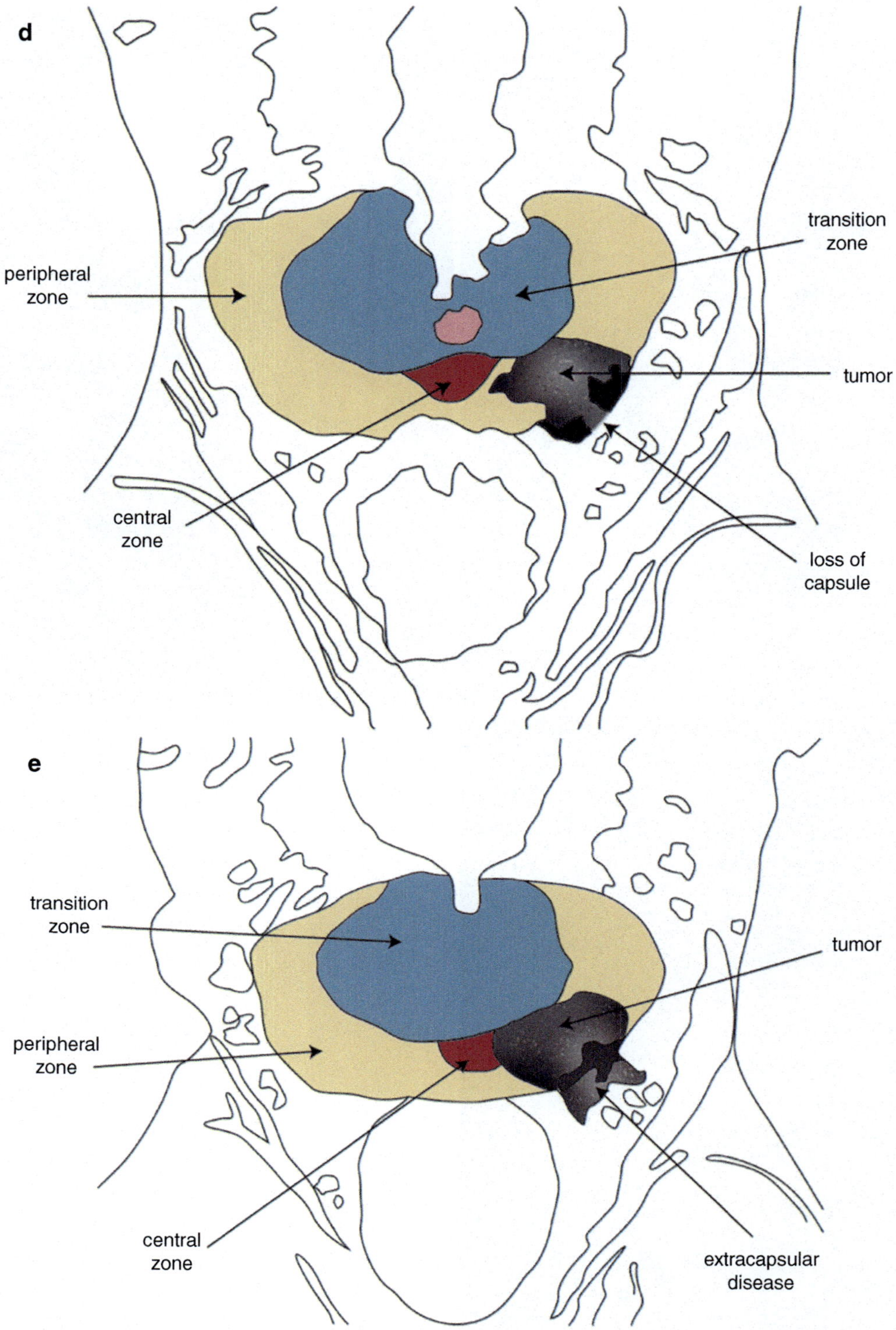

Fig 6.10 (continued)

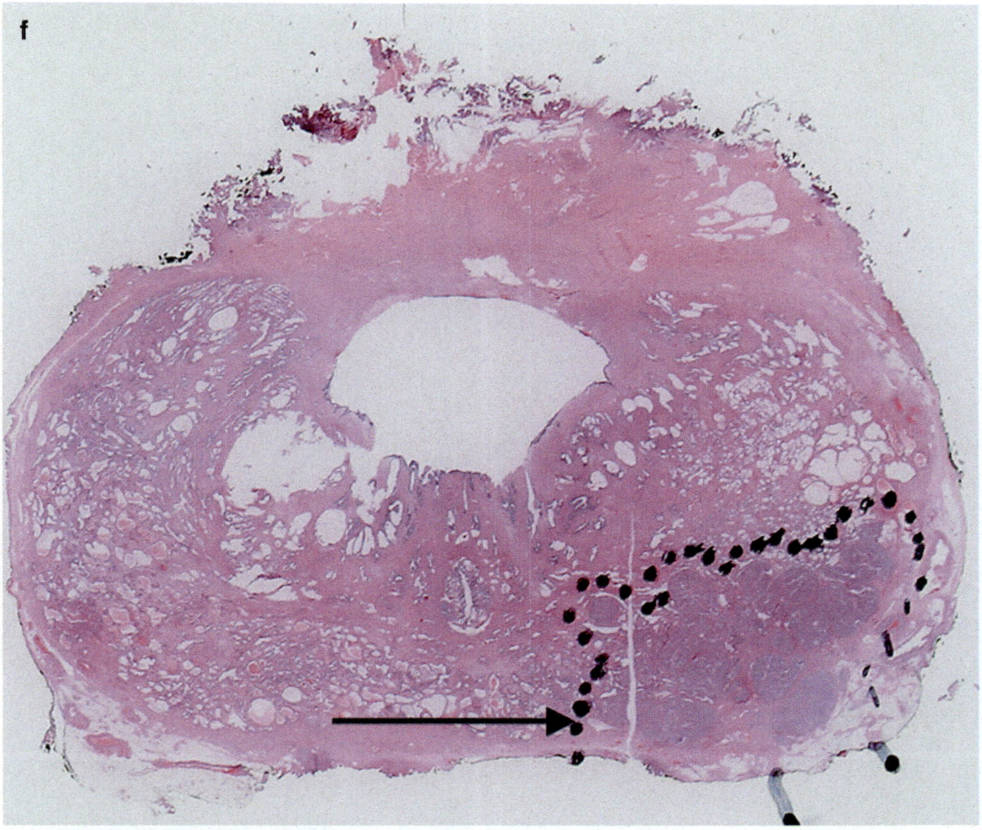

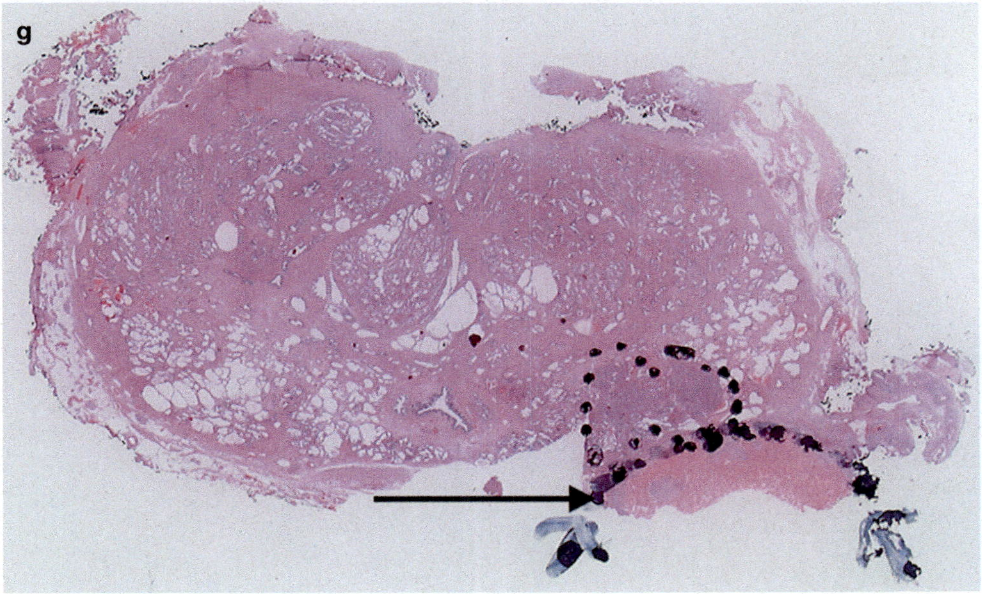

Fig 6.10 (continued)

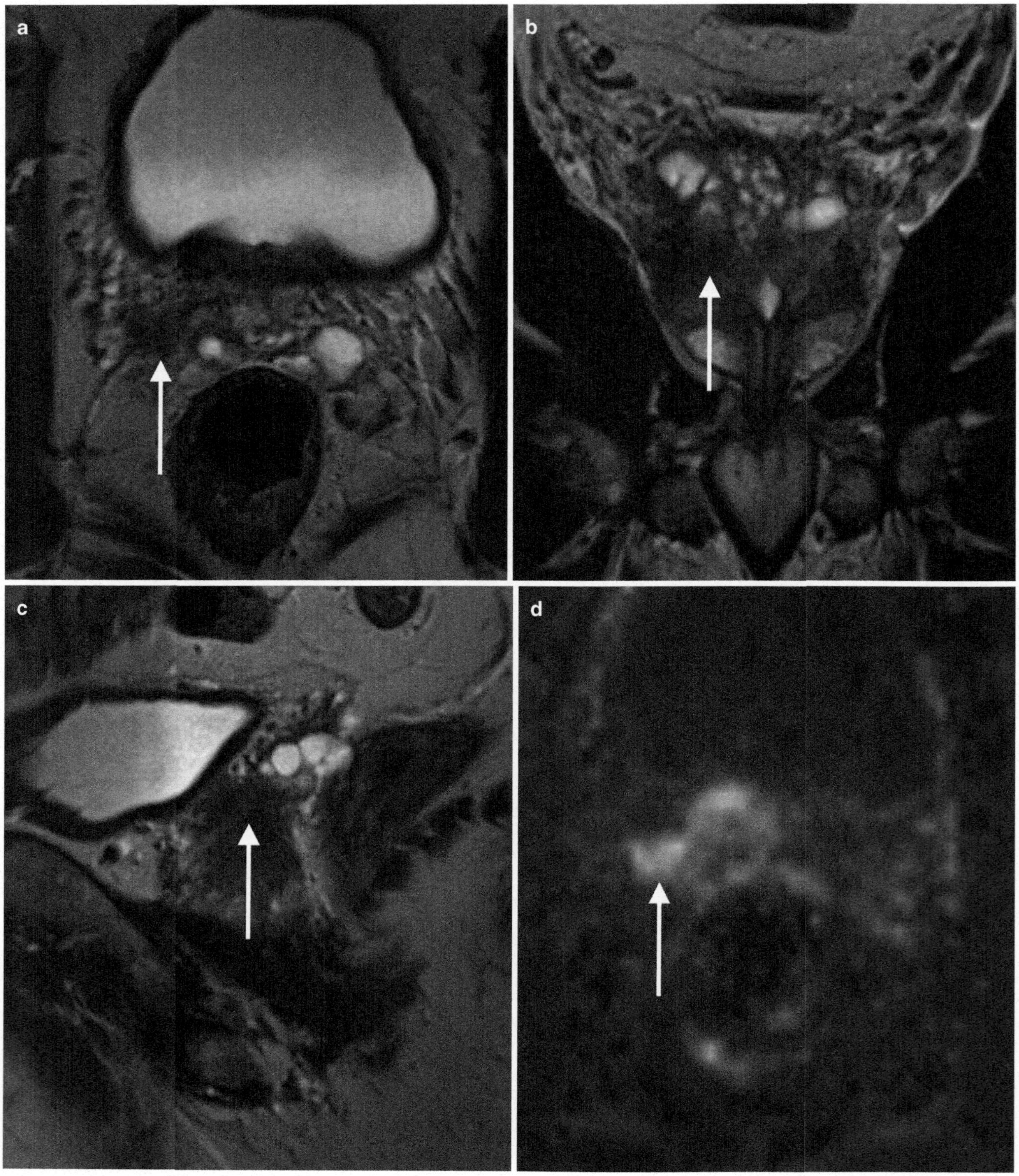

Fig 6.11 Invasion of seminal vesicles (T3b disease) in a 60-year-old patient with a PSA of 4.6 ng/ml. (**a**) Axial, (**b**) coronal, and (**c**) sagittal T2-weighted images show tumoral invasion of the right seminal vesicle extending from a PCa located in the right prostatic base (partially seen as a hypointense lesion in B). The right seminal vesicle presents an ill-defined abnormal hypointensity in its most caudal segment, which also presents restriction to the diffusion in axial DW images (**d**) (*white arrows*). Please note the normal hyperintensity of the rest of the right and the left seminal vesicles. (**e**) Graphic representation. (**f**) Surgical specimen confirmed a pT3b Gleason 4 + 4 PCa with infiltration of the right seminal vesicle (*black arrow*)

e

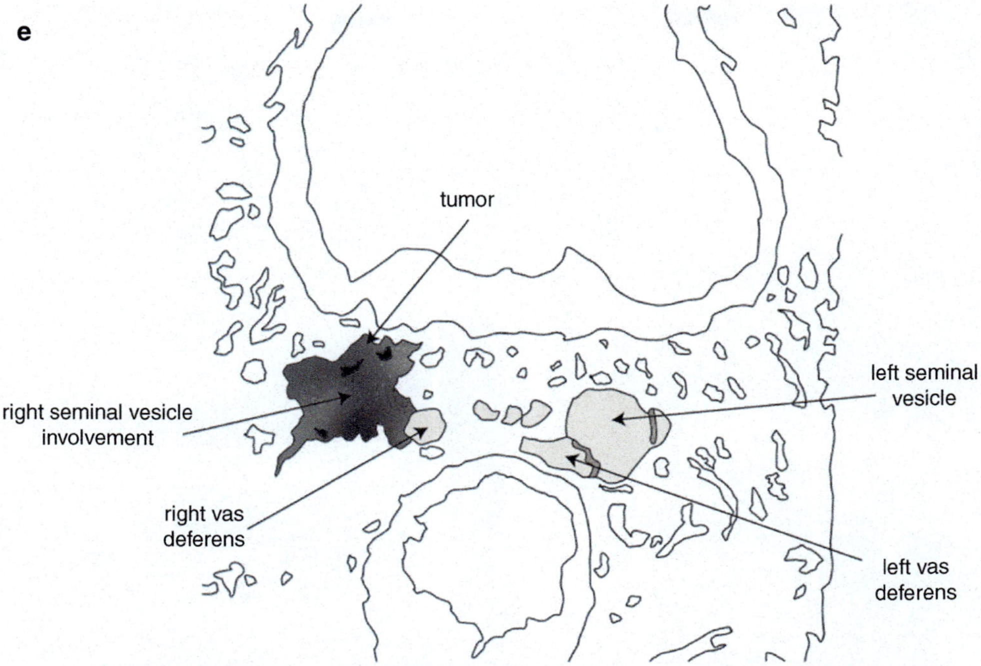

f

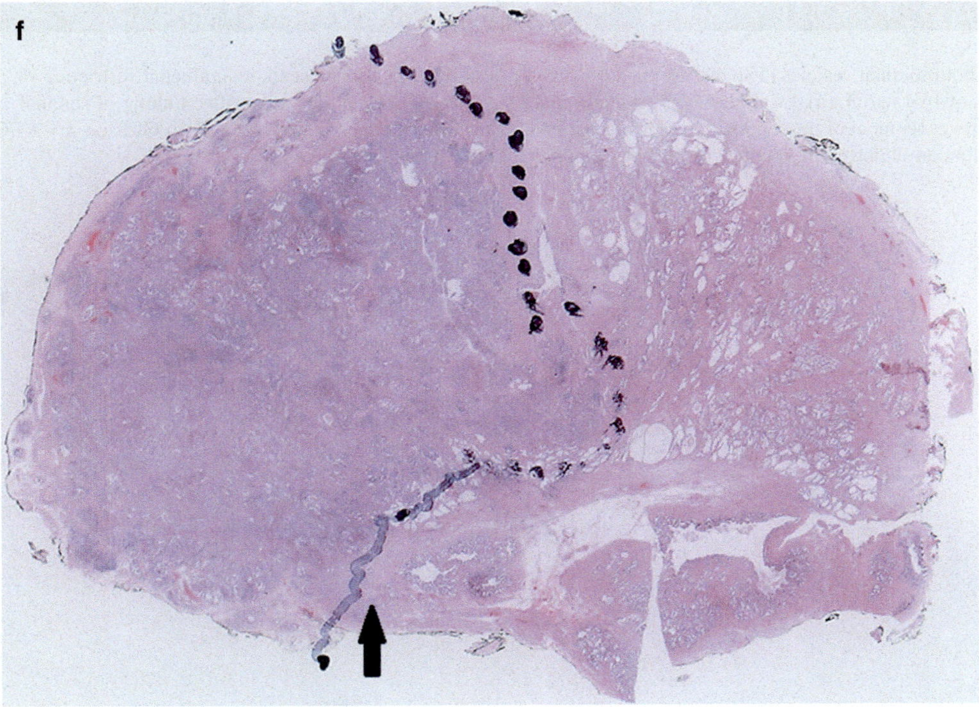

Fig 6.11 (continued)

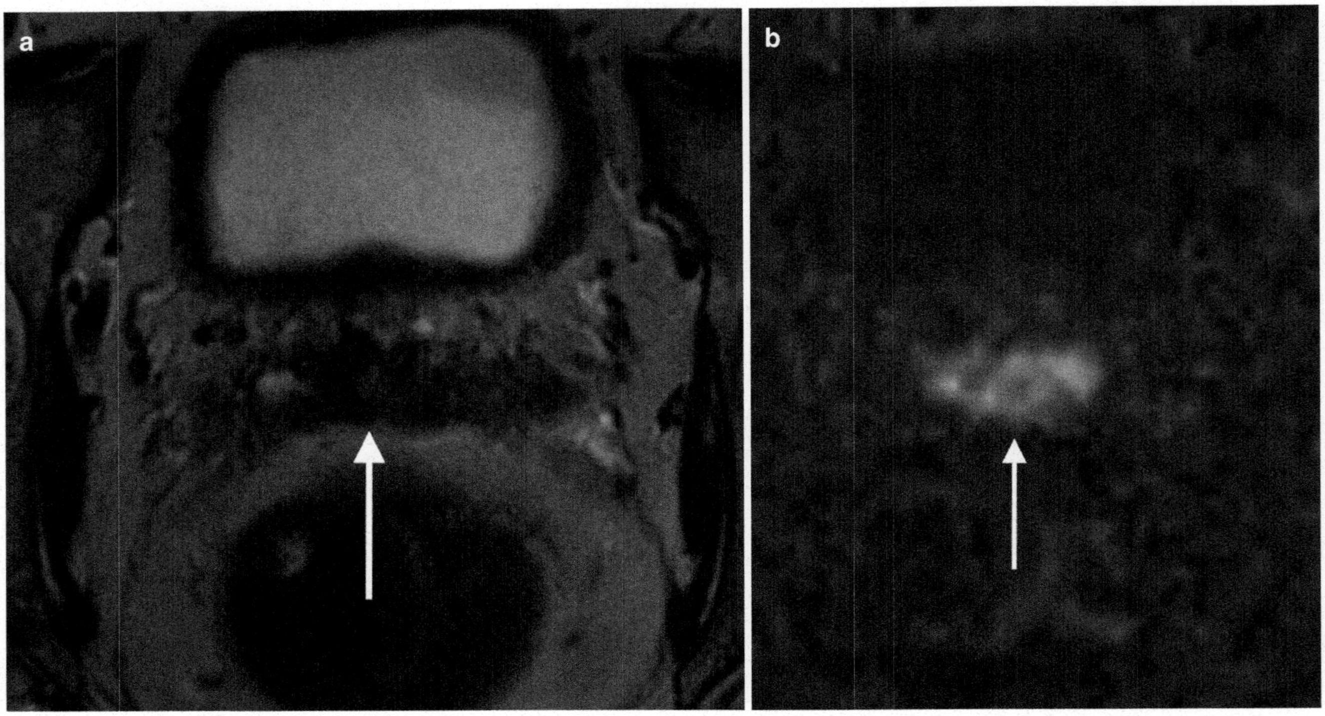

Fig 6.12 Invasion of both seminal vesicles (T3b disease) in a 67-year-old patient with a PSA of 16.1 ng/ml. (**a**) Axial T2-weighted image and (**b**) DW image of the lower segment of the seminal vesicles in a patient with a known PCa show an abnormal hypointensity of both seminal vesicles that also presents a significant restriction of diffusion (*white arrows*). This is a very suggestive finding of seminal vesicle invasion. Surgical specimen confirmed a pT3b Gleason 4 + 4 PCa with infiltration of both seminal vesicles

6.4 Focal Versus Established ECE

It is important to differentiate between focal and established ECE: Focal ECE is defined as a few neoplastic glands outside the prostate and has a better prognosis than established ECE. mpMR is a limited technique for detection of focal ECE. Established ECE is defined as anything more than a few glands. A positive surgical margin in this context is associated with a worse prognosis. The accuracy of mpMR is higher in these cases.

6.5 Sensitivity and Specificity of mpMR for Staging

Rooij et al. have published the most recent meta-analysis concerning the use of mpMRI for local staging of PCa [13]. The authors analyzed the databases from 2000 up to August 2014. This meta-analysis is one of the current pillars for understanding the advantages and limitations of mpMRI as a tool in the management of patients with PCa.

The meta-analysis of Rooij et al. clearly demonstrates that mpMRI is a technique with low sensitivity and high specificity for local staging (Table 6.4). The sensitivity in detection of ECE is influenced by the experience of the reader (being lower for less experienced readers); in contrast, the specificity is more stable and less conditioned by this factor.

All physicians involved in the management of PCa must understand these concepts and apply them in daily practice. For example, consider the case of a patient who has a lesion in the peripheral zone, posterior area, and left lobe, with a Gleason score of 3 + 4 and without mpMR signs of ECE. The surgeon ideally wants to preserve neurovascular bundles. The question is: Can he or she do so in such a case? Because mpMR has low sensitivity for the detection of ECE, it is reasonable, if feasible, to perform an intraoperative frozen section on the left side to confirm the presence of a negative margin. On the right side, because mpMR is a technique with a high predictive negative value for detection of clinically significant PCa, it is reasonable to preserve neurovascular bundles without performing an intraoperative frozen section.

Table 6.4 Results of the meta-analysis by Rooij et al. [13] regarding the sensitivity and specificity of mpMRI for local staging of PCa. ECE, extracapsular extension; SVI, seminal vesical invasion

	Sensitivity	Specificity
ECE	57 (95% CI 0.49–0.64)	91 (95% CI 0.88–0.93)
SVI	58 (95% CI 0.47–0.68)	96 (95% CI 0.95–0.97)
Overall stage T3	61 (95% CI 0.54–0.67)	88 (95% CI 0.85–0.91)

6.6 MR Equipment

The evaluation of ECE requires the use of a field strength of 1.5 T or 3 T. The higher field strength (3 T) provides better results in ECE detection [13].

Likewise, the meta-analysis of Rooij et al. shows that the use of an endorectal coil does not show significant benefit for ECE detection when mpMRI is performed with a field strength of 3 T, although there is a measurable benefit for tumor staging when a field strength of 1.5 T is used. However, improvements in 1.5-T technology are proceeding very quickly, and it is probable that the new 1.5-T equipment has already changed this aspect.

6.7 mpMR Sequences

High technical quality imaging is necessary to provide the most precise information about tumor staging. The high-resolution T2 sequence is required for an adequate PCa tumor local staging. The addition of functional images (DWI/ADC; DCE) improves the detection sensitivity for ECE, SVI, and overall stage T3, particularly in less experienced readers (Figs. 6.7 and 6.10) [12, 13].

Conclusion

Accurate staging of PCa is one of the key points to successful management and treatment. MR is the best imaging tool for evaluation of local staging. However, high image quality is essential, and a dedicated reading is necessary to achieve accurate diagnosis.

Key Points

- Extracapsular extension (ECE) has significant clinical implications regarding the outcome of patients with PCa.
- mpMRI is the best imaging tool for local staging of PCa.
- mpMRI mainly focuses on differentiating T2 from T3 disease on local staging.
- Radiologists and urologists can obtain critical presurgical information from mpMRI regarding the possibility of avoidance of erectile dysfunction and urinary incontinence.
- mpMRI has low sensitivity and high specificity for the detection of ECE in PCa.
- ESUR score for ECE in PCa ranges from low to high risk of ECE in mpMRI for local staging. Radiologists should be familiar with ECE signs on mpMRI and add them, if present, to the report.

References

1. Mikel Hubanks J, Boorjian S, Frank I, et al. The presence of extracapsular extension is associated with an increased risk of death from prostate cancer after radical prostatectomy for patients with seminal vesicle invasion and negative lymph nodes. Urol Oncol. 2014;32(1):26.e1–7.
2. Tollefson M, Karnes R, Rangel L, et al. The impact of clinical stage on prostate cancer survival following radical prostatectomy. J Urol. 2013;189(5):1707–12.
3. Eifler J, Feng Z, Lin B, et al. An updated prostate cancer staging nomogram (Partin tables) based on cases from 2006 to 2011. BJU Int. 2012;111(1):22–9.
4. Ohori M, Kattan M, Koh H, et al. Predicting the presence and side of extracapsular extension: a nomogram for staging prostate cancer. J Urol. 2004;171(5):1844–9.
5. Cooperberg M, Lubeck D, Mehta S, et al. Time trends in clinical risk stratification for prostate cancer: implications for outcomes (data from CaPSURE). J Urol. 2003;170(6):S21–7.
6. Han M, Partin A, Piantadosi S, et al. Era specific biochemical recurrence-free survival following radical prostatectomy for clinically localized prostate cancer. J Urol. 2001;166(2):416–9.
7. Akin O, Riedl C, Ishill N, et al. Interactive dedicated training curriculum improves accuracy in the interpretation of MR imaging of prostate cancer. Eur Radiol. 2010;20(4):995–1002.
8. Fütterer J, Engelbrecht M, Huisman H, et al. Staging prostate cancer with dynamic contrast-enhanced Endorectal MR imaging prior to radical prostatectomy: experienced versus less experienced readers. Radiology. 2005;237(2):541–9.
9. Wibmer A, Vargas H, Donahue T, et al. Diagnosis of Extracapsular extension of prostate cancer on prostate MRI: impact of second-opinion readings by subspecialized genitourinary oncologic radiologists. AJR. 2015;205(1):W73–8.
10. Vargas H, Hötker A, Goldman D, et al. Updated prostate imaging reporting and data system (PIRADS v2) recommendations for the detection of clinically significant prostate cancer using multiparametric MRI: critical evaluation using whole-mount pathology as standard of reference. Eur Radiol. 2015;26(6):1606–12.
11. Le J, Tan N, Shkolyar E, et al. Multifocality and prostate cancer detection by Multiparametric magnetic resonance imaging: correlation with whole-mount histopathology. Eur Urol. 2015;67(3):569–76.
12. Boesen L, Chabanova E, Løgager V, et al. Prostate cancer staging with extracapsular extension risk scoring using multiparametric MRI: a correlation with histopathology. Eur Radiol. 2014;25(6):1776–85.
13. de Rooij M, Hamoen E, Witjes J, et al. Accuracy of magnetic resonance imaging for local staging of prostate cancer: a diagnostic meta-analysis. Eur Urol. 2016;70(2):233–45.

Tumor Recurrence and Follow-Up

7

Joan C. Vilanova, Violeta Catalá, Sandra Baleato, and Joaquim Barceló

Contents

J.C. Vilanova, M.D., Ph.D. (✉) • J. Barceló, M.D
Department of Radiology, Clínica Girona, Institute Catalan of Health-IDI, University of Girona, Lorenzana 36, 17002 Girona, Spain
e-mail: kvilanova@comg.cat; jbarcelo@ressonanciagirona.cat

V. Catalá, M.D., Ph.D.
Department of Radiology, Fundació Puigvert, Cartagena 340, 08005 Barcelona, Spain
e-mail: violetacatala@yahoo.com.ar

S. Baleato, M.D., Ph.D.
Department of Radiology, Hospital Clínico Universitario de Santiago de Compostela (CHUS), 15706 - Santiago de Compostela, A Coruña, Spain
e-mail: baleatorum@hotmail.com

7.1 Introduction

Therapeutic management for prostate cancer has different options: the androgen-deprivation therapy, the classic treatment of prostatectomy and radiotherapy, and the focal therapies, such as high-intensity focused ultrasound, cryoablation, and laser ablation. Moreover, currently active surveillance is an option for monitoring slow-growing prostate cancer.

These therapies are not only a final option but also in salvage solutions if there is a local recurrence. It is therefore essential to detect local recurrence and localize it precisely so that salvage treatment may be undertaken under the best possible conditions [1].

Approximately 30% of patients who underwent radical prostatectomy will develop biochemical recurrence disease [2]. Biochemical failure (i.e., a rising serum PSA in the absence of demonstrable metastases) is accepted as an appropriate end point for defining treatment failure in men with localized prostate cancer.

It is estimated that up to 50% of patients who receive external-beam radiation therapy (EBRT) develop biochemical failure, presumably caused by local recurrence after 5 years [3].

The emergence of novel local therapy options is an additional factor driving the increased interest in a more detailed evaluation of the prostate and prostate bed [4].

Multiparametric MRI plays an important role in assessment of these patients [5] in order to detect or exclude local recurrence in order to facilitate salvage treatment or potentially systemic therapy, ultimately improving the care and lives of patients with prostate cancer [6].

MRI technique to evaluate treated prostate cancer requires similar protocol as the recommendations from the PI-RADS guidelines, but in this setting for tumor recurrence, dynamic contrast-enhanced technique is mandatory as it is useful to differentiate benign tissue from prostate cancer recurrence. Moreover, MR spectroscopy could be an additional tool to combine information [7] from the other functional sequences

J.C. Vilanova et al. (eds.), *Atlas of Multiparametric Prostate MRI*, DOI 10.1007/978-3-319-61786-2_7

in order to improve the complete analysis on MRI for a suspected prostate cancer recurrence [8].

This chapter illustrates an overview from the normal appearances of the prostate and prostatic bed after different kinds of treatment and the multiparametric MRI features from recurrent and residual prostate cancer, as well as the recommendations from the PRECISE panel to standardize the interpretation of MRI for men on active surveillance [9].

7.2 Radical Prostatectomy (Table 7.1)

Radical prostatectomy involves the removal of the entire prostate, the seminal vesicles, and the ampullary portions of the vasa deferentia, with the formation of a vesicourethral anastomosis (Fig. 7.1).

After radical prostatectomy, PSA should be theoretically undetectable. Officially, a patient will be having a biochemical failure when the PSA concentration exceeds 0.2 ng/mL [10].

MRI features of normal postoperative fibrosis include low signal intensity in all sequences in the anterior sphincter and rectal wall (Fig. 7.1). Retained seminal vesicles are observed in approximately 20% of patients after prostatectomy [11]. Recognition of normal residual seminal vesicles is of paramount importance [12], because such recognition prevents biopsies for erroneous suspicion of recurrent tumor (Fig. 7.2). Thus, biochemical failure occurs in about 70% of patients with residual seminal vesicles.

Pelvic lymphadenectomy may be performed, but this is not mandatory. Lymphoceles may occur at the site of lymphadenectomy and are found along the anatomic lymph node chains within the pelvis and the para-aortic region. Lymphoceles should not be confused with other postoperative complications such as urinoma, hematoma, abscess, or necrotic lymphadenopathy. Surgical clips may produce susceptibility artifacts and especially on dynamic contrast gradient-echo sequence [3].

Local recurrence can be suggested with the presence of soft tissue in the prostatectomy bed that is isointense to muscle on T1-weighted images and slightly hyperintense, intermediate signal to muscle on T2-weighted images [13]. Recurrent tumor tends to enhance avidly in the arterial phase and wash out during the venous phase, while granulation tissue shows either no enhancement or mild enhancement in the late phase [14]. Moreover, local recurrence will show high signal on DWI with high b value and low signal on ADC map (Fig.7.3).

Table 7.1 Radical prostatectomy

Normal findings	Recurrence
Low signal intensity fibrosis Retained seminal vesicles Metallic clips Residual prostate Prominent venous plexus Postoperative collections (lymphocele, hematoma, urinoma, abscess)	Nodular soft tissue mass of intermediate signal in prostatic bed Fast and avid enhancement of nodule Focal restricted diffusion Elevated choline on soft tissue

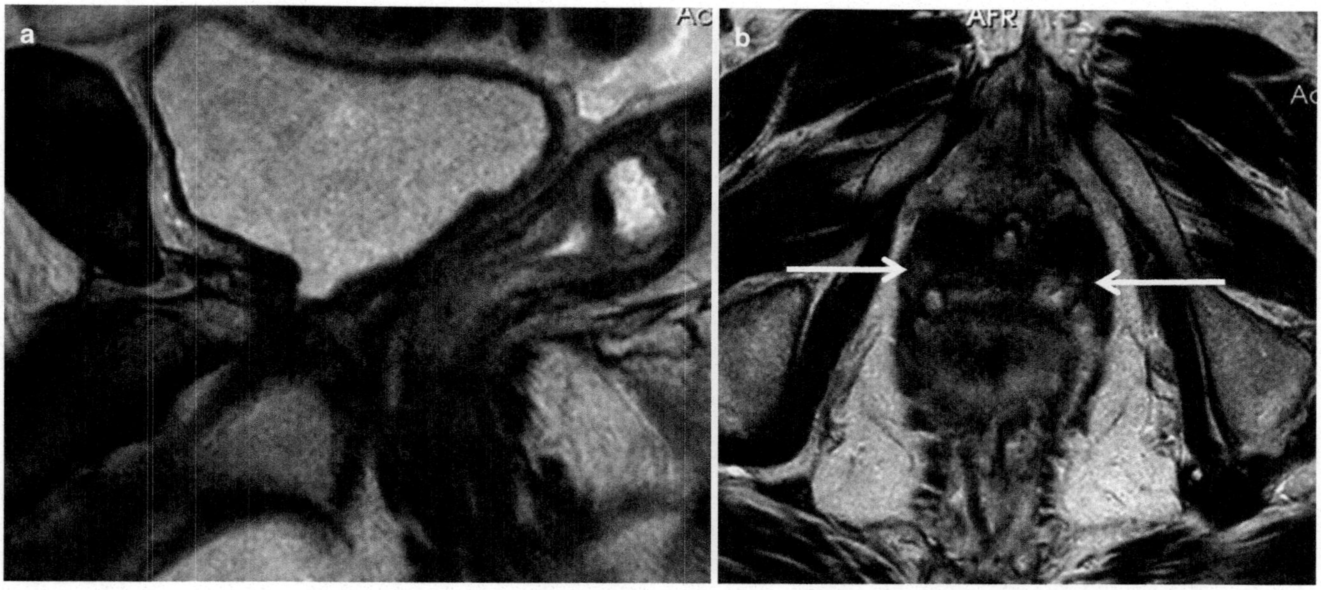

Fig. 7.1 Normal post-prostatectomy bed. (**a**) Sagittal and (**b**) axial T2WI showing the urinary bladder neck pulled down and anastomosed to the membranous urethra. Axial plane shows the anastomosis (*arrows*) with a uniform shape, symmetrical with low signal intensity

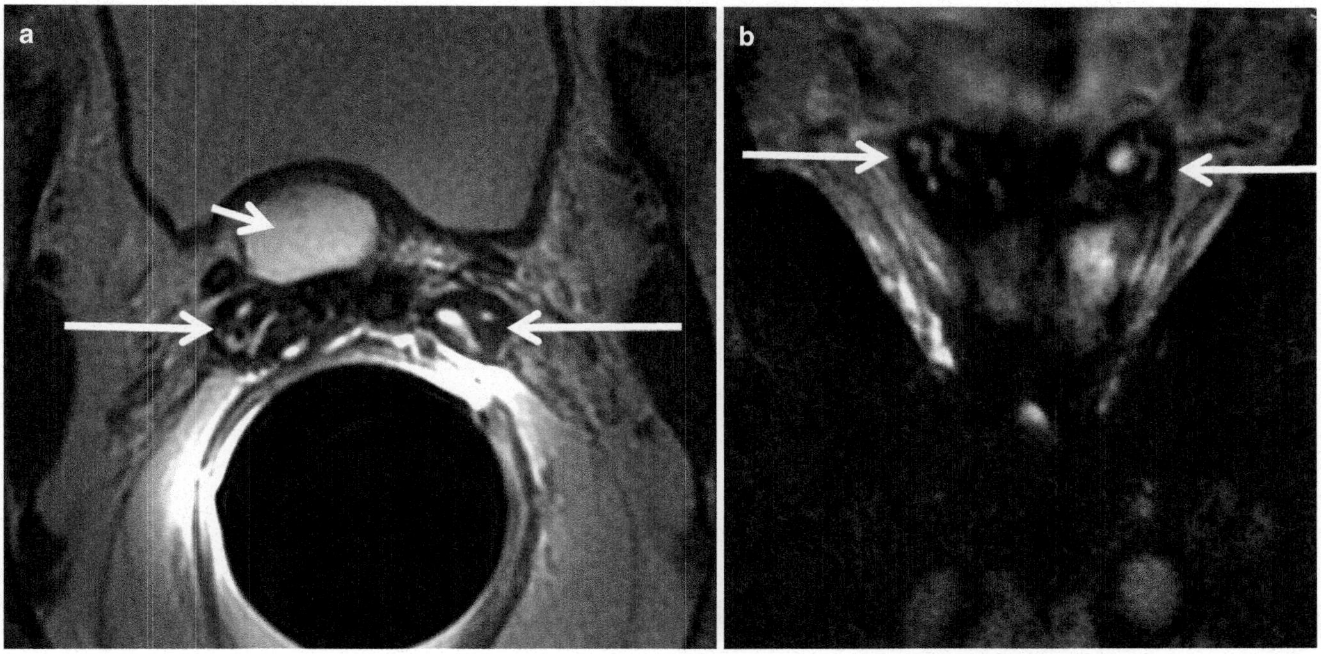

Fig. 7.2 Normal retained seminal vesicles. (**a**) Axial and (**b**) coronal T2WI shows bilateral retained seminal vesicles (*long arrows*), with the typical convoluted tubular appearance of the seminal vesicles. There is also an incidental cyst (*short arrow*) anterior the retained right seminal vesicle in 63-year-old man with a PSA of 0.7 ng/ml

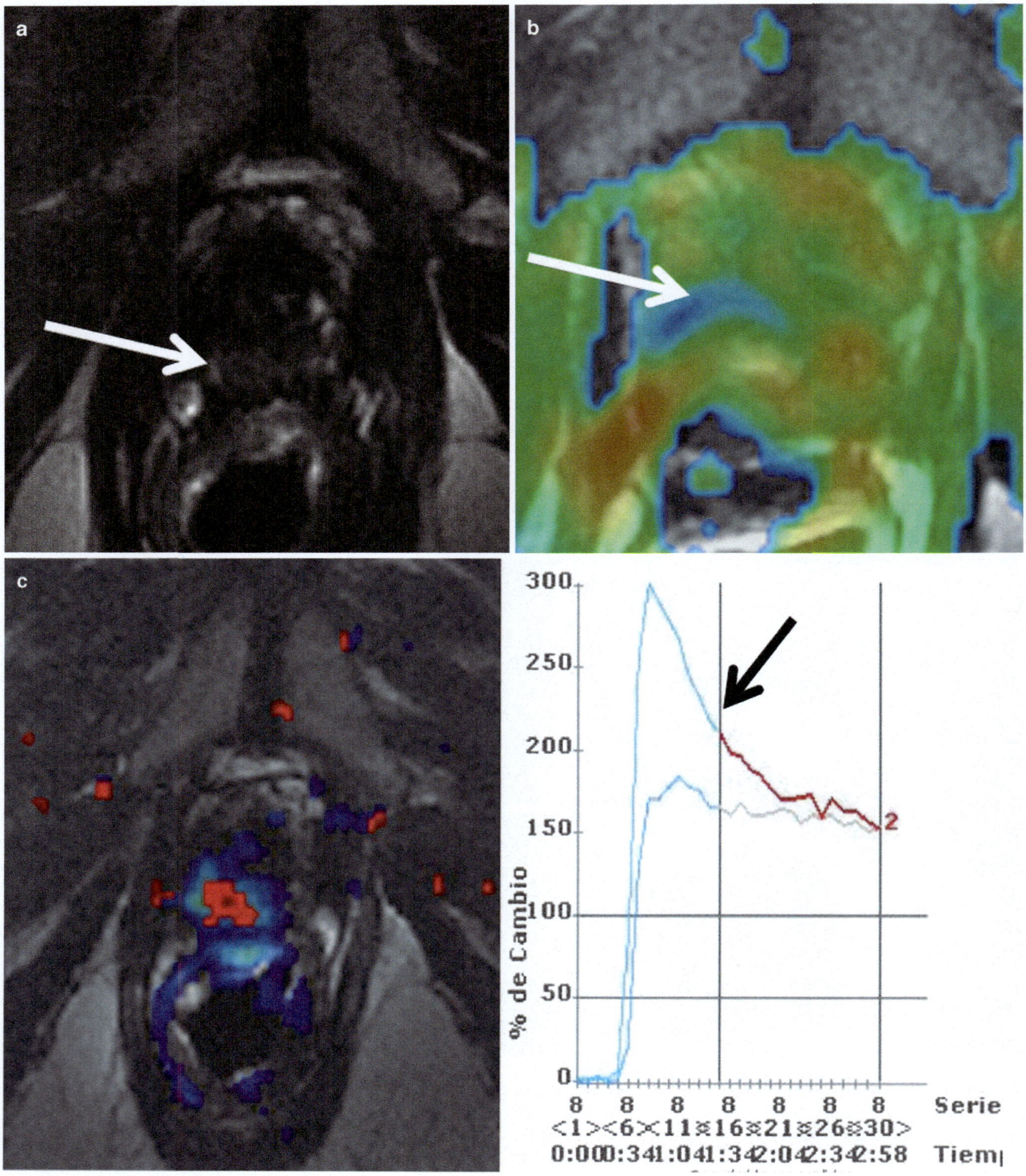

Fig. 7.3 Post-prostatectomy recurrence. (**a**) Axial T2WI, (**b**) ADC color map, and (**c**) DCE on color map and the corresponding time/intensity curve show a soft-tissue mass on T2WI (*arrow*) of intermediate, slight higher signal than muscle in the anastomotic bed. ADC map (**b**) shows restricted diffusion as low ADC value as *blue color* (*arrow*). DCE shows an early uptake and washout pattern on (**c**) (*arrow*), consistent with recurrent disease at the vesicourethral anastomosis

7.3 Radiation Therapy (Table 7.2)

A serum PSA increase after radiotherapy is the best indicator of biologically active tumor [2, 10]. Whenever such an elevation of serum PSA after nadir has taken place, imaging is required to investigate whether this increase is caused by local or systemic recurrent disease. After external-beam radiotherapy (RT), prostatic tissue demonstrates diffuse low signal intensity within all the gland on T2-weighted MR images (Fig. 7.4), which hinder tumor detection. Multiparametric assessment will help to detect recurrence [14] showing higher levels of choline, hypervascularity on DCE [15] and restricted diffusion on DWI, and the corresponding ADC map within a nodular lesion (Fig. 7.5). It is helpful to know the previous location of the lesion to analyze the possible functional changes of the tumor (Fig. 7.6) in order to decide whether there is tumor recurrence [16].

RT may be delivered by means of brachytherapy, in which radioactive sources (seeds or needles) are implanted directly into the prostate gland (Fig. 7.4). The implants might be permanent or temporary. On permanent implants, spectroscopy imaging and DWI might be suboptimal because the metallic seed implants may create susceptibility artifacts and image distortion [17]. Therefore, DCE is a critical sequence in the multiparametric prostate MR exam in order to detect recurrence following permanent brachytherapy [18] and is characterized by an area of rapid contrast enhancement and early washout (Fig. 7.7). Temporary brachytherapy is not affected by susceptibility artifacts because no metallic material is retained; thus, all the multiparametric acquisition can be performed besides DCE, such as DWI and MR spectroscopy, to detect recurrence, with similar findings as described for external RT.

Table 7.2 Radiotherapy

Normal findings	Recurrence
Gland atrophy with diffuse low signal on T2 WI Focal low signal on T2 WI could be due to treated tumor Periprostatic irregularity Inflammatory changes on the pelvis Fatty replacement on bone marrow	Focal and lower signal than normal prostate on T2 WI Fast, avid enhancement and wash out Restricted diffusion

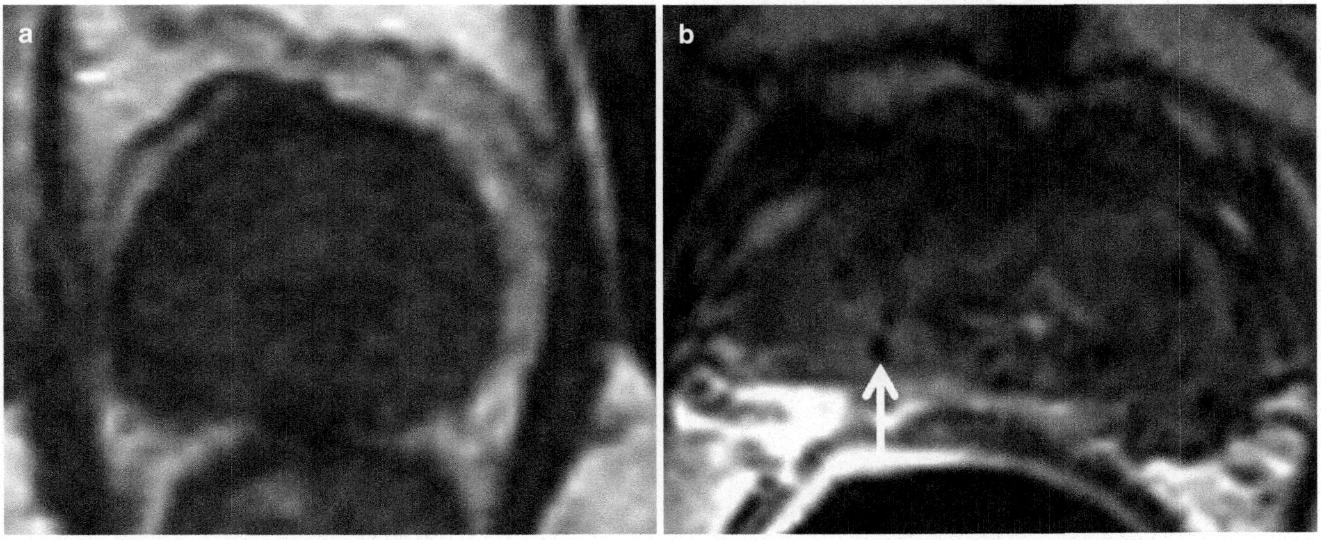

Fig. 7.4 MRI post-external-beam radiotherapy (RT) and brachytherapy. (**a**) Axial T2WI after external-beam RT shows decreased signal intensity throughput prostate, with loss of zonal differentiation. (**b**) Axial T2WI shows multiple radioactive seeds (*arrow*) implanted in the prostate with decreased signal intensity throughout the prostate which makes difficult to distinguish a tumoral lesion

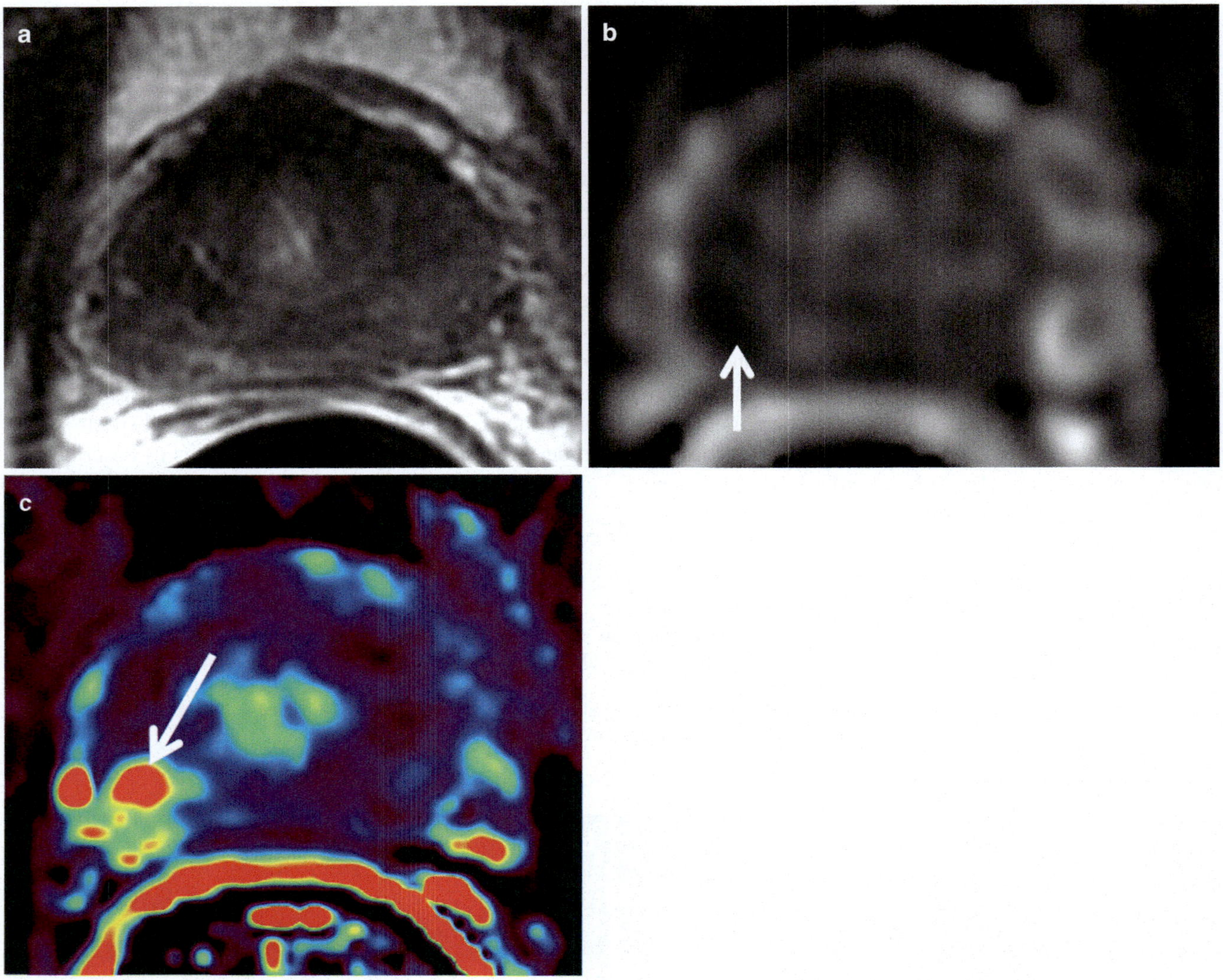

Fig. 7.5 Cancer recurrence post-external-beam radiotherapy (RT). (**a**) Axial T2WI after external-beam RT shows diffuse decreased signal without clear nodular lesion. (**b**) Axial ADC map shows marked low signal intensity in the right peripheral zone (*arrow*) with early and avid enhancement pattern on the axial dynamic contrast enhancement sequence on color map (**c**) (*arrow*), corresponding to a recurrent mass, which was biopsy-proven prostate cancer recurrence

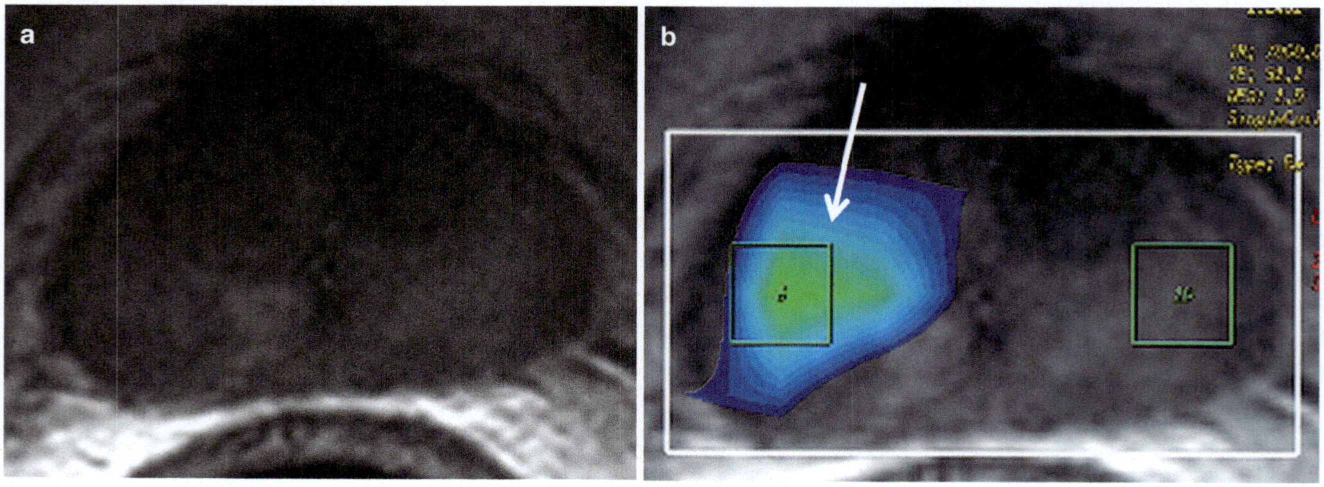

Fig. 7.6 Cancer recurrence post-external-beam radiotherapy (RT). (**a**) Axial T2WI after external-beam RT shows diffuse decreased signal with slight bulging on the right side without clear nodular lesion. (**b**) Axial color map postprocess of spectroscopy acquisition shows higher levels of choline within the right side demonstrated as color green, due to recurrence and proven on biopsy

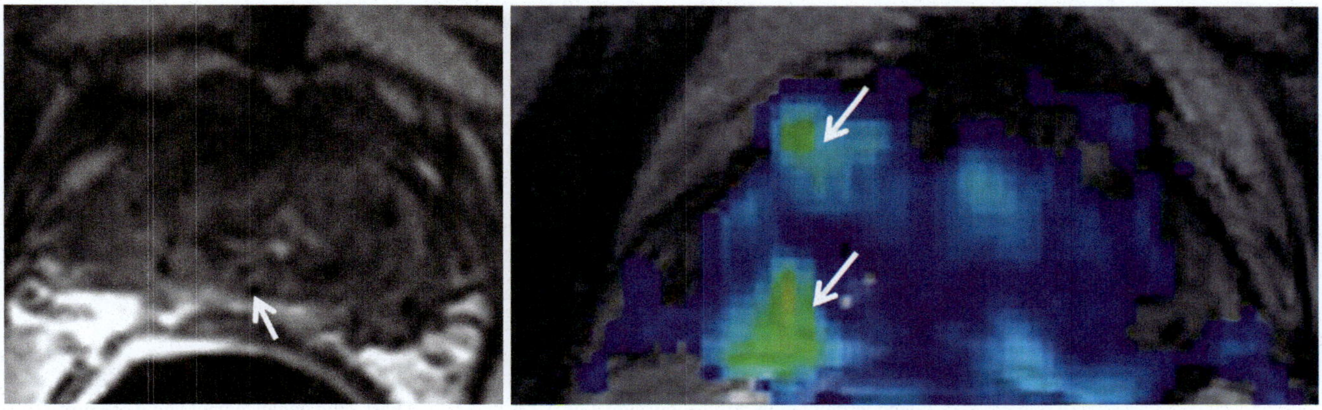

Fig. 7.7 Cancer recurrence post-brachytherapy. Axial T2WI (*left*) shows multiple radioactive seeds (*arrow*) implanted in the prostate with decreased signal intensity throughout the prostate which makes difficult to distinguish a tumoral lesion. The corresponding axial dynamic contrast enhancement sequence (*right*) shows early and avid enhancement pattern in the right peripheral zone on two nodular lesions (*arrows*) corresponding to recurrent tumors, which were biopsy-proven prostate cancer recurrence

7.4 Androgen-Deprivation Therapy (Table 7.3)

The MR findings after androgen-deprivation therapy show diverse findings depending on the type (single therapy or combined agents) and duration of therapy [3]. The findings range from no changes with short-duration monotherapy to homogeneously reduced signal on T2-weighted images and decrease in prostate volume and size of the seminal vesicles. It is difficult to differentiate benign and malignant prostate tissue although the features of focal lower signal on T2-weighted images (Fig. 7.8), choline levels (Fig. 7.9), restricted diffusion, and hypervascularity (Fig. 7.8) can be combined. Functional sequences (DWI, DCE, and spectroscopy) are useful to monitorize treatment (Fig. 7.9) which are more accurate to evaluate response than the morphological sequences such as T2WI. Benign, inflammatory changes could be erroneously interpreted as recurrence on T2WI (Fig. 7.9).

Table 7.3 Androgen-deprivation therapy

Normal findings	Recurrence
Gland atrophy with diffuse low signal on T2 WI No periprostatic irregularity No inflammatory changes on the pelvis No fatty replacement on bone marrow	Fast, avid enhancement and wash out Restricted diffusion Elevated choline

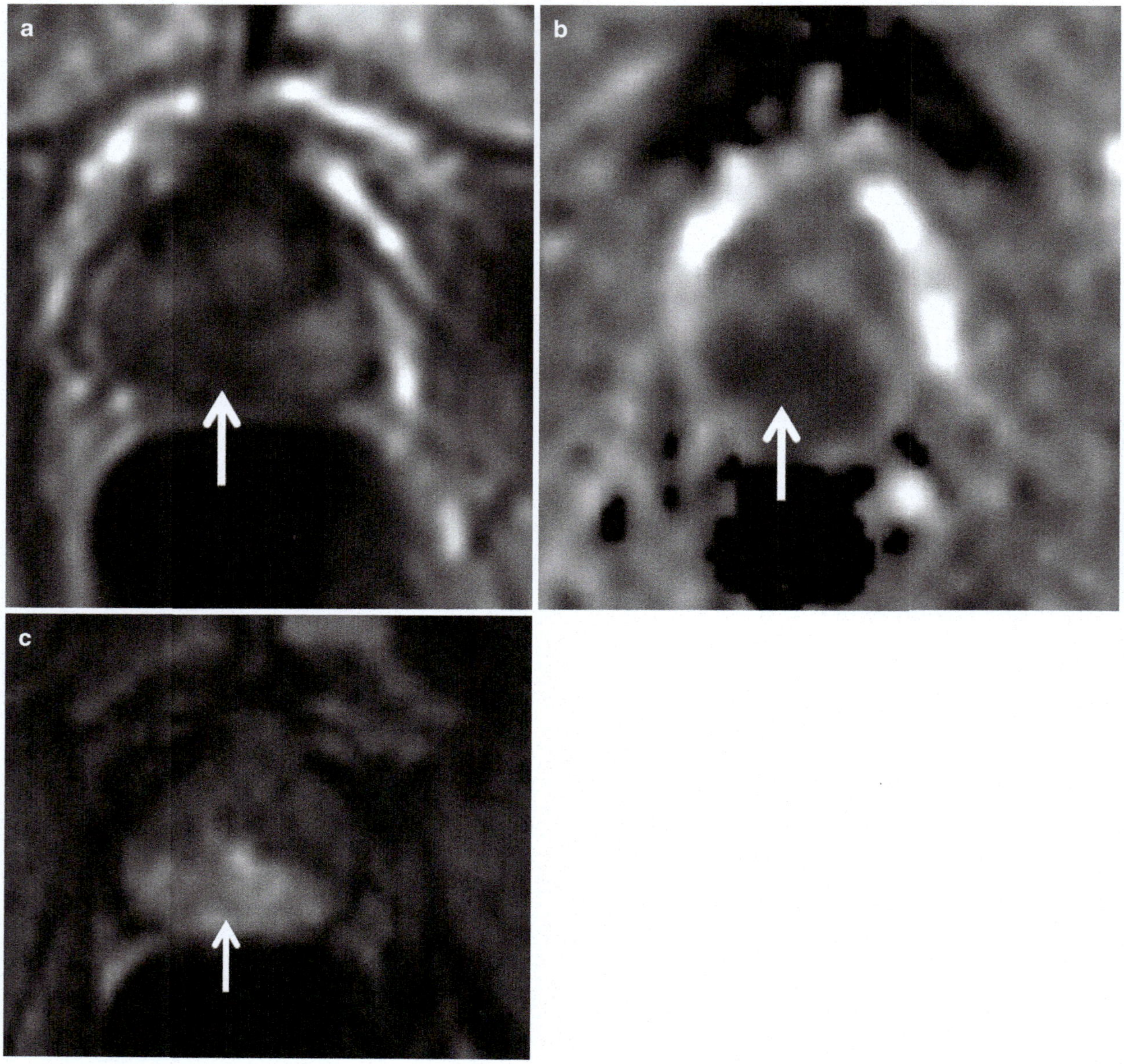

Fig. 7.8 Recurrent tumor after androgen-deprivation therapy (ADT). (**a**) Axial T2WI after ADT shows heterogeneous low signal intensity mainly in the right peripheral zone (*arrow*). (**b**) The lesion becomes more conspicuous on axial ADC map (*arrow*) and also on dynamic contrast enhancement acquisition (**c**) (*arrow*)

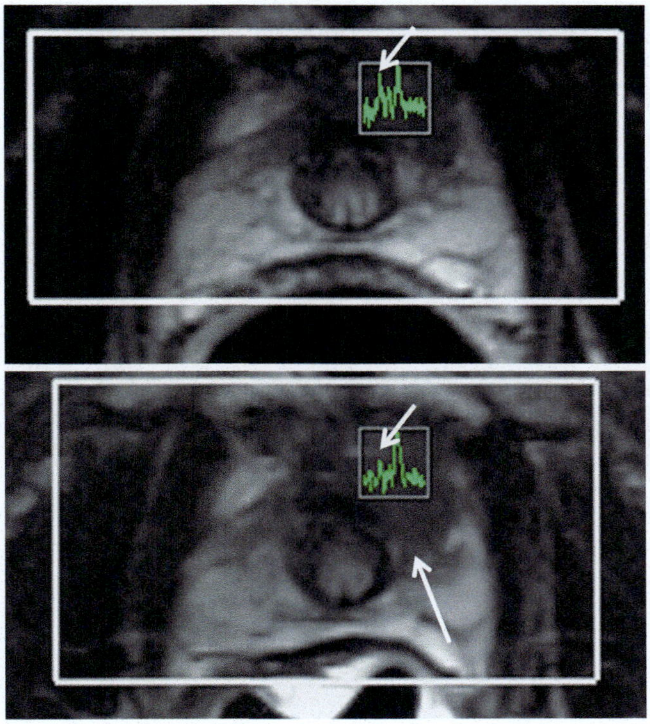

Fig. 7.9 Follow-up after androgen-deprivation therapy (ADT). Axial T2WI before ADT (*upper*) shows high level of choline (*arrow*) within a focal low signal intensity tumoral lesion. Six months after therapy (*below*), the PSA levels were significantly lower, and the T2WI shows lower level of choline peak (*short arrow*) within a longer extension of the lesion (*long arrow*), which is due to nontumoral changes of the lesion

7.5 Focal Therapies (Table 7.4)

7.5.1 Cryotherapy

Cryotherapy consists of the ablation of tissue by extremely cold temperature. No specific changes can be established after cryotherapy [19], which depends on the extent of the treatment and location of the lesion (Fig. 7.10). Expected normal findings might show heterogeneous enhancement with areas of necrosis and thickening of the prostatic boundary (Fig. 7.11), urethra, and rectal wall. Recurrent tumor could show intermediate signal on T2-weighted images, restricted diffusion, metabolic changes [20], and marked enhancement (Fig. 7.12).

Table 7.4 Focal therapies

Normal findings	Recurrence
Atrophy Necrosis Thickening within the treatment boundary	Fast, avid enhancement and wash out Restricted diffusion Higher level of choline

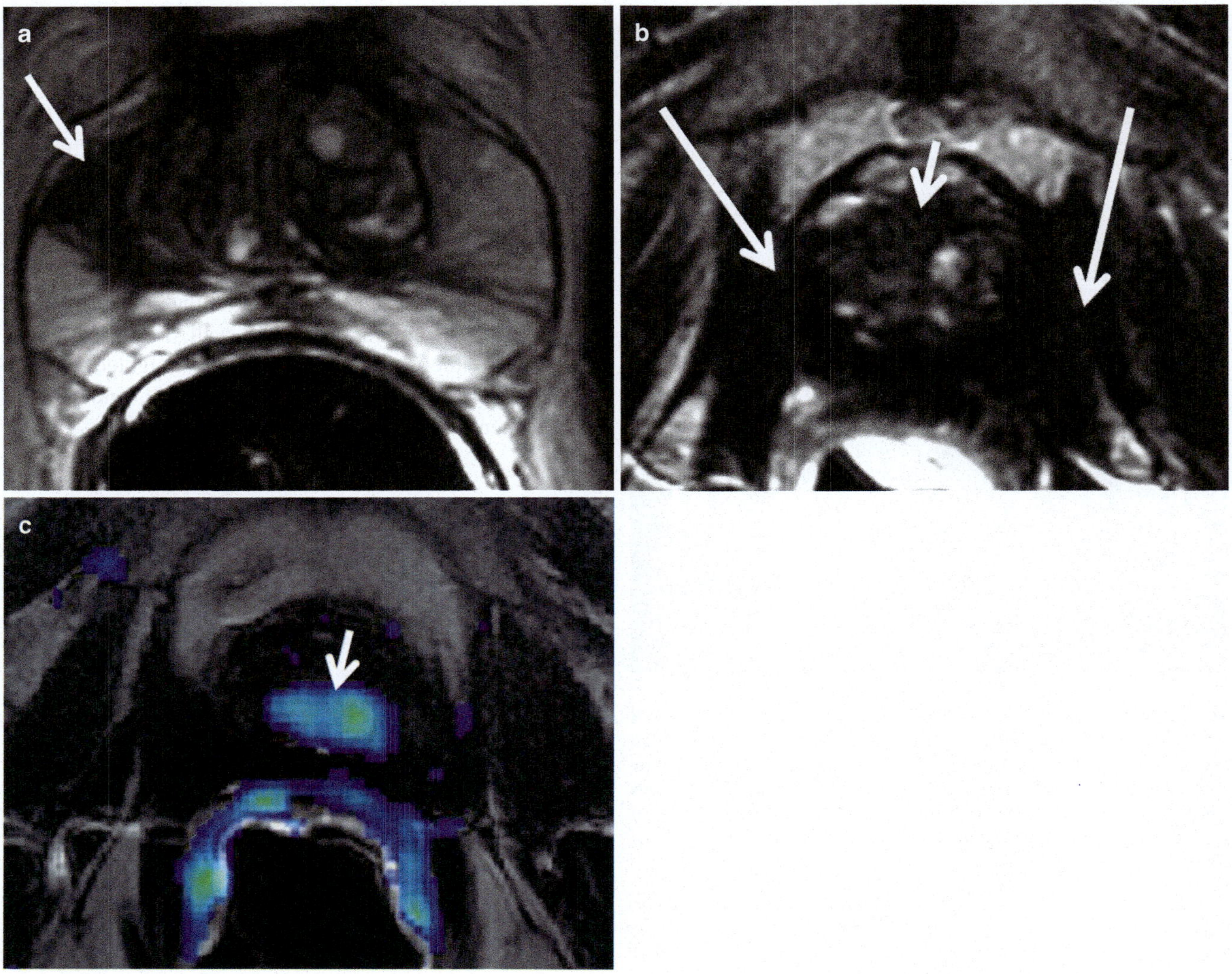

Fig. 7.10 Post-cryotherapy changes. (**a**) Axial T2WI previous to cryotherapy shows the prostate tumor on the right anterior horn of the peripheral zone (*arrow*). (**b**) Axial T2WI after cryotherapy shows atrophy of the peripheral zone, thickened prostatic capsule (*arrows*), and lower volume of the transition zone with diffuse uptake of contrast on dynamic sequence (**c**) (*arrow*)

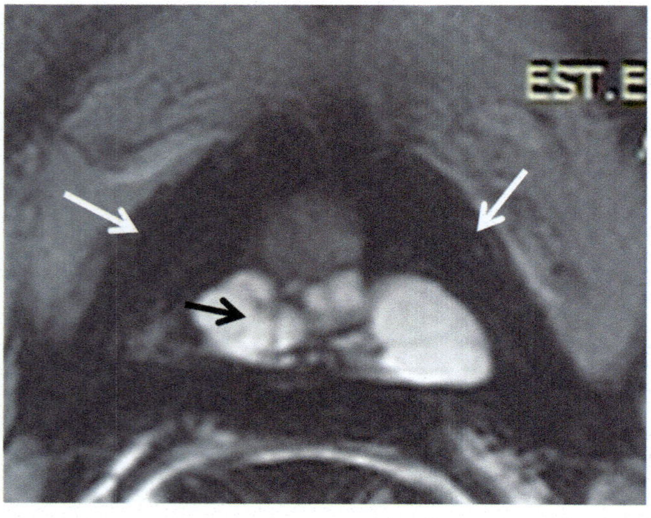

Fig. 7.11 Post-cryotherapy changes. Axial T2WI after cryotherapy shows thickened prostatic capsule, fibrosis (*arrows*) with decreased volume of the prostate, and necrotic tissue within the gland (*black arrow*)

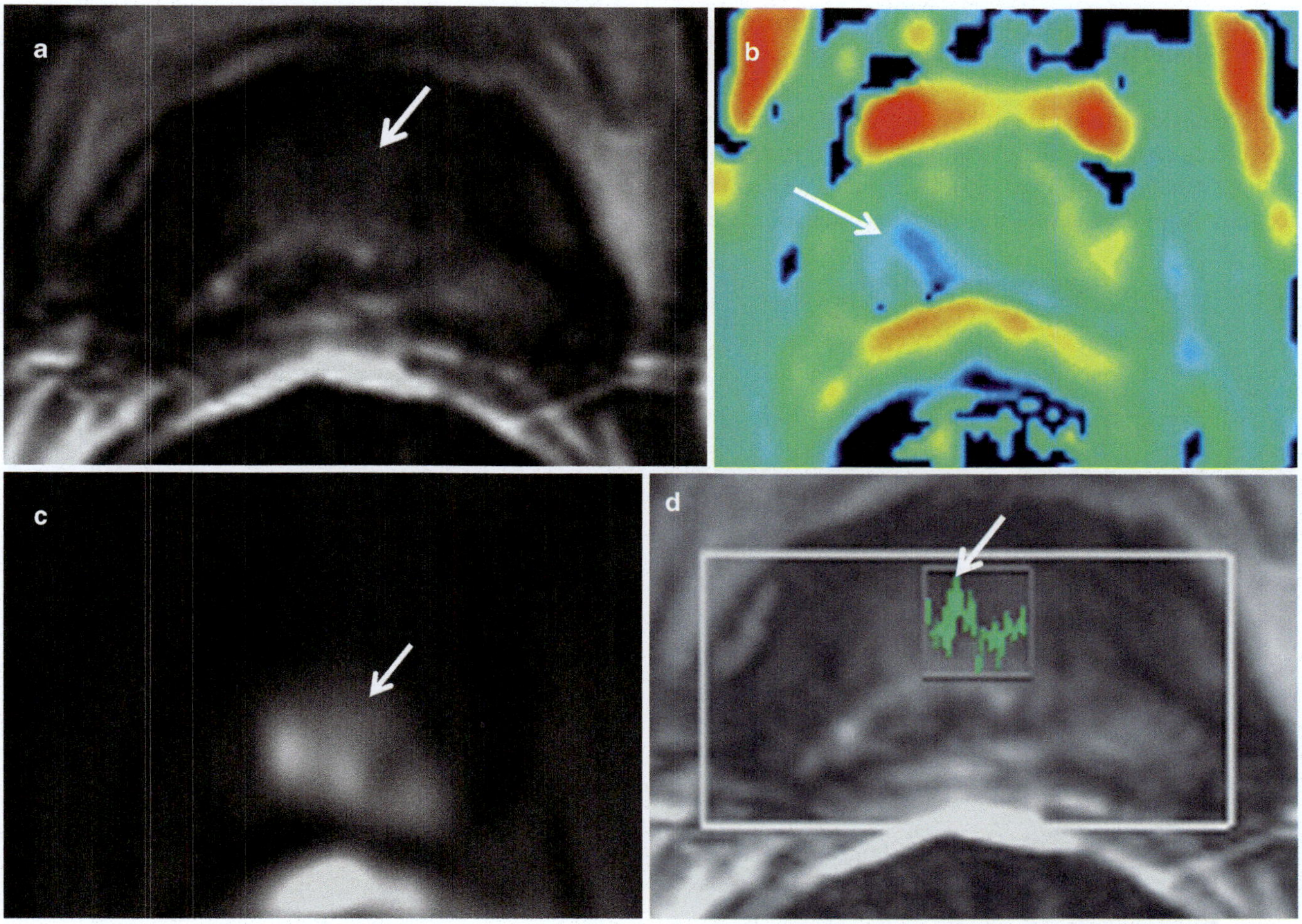

Fig. 7.12 Recurrence post-cryotherapy. (**a**) Axial T2WI after cryotherapy shows an intermediate signal intensity area within the prostate gland (*arrow*), with lower ADC values on color map (**b**), represented as *blue color* (*arrow*), early and avid enhancement (*arrow*) on dynamic sequence (**c**), and high choline peak (*arrow*) on spectroscopic imaging (**d**) due to recurrent tumor

7.5.2 High-Intensity Focused Ultrasound (HIFU)

HIFU causes necrosis due to heat that can generate cavitation effect, atrophy of the gland, or periprostatic thickening without enhancement (Fig. 7.13). DCE and DWI seem to be the most helpful sequences to analyze recurrence [21], especially as it can show tumor recurrence as nodules with early enhancement (Fig. 7.14). Reactive enhancing regions of prostate tissue related to the treatment may be difficult to distinguish from residual viable tumor, particularly at the margins of a treated lesion. A short time to peak enhancement and early wash out can be present in cases of recurrence.

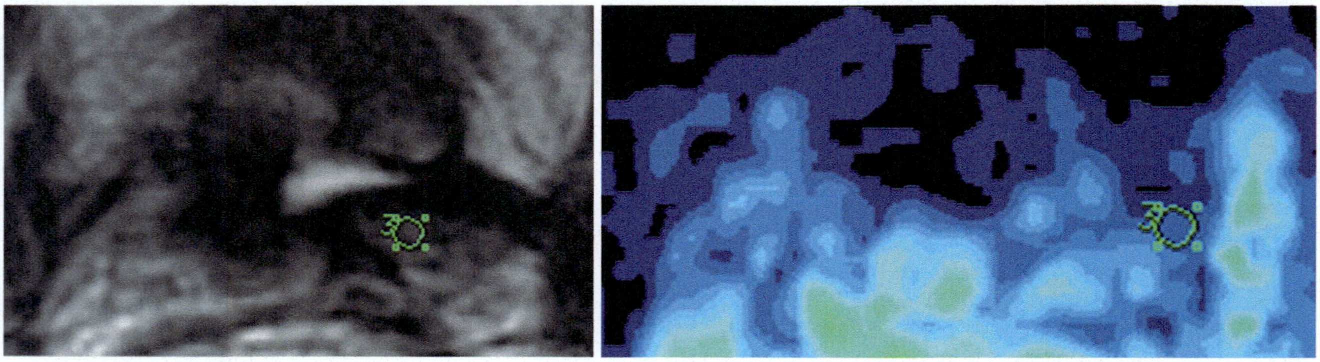

Fig. 7.13 Post-high-intensity focused ultrasound (HIFU) changes. Axial T2WI (*left*) after HIFU treatment shows atrophy of the transition zone without focal contrast enhancement pattern within a region of interest (*circle*) evaluated on the right side; related to benign changes and without focal recurrence

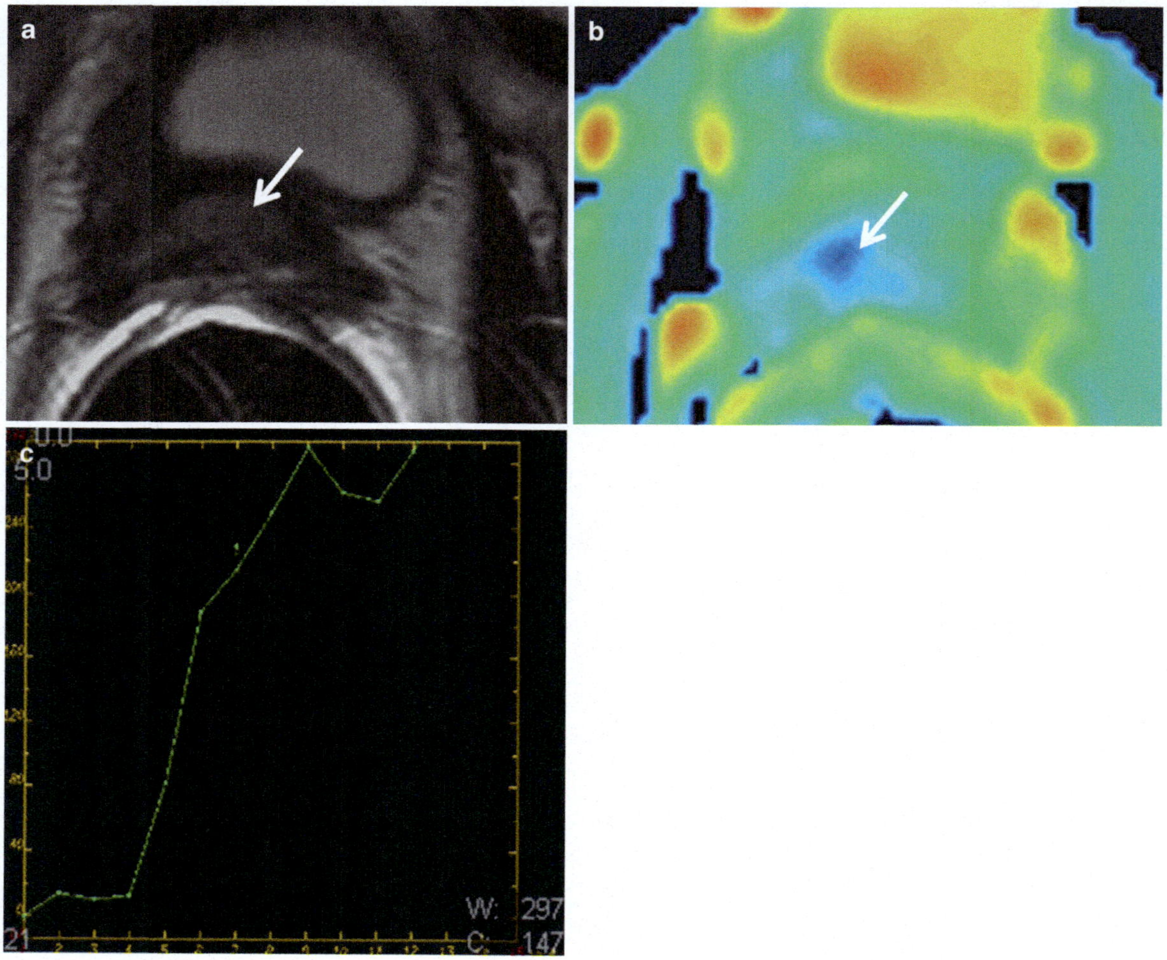

Fig. 7.14 Recurrence post-high-intensity focused ultrasound (HIFU). (**a**) Axial T2WI after HIFU treatment shows an intermediate signal intensity zone (*arrow*) with lower ADC values on color map (**b**), represented as *blue color* (*arrow*), and early and avid enhancement on dynamic sequence in the time/intensity curve (**c**) due to recurrent tumor

7.5.3 Laser Therapy

Laser therapy, photodynamic therapy, uses a laser light of specific wavelength in the presence of oxygen. It can be seen necrotic areas with marked irregularity at the treatment boundary [22], especially after DCE and with areas of enhancement (viable tissue) interposed between necrotic areas [23].

7.6 Active Surveillance

Active surveillance of prostate cancer is a management strategy for low-risk and localized prostate cancer, in order to follow-up the disease progression to delay standard active treatment (radical prostatectomy and radiotherapy). This strategy involves regular follow-up testing for serum PSA, digital rectal examination, and repeat prostate biopsy. PSA kinetics do not reliably predict progression, and biopsy is an invasive procedure associated with considerable morbidity. Therefore, mpMRI has become an increasing commonly used imaging tool for active surveillance. For this purpose, the PRECISE recommendations have been developed to facilitate data collection and assess the MRI findings in men on active surveillance [9]. The PRECISE checklist outlines key information that should be reported on MRI at baseline or follow-up including clinical variables and MRI data, such as volume, ADC values, and imaging appearance on different sequences (Fig. 7.15). MRI report after a baseline MRI report should include an assessment of the likelihood of significant radiologic progression from the baseline MRI scan, on a 1–5 scale, along with a description of the change that has given rise to that assessment (Table 7.5).

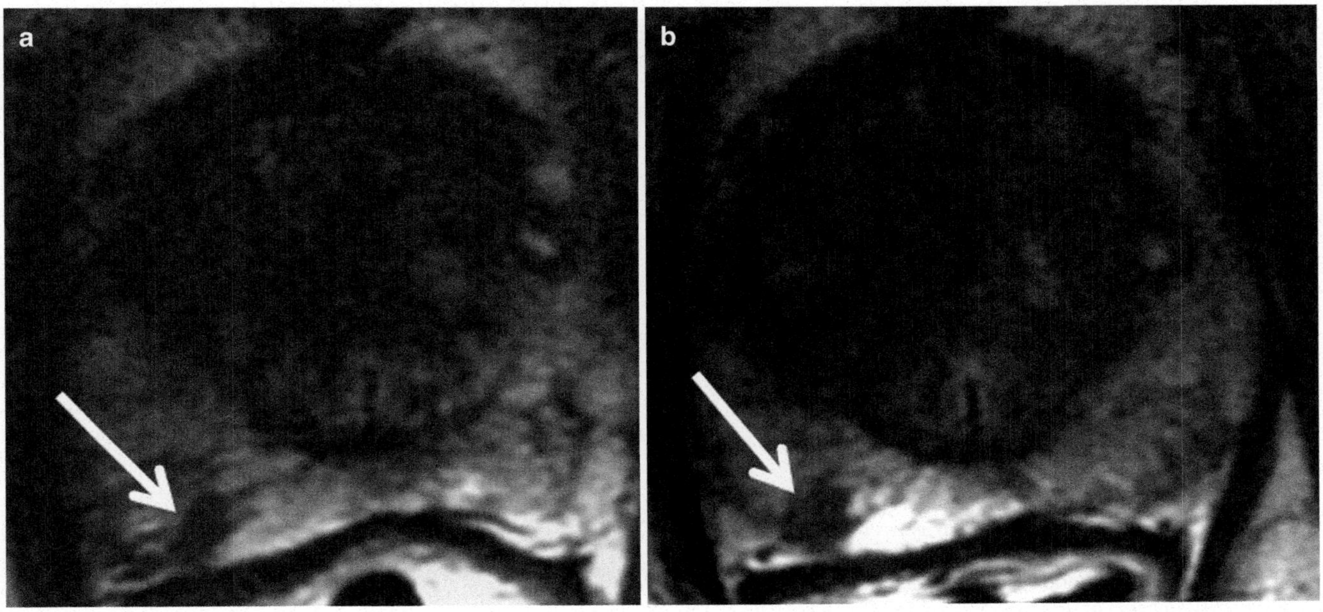

Fig. 7.15 Active surveillance progression. (**a**) Axial T2WI previous to biopsy, showing a lesion on the right side of the apex (*arrow*). The targeted biopsy result revealed a Gleason score 3 + 3 (10%) cancer. (**b**) Axial T2WI after 2-year follow-up shows a slight increase in size of the lesion with spiculated margins (*arrow*), which also showed a mild decreased ADC value. The follow-up target biopsy revealed a Gleason score 3 + 4 (15%) cancer, which was confirmed on the prostatectomy specimen

Table 7.5 Assessment of likelihood of MRI progression in men on active surveillance

Likert scale	Assessment of likelihood of MRI progression
1	Resolution of previous features suspicious on MRI
2	Reduction in volume and/or conspicuity of previous features suspicious on MRI
3	Stable MRI appearance: no new focal/diffuse lesions
4	Significant increase in size and/or conspicuity of features suspicious for prostate cancer
5	Definitive radiologic stage progression

Conclusion

Multiparametric MRI of the prostate provides significant information following different therapies on prostate cancer: radical prostatectomy, radiation therapy-brachytherapy, androgen-deprivation therapy, and focal therapies. The MRI findings of recurrent prostate cancer require the analysis of the different sequences, especially DWI and DCE. Moreover, the current approach to follow-up low-risk and localized prostate cancer with active surveillance requires to assess the changes on MRI to determine the presence of significant disease over time.

Key Points

- mpMRI provides significant information following different therapies on prostate cancer: radical prostatectomy, radiation therapy-brachytherapy, androgen-deprivation therapy, and focal therapies.
- The mpMRI findings of recurrent prostate cancer require the analysis of the different sequences, especially DWI and DCE.
- Current approach to follow-up low-risk and localized prostate cancer with active surveillance requires to assess the changes on MRI to determine the presence of significant disease over time.

References

1. Martino P, Scattoni V, Galosi A, Consonni P, Trombetta C, Palazzo S, et al. Role of imaging and biopsy to assess local recurrence after definitive treatment for prostate carcinoma (surgery, radiotherapy, cryotherapy, HIFU). World J Urol. 2011;29:595–605.
2. Fütterer JJ. Imaging of recurrent prostate cancer. Radiol Clin N Am. 2012;50(6):1075–83.
3. Vargas HA, Wassberg C, Akin O, Hricak H. MR imaging of treated prostate cancer. Radiology. 2012;262(1):26–42.
4. Wassberg C, Akin O, Vargas HA, Shukla-Dave A, Zhang J, Hricak H. The incremental value of contrast-enhanced MRI in the detection of biopsy-proven local recurrence of prostate cancer after radical prostatectomy: effect of reader experience. AJR Am J Roentgenol. 2012;199(2):360–6.
5. Panebianco V, Barchetti F, Grompone MD, Colarieti A, Salvo V, Cardone G, et al. Magnetic resonance imaging for localization of prostate cancer in the setting of biochemical recurrence. Urol Oncol. 2016;34(7):303–10.
6. De Visschere PJ, De Meerleer GO, Fütterer JJ, Villeirs GM. Role of MRI in follow-up after focal therapy for prostate carcinoma. AJR Am J Roentgenol. 2010;194(6):1427–33.
7. Vilanova JC, Luna-Alcalá A, Boada M, Barceló J. Multiparametric MRI. The role of MRI techniques in the diagnosis, staging and follow up of prostate cancer. Arch Esp Urol. 2015;68(3):316–33.
8. Catalá V, Vilanova JC, Gaya JM, Algaba F, Martí T. Multiparametric magnetic resonance imaging and prostate cancer: what's new? Radiologia. 2017;59(3):196–208.
9. Moore CM, Giganti F, Albertsen P, Allen C, Bangma C, Briganti A, et al. Reporting magnetic resonance imaging in men on active surveillance for prostate cancer: the PRECISE recommendations-a report of a European School of Oncology Task Force. Eur Urol. 2017;71(4):648–55.
10. Professionals S-O. Uroweb - European Association of Urology (EAU) [Internet]. Uroweb. 2017. http://uroweb.org/. Cited 8 April 2017.
11. Theodorescu D, Lippert MC, Broder SR, Boyd JC. Early prostate-specific antigen failure following radical perineal versus retropubic prostatectomy: the importance of seminal vesicle excision. Urology. 1998;51(2):277–82.
12. Sella T, Schwartz LH, Hricak H. Retained seminal vesicles after radical prostatectomy: frequency, MRI characteristics, and clinical relevance. AJR Am J Roentgenol. 2006;186(2):539–46.
13. Murphy G, Haider M, Ghai S, Sreeharsha B. The expanding role of MRI in prostate cancer. AJR Am J Roentgenol. 2013;201(6):1229–38.
14. Barchetti F, Panebianco V. Multiparametric MRI for recurrent prostate cancer post radical prostatectomy and postradiation therapy. Biomed Res Int. 2014;2014:316272.
15. Sciarra A, Panebianco V, Salciccia S, Osimani M, Lisi D, Ciccariello M, et al. Role of dynamic contrast-enhanced magnetic resonance (MR) imaging and proton MR spectroscopic imaging in the detection of local recurrence after radical prostatectomy for prostate cancer. Eur Urol. 2008;54(3):589–600.
16. Roy C, Foudi F, Charton J, Jung M, Lang H, Saussine C, et al. Comparative sensitivities of functional MRI sequences in detection of local recurrence of prostate carcinoma after radical prostatectomy or external-beam radiotherapy. AJR Am J Roentgenol. 2013;200(4):W361–8.
17. Lopes Dias J, Lucas R, Magalhães Pina J, João R, Costa NV, Leal C, et al. Post-treated prostate cancer: normal findings and signs of local relapse on multiparametric magnetic resonance imaging. Abdom Imaging. 2015;40(7):2814–38.
18. Boonsirikamchai P, Choi S, Frank SJ, Ma J, Elsayes KM, Kaur H, et al. MR imaging of prostate cancer in radiation oncology: what radiologists need to know. Radiographics. 2013;33(3):741–61.
19. Kalbhen CL, Hricak H, Shinohara K, Chen M, Parivar F, Kurhanewicz J, et al. Prostate carcinoma: MR imaging findings after cryosurgery. Radiology. 1996;198(3):807–11.
20. Kurhanewicz J, Vigneron DB, Hricak H, Parivar F, Nelson SJ, Shinohara K, et al. Prostate cancer: metabolic response to cryosurgery as detected with 3D H-1 MR spectroscopic imaging. Radiology. 1996;200(2):489–96.
21. Rouvière O. Imaging techniques for local recurrence of prostate cancer: for whom, why and how? Diagn Interv Imaging. 2012;93(4):279–90.
22. Woodrum DA, Kawashima A, Gorny KR, Mynderse LA. Prostate cancer: state of the art imaging and focal treatment. Clin Radiol. 2017;72:665–79.
23. Oppenheimer DC, Weinberg EP, Hollenberg GM, Meyers SP. Multiparametric magnetic resonance imaging of recurrent prostate cancer. J Clin Imaging Sci. 2016;6:18.

The manufacturer's authorised representative in the EU is Springer Nature Customer Service Centre GmbH, Europaplatz 3, 69115 Heidelberg, Germany. If you have any concerns regarding our products, please contact ProductSafety@springernature.com

Printed and bound by CPI Group (UK) Ltd, Croydon, CR0 4YY
22/09/2026
02221077-0003